T0271337

Tribo-Behaviors of Biomaterials and Their Applications

Tribo-Behaviors of Biomaterials and Their Applications enables the reader to make an informed choice in the selection of biomaterials that aid the creation of safe and long-lasting surgical devices. Looking at metals, ceramics, and polymers with craniofacial, cardiovascular, spinal, dentistry, and orthopedic applications, this book is an essential guide to tribology in biomaterials.

Handling wear within biodevices is a pressing issue due to the continuous friction and corrosion within the body. It is further complicated by the involvement of body fluids, which can lead to revision surgery to relieve pain. In order to lessen this, engineers can choose a biomaterial better suited to the application. Including detailed discussion of the properties of each biomaterial, this book covers the behaviors of implants, along with the methods and standards applied to devices. It has chapters on metals, ceramics, and polymers. It also covers body fluid lubrication and the physiological effects they have on implants, along with their tribo-corrosion behaviors.

This book will be of interest to engineers and researchers in the field of biomechanical engineering, biomedical engineering, materials science, and manufacturing engineering, alongside all those researching tribology and nanocomposites.

Tribo-Behaviors of Biomaterials and Their Applications

Fundamentals, Recent Advancements, and Future Trends

Edited by Jawahar Paulraj, Prasun Chakraborti,
V. Anandakrishnan, and S. Sathishkumar

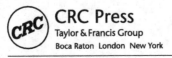

CRC Press
Taylor & Francis Group
Boca Raton London New York

CRC Press is an imprint of the
Taylor & Francis Group, an **Informa** business

Designed cover image: Shutterstock

First edition published 2025
by CRC Press
2385 NW Executive Center Drive, Suite 320, Boca Raton FL 33431

and by CRC Press
4 Park Square, Milton Park, Abingdon, Oxon, OX14 4RN

CRC Press is an imprint of Taylor & Francis Group, LLC

© 2025 selection and editorial matter, Jawahar Paulraj, Prasun Chakraborti,
V. Anandakrishnan, and S. Sathishkumar; individual chapters, the contributors

ISBN: 978-1-032-47056-6 (hbk)
ISBN: 978-1-032-47156-3 (pbk)
ISBN: 978-1-003-38484-7 (ebk)

DOI: 10.1201/9781003384847

Typeset in Times
by Apex CoVantage, LLC

Contents

Preface

This book on tribological behaviors of biomaterials and their applications offers in-depth insights into the tribology and tribo-corrosion attributes of diverse biomaterials. Implant interventions play a crucial role in facilitating comfortable access to the human body, particularly for those facing challenges with natural bodily systems. Over the past century, a myriad of organic and inorganic engineering materials have significantly influenced various biomedical applications, encompassing areas such as hip implants, scapula implants, limb implants, dental implants, vertebrae implants, talus implants, sternum implants, craniofacial implants, cardiovascular implants, bone plates, and its fixation with pins and screws.

Material selection for these applications is rigorously guided by factors such as the specific medical application, surgical methods employed, patient's age, and the intended usage. This book extensively illustrates the profound tribo-resistance characteristics, tribo-resistance improvement methods for different biomaterials, providing a comprehensive understanding of their performance in diverse medical contexts.

Chapters 1 and 2 are structured to offer a foundational overview of the pivotal role played by biomaterials and their tribological behaviors in human health. The preliminary focus is on assessing the tribological behaviors of the core system before implantation, a crucial step in significant procedures. Chapter 3 delves into a detailed description of the tribology assessment, encompassing various standards and regulations.

Chapter 4 provides extensive information on the tribological nature of various bioimplants, while Chapter 5 explores their tribo-corrosion behaviors. The surface characteristics and their responses are shown to have notable implications for the durability of implants. Chapter 6 is dedicated to discussing the tribo-surface behaviors of biomaterials and methods for their improvement.

Over the past seven decades, three predominant materials—metals, ceramics, and polymers—have played a superior role in the biomaterials industry. The indispensable contribution of nonconventional fabrication methods in the biomaterials field is emphasized for creating complex structured bioimplants, enhancing recovery rates in afflicted communities. Chapter 7 highlights the influences of metal-based additive manufacturing on the fabrication of wear-resistant medical implants. Chapter 8 focuses on ceramics, with their wear resistivity characteristics, as feasible substances for bioimplants.

Polymers are evolving as highly valuable materials for various medical applications due to their strength, light weight, esthetics, and easy fabrication. The overviews of polymer-based biomaterials are thoroughly discussed in Chapter 9. Chapter 10 specifically investigates ultra-high-molecular-weight polyethylene (UHMWPE) for various wear-resistant bioimplant applications.

Post-implantation, the emission of wear debris becomes a serious problem, profoundly impacting the host body and disrupting the equilibrium of human health.

Addressing this concern, Chapter 11 illustrates wear mechanisms, the implications of wear debris on artificial hip joints, and remedial actions to enhance the longevity of implants. Similarly, the impact of coatings on medical implant surfaces and their role in improving wear resistance are detailed in Chapter 12.

In the modern era, the text acknowledges the countless contributions of machine learning algorithms. Chapter 13 specifically discusses various machine learning algorithms in the realm of metal-based additive manufactured wear-resistant bio-implants. This comprehensive content caters to a broad audience, ranging from fundamental to advanced levels, making it particularly valuable for academic and scientific researchers, postgraduate students, and professionals engaged in this esteemed field.

Editors

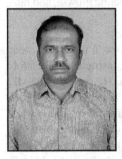

Jawahar Paulraj, PhD, is a member of the Faculty in the Mechanical Engineering Department, National Institute of Technology Agartala, an institute of national importance in Tripura, India, and has 17 years of academic and research experience. He earned a bachelor's degree in mechanical engineering in 1999 at Manonmaniam Sundaranar University, Tamil Nadu, India, a master's degree in production engineering in 2001 at Annamalai University, Tamil Nadu, India, and a PhD in metallurgical and materials engineering in 2007 at the Indian Institute of Technology Madras, Tamil Nadu, India. He has published more than 50 research articles in reputed international journals and at international conferences and has published three chapters in peer-reviewed books. Dr. Jawahar has ongoing/completed research projects worth Rs. 62 lakhs in the fields of polymer composites and the friction stir welding of nonferrous metals/alloys. His areas of interest include tribology, nanocomposites, polymer composites, elastomeric composites, friction stir welding of nonferrous alloys, and metal casting.

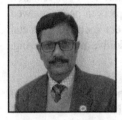

Prasun Chakraborti, PhD, is the senior-most Professor in the Department of Mechanical Engineering at the National Institute of Technology Agartala, an institute of national importance in Tripura, India. He earned a PhD in machine design at the Indian Institute of Technology, Kharagpur, and an MTech in the design of mechanical equipment at IIT Delhi. With an extensive career spanning nearly 40 years of teaching and research experience, Professor Chakraborti has a rich background in academics and research and as a professional. His contributions extend beyond academia, as he has successfully led various projects at the National Institute of Technology Agartala and has collaborated with renowned funding agencies. Under his guidance, 11 PhD scholars and more than 20 postgraduate scholars have completed their thesis, as Professor Chakraborti has helped to shape the next generation of researchers. Professor Chakraborti's commitment to academic enrichment is further demonstrated through his active participation in numerous workshops, faculty development programs, and conferences over the last three decades. He also has organized several events, showcasing his leadership in academics through the formation of two dozen academic and research memorandums of understanding (MoUs) with premier institutions in India and abroad. His scholarly pursuits are evident through the presentation of keynote lectures at several national and international conferences, coupled with the publication of more than 75 articles in peer-reviewed international journals.

Beyond his academic and research endeavors, Professor Chakraborti plays a pivotal role in the scholarly community by serving as an editorial board member and reviewer for various journals and PhD theses. His multifaceted contributions underscore his commitment to advancing knowledge, fostering academic growth, and nurturing the talents of aspiring scholars.

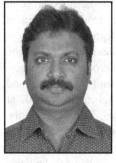

V. Anandakrishnan, PhD, is a Professor in the Department of Production Engineering, National Institute of Technology Tiruchirapalli, Tamil Nadu, India. He earned a BSME in 1999 at Bharathidasan University, Tiruchirappalli, Tamil Nadu, and an ME and PhD in production engineering at Annamalai University, Tamil Nadu, India, and the National Institute of Technology, Tiruchirappalli, Tamil Nadu, India, in 2001 and 2010, respectively. Currently he is the Associate Head of the Center of Excellence in Manufacturing at the National Institute of Technology, Tiruchirapalli, Tamil Nadu, India. He has completed research/consultancy projects worth Rs. 40 lakhs in the field of metal additive manufacturing and unconventional manufacturing processes for DRDO laboratories. He has produced six PhD degrees and is currently guiding eight PhD scholars. He has delivered more than 125 guest lectures at various engineering colleges. He has also published more than 100 research articles in reputed international journals and published 8 chapters in peer-reviewed books. His research interests include materials design, powder metallurgy, metal forming, unconventional manufacturing processes, metal additive manufacturing, tribology, automation, robotics, and CNC technology.

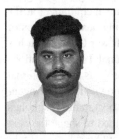

S. Sathishkumar is a PhD Research Scholar in the Department of Mechanical Engineering at the National Institute of Technology, Agartala (Ministry of Education, Government of India). He earned a BE in mechanical engineering and an ME in engineering design at Anna University in Tamil Nadu, India, and an MBA in the operation management division at the University of Madras. He previously held the position of Assistant Professor at Chennai's Vel Tech Rangarajan Dr. Sagunthala Research and Development Institute of Science and Technology. He has presented more than ten research articles at national and international conferences and has published more than 20 research articles in various reputed national and international publications. Additionally, he serves as one of the editors of the Futuristic Trends in Mechanical Engineering book series. In 2018, he received the Research Excellence Award from the Institute of Scholars (InSc) and obtained a lifetime membership in the Indian Society for Technical Education (MISTE), ISRD, and IAENG. He also has contributed as a reviewer and editorial member at various reputed high-impact factored international journals. His research interests include solid mechanics, polymer composites, biomaterials, tribology, fatigue, and material characterization.

Contributors

Kumaravel A
K.S. Rangasamy College of Technology
Tiruchengode, Tamil Nadu, India

T Archana Acharya
Vignan's Institute of Information
Technology
Visakhapatnam, Andhra Pradesh, India

Shirisha Bhadrakali Ainapurapu
Vignan's Institute of Information
Technology
Visakhapatnam, Andhra Pradesh, India

Gülşah Akincioğlu
Duzce University
Duzce, Turkey

S Arulvel
Vellore Institute of Technology
Vellore, Tamil Nadu, India

Kemal Çetin
Necmettin Erbakan University
Konya, Turkey

Prasun Chakraborti
National Institute of Technology
Agartala, Tripura, India

Bharat Kumar Chigilipalli
Vignan's Institute of Information
Technology
Visakhapatnam, Andhra Pradesh,
India

Borra N Dhanunjayarao
Aditya Engineering College
Surampalem, Andhra Pradesh, India

R Govindan
Saveetha Institute of Medical and
Technical Sciences
Chennai, Tamil Nadu, India

S Indiran
King Mongkut's University of
Technology
North Bangkok, Thailand

P Jawahar
National Institute of Technology
Agartala, Tripura, India

Ananthakumar K
Karpagam College of Engineering
Coimbatore, Tamil Nadu, India

V Kanchana
Sree Sastha Institute of Engineering
and Technology
Chennai, Tamil Nadu, India

Jayakrishna Kandasamy
Vellore Institute of Technology
Vellore, Tamil Nadu, India

Ravi Kumar Kottala
MVGR College of Engineering
Vizianagaram, Andhra Pradesh, India

Dhanunjay Kumar Ammisetti
Lakireddy Bali Reddy College of
Engineering
Mylavaram, Andhra Pradesh, India

GS Lekshmi
Lodz University of Technology
Lodz, Poland

Baskaran M
K.S. Rangasamy College of Technology
Tiruchengode, Tamil Nadu, India

Arunakumari Mavuri
Vignan's Institute of Information
    Technology
Visakhapatnam, Andhra Pradesh, India

BS Mohan Kumar
Rajalakshmi Engineering College
Chennai, Tamil Nadu, India

Mohanram Murugan
Vellore Institute of Technology
Vellore, Tamil Nadu, India

M Muthusivaramapandian
National Institute of Technology
Agartala, Tripura, India

R Padmavathi
Vel Tech Multi Tech Dr. Rangarajan
    Dr. Sakunthala Engineering
    College
Chennai, Tamil Nadu, India

Anbumathi Palanisamy
National Institute of Technology
Warangal, Telangana, India

Ravivarman R
National Institute of Technology
Agartala, Tripura, India

R Prayer Riju
Vellore Institute of Technology
Vellore, Tamil Nadu, India

D Dsilva Winfred Rufuss
Vellore Institute of Technology
Vellore, Tamil Nadu, India

Sathish S
Madras Institute of Technology
Anna University
Chennai, Tamil Nadu, India

Koray Şarkaya
Pamukkale University
Denizli, Turkey

P Sathishkumar
King Mongkut's University of
    Technology
North Bangkok, Thailand

S Sathishkumar
National Institute of Technology
Agartala, Tripura, India

Momina Shanwaz Mohammad
National Institute of Technology
Warangal, Telangana, India

Perugu Shyam
National Institute of Technology
Warangal, Telangana, India

Suchart Siengchin
King Mongkut's University
    of Technology
North Bangkok, Thailand

S Thiruvengadam
Rajalakshmi Engineering College
Chennai, Tamil Nadu, India

Anandakrishnan V
National Institute of Technology
Tiruchirappalli, Tamil Nadu, India

1 Biomaterials and Health

Anbumathi Palanisamy
National Institute of Technology
Warangal, Telangana, India

1.1 INTRODUCTION

Biomaterials are synthetic or natural materials that are used in medical applications to support, replace, or enhance crucial biological functions (Ratner & Bryant, 2004). Biomaterials are engineered into specific dimensions and shapes to emulate the biological part that is being supported, replaced, substituted (Ratner & Bryant, 2004). Biomaterials science and engineering have a modern well studied history since the 1940s (Ratner, 2019). Since then, the field has grown with the development of numerous natural, synthetic materials and products that have enhanced quality of life (Ishihara, 2015; Learmonth et al., 2007). Surface modification of the materials to enhance their biocompatibility has supported the biological integration of the biomaterials (Ishihara, 2015; Ratner & Bryant, 2004). When implanted, all the biomaterials elicit immune and tissue responses (Anderson, 2001). Most synthetic materials used as biomaterials elicit nonspecific responses upon implantation, which requires specific surface engineering to avoid unwanted reactions including thrombosis, inflammation, and foreign body response (Vancso et al., 2022). During implantation, surface gets the first contact with the local host environment; hence surface engineering of the implants and artificial joints not only improves biocompatibility but also contributes to improving material performance and design. Biological properties such as osteointegration, cell adhesion, and proliferation are promoted toward healing (Bandyopadhyay et al., 2023).

Tribology deals with the science and engineering of interacting surfaces, including friction, lubrication, and wear of material parts (Dowson, 2012; Neu et al., 2008). Friction, wear, and lubrication are important phenomena that are ubiquitous in diverse biological systems (Angelini et al., 2012; Neu et al., 2008). Biotribology, introduced in the 1970s, plays a vital role in designing artificial joints, in implant materials, in developing synthetic cartilage, and in lubricants for health and medical applications (Dowson, 2012). Biological research in this domain focuses on understanding the molecular basis of lubrication, the mechanical and biochemical regulation of lubricating molecules, the wear process of natural articular cartilages in disease progression especially degenerative diseases such as osteoporosis (Angelini et al., 2012; Neu et al., 2008). Skin and articular cartilage are two of the most widely studied tissues in biotribology, and saliva is the natural lubricant that protects the oral cavity, supports mastication, and further helps in transportation of the masticated food (Dowson, 2012). For instance, the

DOI: 10.1201/9781003384847-1

friction and lubrication characteristics of human skin across multiple locations of the body have been extensively studied (Adams et al., 2007). Materials research in this domain focuses on exploring tribological properties of the individual materials, polymer blends, designed artificial joints, and implants and proposed designs are explored (Georgescu et al., 2021; Osaheni et al., 2020). Recently, the tribology of tissue engineering scaffolds was also explored, specifically for ligament and cartilage tissue engineering applications (Freed et al., 2009; Neu et al., 2008). Biotribological studies have been gaining momentum since the 1970s due to the interest in biomaterials engineering to develop artificial joints and implants that are compatible and long-lasting after implantation. Specifically, in the design of the acetabular component (the shell with its lining material), tribological studies to develop joints with low friction and that are resistant to wear become very crucial (Dowson, 2012; Ratner et al., 2013). Tribological performance plays a crucial role in artificial joint replacement devices, orthopedic implants, orthodontic or dental implants, contact lenses, and drug delivery systems (Dowson, 2012). In biological systems, tribology is crucial in the functioning of eye, skin, teeth, and joints (Angelini et al., 2012). Tribology in biomaterial device manufacturing is a rapidly expanding field that studies and improves the interfaces in relative motion (Shekhawat et al., 2021). Figure 1.1 provides an overall visual representation of different biomedical devices used in the field of medicine. It showcases a range of devices that aid in medical diagnosis, treatment, and patient care.

The principles of the biomechanics of each joint, namely knee joint, hip joint, shoulder joint, elbow joint, etc., also play a huge role in designing and developing specific implant materials and respective total artificial joint prosthesis (Brockett, 2023). Biomechanics involves analysing forces, motions, sliding friction and stresses that occur within each joint and their surrounding tissues including bone, cartilage, and soft muscles (Angelini et al., 2012; Brockett, 2023). At the cellular level, there are mechanochemical signalling pathways that sense, transmit, and respond to stress stimuli by altering cellular forces, elasticity, etc. Contact and friction are sensed through such mechanotransduction pathways which determines the cell fate decision of the cells and tissues that are in contact (Angelini et al., 2012). Wear and frictional analysis are performed on different types of artificial joint prosthetic devices to examine wear rates and friction coefficients (Hasan Basheet et al., 2022). Combined experimental and computational simulation tools are developed for extensive testing of patients' active lifestyle to reduce the failure of the artificial joints developed (Abdelgaied et al., 2018). Computational models are also built to explore the tribological behaviors of the artificial joints designed (Mukherjee et al., 2020; Yin et al., 2007). Such models provide additional insights into designing the artificial joints before the production or implantations process.

In this chapter, the biotribological characteristics of friction, lubrication, wear, and their associated impacts are discussed. Understanding these characteristics, which contribute to better designed artificial joints and implants, eliminates the crude trial-and-error-based design approaches. Investigation and optimization of biotribological properties are vital for advancing the field of

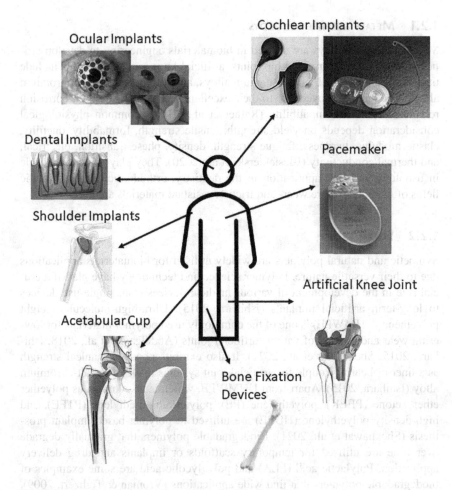

FIGURE 1.1 Overview of various biomedical devices.

medicine, improving patient outcomes, and creating innovative biomaterials and medical devices that are better suited to the dynamic and complex biological environments within the human body.

1.2 DIFFERENT CLASSES OF BIOMATERIAL

Biomaterials can be classified into diverse groups based on their chemical composition and applications. Some of the important classes that find application in the field of medicine and biotribology, along with their specific functional roles and applications, are discussed in this section. Biotribology has increased the interest in soft and low elastic biomaterials, which are utilized to develop applications related to biological tissues such as menisci, tendons, contact lenses, eyelids, synovial membranes, and articular cartilage (Dowson, 2012).

1.2.1 METALS AND METAL ALLOYS

Metals and metal alloys are utilised in biomaterials engineering to develop artificials joints such as artificial hip joints, artificial knee joints. Examples include titanium, stainless steel, nickel titanium alloys, and nitinol and copper chromium alloys. They are employed due to their excellent mechanical strength, corrosion resistance, and biocompatibility (Ratner et al., 2013). Common physiological consideration depends on yield strength, tensile strength, formability, ductility, elastic modulus, hardness, fatigue strength, density, phase transition, electrical, and thermal conductivity (Biesiekierski et al., 2020). They play a significant role in tribology and find application in the dentistry, orthodontic, and orthopedic fields of medicine where wear- and friction-resistant materials are necessary.

1.2.2 POLYMERS

Synthetic and natural polymers are widely utilised for biomaterials applications due to their versatile nature. Polymer science and technology have played a crucial role in the development of various medical devices from single-use devices to long-term artificial implants (Ishihara, 2015). Ultra-high-molecular-weight polyethene (UHMWPE) is one of the commonly used polymer materials for lowering wear and friction of various artificial joints (Abdelgaied et al., 2018; Ishihara, 2015; Shekhawat et al., 2021). It also exhibits good mechanical strength as a liner or bearing couple for artificial joint systems made of cobalt-chromium alloy (Ishihara, 2015). Apart from UHMWPE, which is also known as polyether ether ketone (PEEK), polyethylene (PE), polytetrafluoroethylene (PTFE), and high-density polyethylene (HDPE) are utilised in polymer-based implant prosthesis (Shekhawat et al., 2021). Biodegradable polymers that gradually degrade over time are utilised for temporary scaffolds or implants and drug delivery application. Polylactic acid (PLA) and polyglycolic acid are some examples of biodegradable polymers that find wide applications (Vroman & Tighzert, 2009). Hydrogels and soft hydrogel materials, such as polyacrylamide or polyethylene glycol polyvinyl alcohol, find a wide variety of applications including ocular, controlled drug delivery, and soft tissue engineering due to their increased biocompatibility (Bhamra et al., 2019; Kirchhof et al., 2015; Qin et al., 2019). Osteolysis after total hip replacement surgery decreased significantly because of the usage of highly cross-linked ultra-high-molecular-weight polyethylene (HXLPE) and porous coating for cementless fixation (Yamamoto et al., 2016). Moderately cross-linked polyethylene materials are preferred in joint prosthesis due to their wear-resistant properties (Fisher, 2012).

1.2.3 CERAMICS

Biomaterials that are made of nonmetallic inorganic compounds are utilized to develop medical devices and implants. These are a unique class of materials with excellent mechanical strength, stiffness, biocompatibility, biological inertness, wear resistance, corrosion resistance, nontoxicity, and osteointegration. Some biomaterials such as hydroxyapatite (HA) or tricalcium phosphate (TCP) are biologically active, and they can bond with the natural bone and promote osteointegration toward bone remodelling and regeneration. Clinical and radiographic outcomes of revision hip and knee arthroplasty by using HA+ beta-TCP with bone graft impaction were observed to be effective (Kowalczewski et al., 2010). Ceramic-on-ceramic joints find application in hip joint arthroplasty (Hasan Basheet et al., 2022).

1.2.4 COMPOSITES

Composites are a combination of different types of materials that are used together to leverage their individual properties. Compared to the devices of implants made from individual materials, composite materials aim to harness the benefits of all of their material components (Dunlop & Fratzl, 2010; Lakes, 2003). Composite has a matrix phase or bulk phase, which provides the mechanical strength, along with reinforcement phase as fillers in various geometries (Jesson & Watts, 2012). The matrix phase, which provides the specific mechanical strength, stiffness, toughness, and wear resistance, can be made of polymer, metal, or ceramic biomaterials (Affatato et al., 2015). A polymer matrix made of biodegradable polymer with reinforced fibres, particles of polymers, ceramics, and metals have enhanced mechanical properties along with wide range of applications in tissue engineering, drug delivery systems, and temporary implants development (Armentano et al., 2010; Habraken et al., 2007). A ceramic matrix can be combined with metal, polymer, and ceramic reinforcement materials. The resulting composites exhibit improved toughness, wear resistance, fracture resistance, and thermal stability, which are suitable for dental and orthopedic applications (Dunlop & Fratzl, 2010; Krishnakumar & Senthilvelan, 2021). A metal matrix can be reinforced with ceramic fibres, carbon fibres, or other metals. Metal matrix composites, due to their high stress tolerance, strength, and corrosion resistance abilities, find applications in load-bearing implant development in orthopedic and orthodontic devices (Dutta et al., 2020; Pramanik et al., 2017). Engineering specific properties for specific biomaterial or specific application is possible through the engineering of the composition of the composites.

1.2.5 NATURAL MATERIALS

These materials are derived directly from biological sources such as collagen, chitosan, silk, and gelatine. Because of their biological sources, they have improved biocompatibility and safety. These materials are most commonly utilized in tissue engineering and regenerative medicine applications. Natural materials, such as hyaluron, which is present in the vitreous humour, skin, and cartilage, provide good friction resistance due to its viscoelastic properties (Dowson, 2012).

1.2.6 BIOMIMETIC MATERIALS

Biomimetic materials are designed to mimic the structure and shape of the biological organ or tissue that requires replacement. Their finer qualities, such as their surfaces, are engineered to resemble the natural surface of the tissues and vessels. Biological tissue's specific properties such as specific elasticity and conductivity are engineered to suit individual applications.

The choice of materials utilised depends on the specific application (Biesieki-erski et al., 2020). There is an increased requirement for finding or developing suitable materials with low friction, wear, and durability for specific joint prosthe-sis (Shekhawat et al., 2021). Material properties, such as biocompatibility, deg-radation characteristics, mechanical and thermal properties, along with biologi-cal interaction behaviours, are key because immune responses play a central role in the design and development of medical devices and artificial implants. The devices and implants thus developed must adhere or comply to safety norms and regulations set by the quality and safety assurance institutions, such as ISO, FDA, IMA, PMDA, etc. Thus biomedical engineers and device manufacturers have to carefully select the material and diligently design for specific applications.

1.3 DESIGN AND PRODUCTION STRATEGIES

The development of biomaterial and surgical techniques for total hip preplacement and total knee replacement has received increased attention globally (Yamamoto et al., 2016). New-generation artificial joint design focuses on developing high lubrication surfaces to mimic the natural mechanisms of the human system (Ishihara, 2015; Vancso et al., 2022). Lowering friction and lowering wear are essential design criteria for all artificial joints (Ishihara, 2015). There is a lack of understanding of the mechanism of synovial joint lubrication, which limits fric-tion studies to select materials and design with low friction (Dowson, 2012).

The conventional bearing design utilises metal on polymer (MoP), which com-prises a metal femoral head fixed with a liner of polyethylene (PE) acetabular cup. Apart from this, metal on metal (MoM), ceramic on polymer (CoP), and ceramic on metal (CoM) are the most commonly available joint prothesis material com-binations with improved properties. Commonly utilized biomaterials for these designs includes polyethylene (UHMWPE, PEEK, and cross-linked polyethylene), titanium alloys (Ti), cobalt-chromium-molybdenum (CoCrMo), alumina (Al_2O_3), zirconia (ZrO_2), stainless steel (SS), etc. (Shekhawat et al., 2021). Low-friction polymer poly-tetra-fluoroethylene (PTFE) have also been employed for acetabular cups (Dowson, 2012).

It is necessary to lower the wear of the acetabular liner made of ultra-high-molecular-weight polyethene for long-lasting artificial hip joints. Using pho-toinduced polymerization an articular cartilage mimicking technology was developed as a nanoscale surface modification to increase hydrophilicity by grafting poly (2-methacryloyloxyethyl phosphorylcholine) (MPC) onto highly cross-linked UHMWPE. Thus grafting decreased the wear of X-UHMWPE and assisted in engineering highly lubricated surfaces on artificial hip joints (Ishihara, 2015).

Biomaterials such as silicone rubbers, hydrogels, and poly urethane with low modulus are considered for cartilage repair materials. These materials ensure low wear, satisfactory lubrication, and durability (Dowson, 2012). Hyaluron injections, γ-globulins, and phospholipids to preserve the low frictions were found to be effective (Dowson, 2012). Electrohydrodynamic film thickness equations can be employed to understand steady-state and dynamic viscoelastic conditions and the film thickness necessary for designing artificial joints mimicking the local biological environment. an optimal fluid–film lubrication regime can be identified for better designs (Dowson, 2012).

The AMTI Orth-POD machine was utilised for testing composite-on-composite artificial hip joints for pin-on-disk wear of composite ceramic materials (for calcia-magnesia-alumina-silica of self-mated ceramics) synthesized via coprecipitation technique. Both dry and wet wear tests were conducted under physiologically relevant conditions for 5000 cycles with a sliding velocity 81.4487 mm/s under normal load of 50 N. The coefficient of friction was observed to decrease with an increase in alumina concentration (Hasan Basheet et al., 2022). Thus it is possible to test the wear and frictional characteristics for changing ratios of biomaterials in ceramic and composite biomaterials.

1.4 PRECLINICAL STUDIES AND CLINICAL REQUIREMENTS

Preclinical and clinical studies are absolutely necessary before introducing the newly developed biomaterials and artificial implant devices into human hosts. Preclinical studies involve extensive laboratory testing of the implants through analytical methods and simulations. Repetitive cycles of mechanical loading, motion, and stress are applied from weeks to months to predict the wear and friction behaviour of the materials developed. The observed mechanical wear is attributed to tribo-corrosion (Dowson, 2012). Preclinical wear simulation for 3 sigma curved total knee joint (TKJ) (DePuy, UK) was performed through comprehensive experimental and computational simulation to study the wear trend of different daily activities including walking, deep squats, and ascending stairs kinematic conditions. This mimicked the conditions similar to the load bearing under realistic conditions. Wear parameters of the moderately cross-linked ultra-high-molecular-weight polyethene-bearing material with input parameters of elastic modulus and Poisson's ratio to reflect mechanical stress were studied to explore the wear trends of the TKJ (Abdelgaied et al., 2018). Such studies will help in preclinical optimization of different materials, designs toward developing patient-specific artificial joints (Abdelgaied et al., 2018). Similarly, Shekhawat et al. elaborately reviewed the wear analysis for various polymer-, ceramic-, and metal-based prosthetic materials along with their production route and wear testing equipment and the resulting outcomes (Shekhawat et al., 2021).

In vivo experiments with mouse cornea were performed through a portable microtribometer with a smooth glass probe to measure the friction coefficient. Before and after the experiment, the eye is gently wiped with a fluorescent dye to support cell imaging, and no corneal damage was observed on any of the corneas tested. The mouse was provided continuous inhalational anaesthetic during the course of the experiments and imaging process and observed later in a pathogen-free isolation cage until they resumed normal activity as per regulatory guidelines. The average friction coefficient of 0.06 was observed with no measurable damage of the cornea (Angelini et al., 2012). Thus various systematic preclinical and clinical procedures were performed to evaluate the tribological performance of various prostheses.

1.5 BIOMATERIALS AND TRIBOLOGICAL BEHAVIOR

The choice of biomaterial and tribology are interconnected because it influences virtually all the features of the implants and of the artificial joint prosthesis manufactured including dimensions, wear, lifespan, and cost (Biesiekierski et al., 2020). Wear affects the performance and life time of the orthopedic joints and implants (Hasan Basheet et al., 2022). Figure 1.2 provides an overview and highlights the importance of considering both biotribological properties and biomaterial selection when designing medical devices.

In an effort to develop biomimetic tribological materials, a study focused on increasing lubrication utilized poly (vinyl alcohol) (PVA) and zwitterionic polysulfobetaine (PMEDSAH). Both were blended to develop hydrogel form. The presence of PMEDSAH contributed to increase the lubrication, and PVA provided the essential mechanical strength. Apart from increased lubrication, the friction behav-

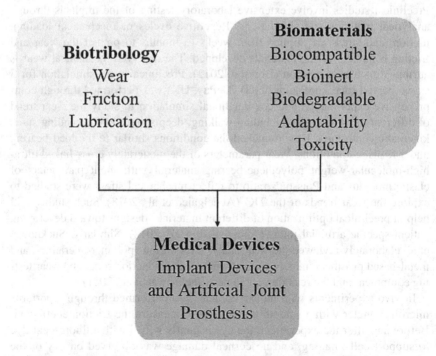

FIGURE 1.2 Influence of both biotribological properties and biomaterial selection for designing various medical devices.

iors closely resembled that of articular cartilage. Such materials can have wide applications including articular cartilage repair, ligament replacement, ophthalmic materials development, meniscal repair, and vascular craft (Osaheni et al., 2020). Similarly, blends of polybutylene terephthalate (PBT) and polytetrafluoroethylene (PTFE) developed exhibited materials with linear wear rate and low friction (Georgescu et al., 2021). Thus numerous unique polymer blends were explored for their low frictional and low wear properties (Jozwik et al., 2019).

$Ti_3C_2T_x$MXene is a unique 2D polymer composites with a lot of applications in energy storage, electromagnetic interference shielding, biomedicine due to its turntable surface and corrosion-resistant properties (Amin et al., 2022). $Ti_3C_2T_x$-MXene/bacterial cellulose (BC) composite films were fabricated by an in situ biosynthesis method. This scalable method enabled developments of ultrathin, strong and highly flexible MXene/bacterial cellulose (BC) composites with electromagnetic interference shielding properties (Wan et al., 2021). Moderately cross-linked polyethylene in the knee joints can reduce wear under high kinematic demand and normal conditions (Fisher, 2012). Thus the tribological characters of biomaterials are continuously explored to find materials that complement specific applications.

1.6 TRIBOLOGY IN JOINT PROSTHESIS

Replacement of worn, damaged, or disease-prone human joints is one of the greatest medical advancements in the history of medicine and humankind. Tribological principle-based studies resulted in the development of long-lasting joint replacements (Dowson, 2012; Shekhawat et al., 2021). Synovial joints functions similarly to bearings during motion and mechanical movement. The surface of the synovial joints is lubricated by synovial fluid synthesized locally by synovial cells and stored in the lining of fibrous capsule surrounding the joints (Dowson, 2012; Shekhawat et al., 2021). The hydrodynamic properties and synovial film thickness for knee and hip joints were estimated through various studies (Dowson, 2012). In vivo studies reveal that the contact stresses in joints of humans, sheep, dogs, and cats lie in the range from 0.5–5 MPa, which is in a comparable range of the cartilage aggregate modulus 0.5–1 MPa (Angelini et al., 2012). In normal joints, the articulating cartilage liner and the nearby muscles result in conformal contact, whereas in artificial joints, point contact arrangements are designed (Shekhawat et al., 2021). The joint contact pressure is supported by interstitial fluid pressure under normal stress, which increases the load capacity while reducing matrix stress and friction (Angelini et al., 2012; Park et al., 2003). Such studies were helpful in developing a synthetic-materials-based lubricant surface while designing various joint prosthetic implants.

The hip joint is one of the greatest load-bearing joints in humans. Age-related osteoarthritis and age-independent rheumatoid arthritis results in cartilage tissue wear, which increases pain and restricts movement (Shekhawat et al., 2021). Total hip arthroplasty (THA) with a cemented and uncemented artificial hip joint is one of the most effective treatments for severe arthritis patients and youngsters who need total hip arthroplasty. Both have been observed to provide good fixation with long-term support and quality of life, though recently uncemented prostheses are preferred globally (Karachalios et al., 2020; Learmonth et al., 2007).

Total ankle replacement has low clinical success compared to other total replacement surgeries. Metal-bearing components are fixed to the tibia and talus bone along with the polyethylene insert in between. This also requires several cointerventions such as fixation of the syndesmosis or subtalar fusion to mimic the complex anatomy and biomechanics of the ankle joint (Brockett, 2023). Joint replacement surgeries and prosthesis are developed for the repair and replacement of hip, knee, ankle, shoulder, elbow, wrist, and finger joints. Thus studying the friction, wear, and lubrication of the joint prosthesis has a significant impact on the long-term success of the implant devices.

1.7 DENTAL TRIBOLOGY

The wear and friction of natural teeth are calculated prior to finding suitable biomaterials. The bite forces of teeth are known to vary in the range of 30–850 N. The coefficient of friction for the enamel-on-enamel is in the range of 0.2–0.6 when dry and 0.03–0.6 in the presence of saliva, which is the natural lubricant of the oral cavity. Enamel is the hardest tissue in the body (Dowson, 2012). Wear in the oral cavity is abrasive and corrosive, and it takes place at rates of 10–50 µm/ year equating to the dimensionless wear factor of 10^{-4}–10^{-3}. Wear factors covering a wide range 10^{-4}–10^{-1} are achieved by most restorative dentistry materials (Dowson, 2012). Thus the tribological characteristics of natural teeth and the oral cavity have led to the development of biomaterials and implants with appropriate wear, friction, and chewing and bruising forces.

Various materials, including 316L steel, NiCrMo alloy, technically pure titanium (ASTM-grade 2), and Ti6Al4V ELI alloy (ASTM-grade 5), were tested for friction and wear (Walczak & Drozd, 2016). Understanding the wear and friction properties of biomaterials that can be utilized to develop dental implants will assist in developing implants with appropriate restorative properties. Dental tribology is a growing area of research with high market potential in the field of biomaterials and implant development.

1.8 OCULAR TRIBOLOGY

The cornea is a natural tribological system that is made of epithelial cell linings (Angelini et al., 2012). Blinking involves the motion of the eyelid over the cornea that occurs 5–30 times per minute is an example of soft tissue tribology. When contact lenses are worn, the tear film between eyelid and lens and the tear film between the lens and cornea present two separate tribological regions (Dowson, 2012). In vivo and in vitro experiments show that the frictional constant is in the order of 0.03–0.06 for interacting corneal cells (Angelini et al., 2012; Dowson, 2012). Boundary lubrication is the focus of recent modelling studies of contact lenses toward increasing comfort and maintaining lubricity during extended wear (Angelini et al., 2012; Dunn et al., 2013; Kamiyama & Khonsari, 2000). Acrylic materials, hydrogels, and silicone polymers find huge application in ocular prosthesis (Aghamollaei et al., 2019; Bhamra et al., 2019; Dowson, 2012; Kirchhof et al., 2015; Lloyd et al., 2001; Qin et al., 2019; Rokaya et al., 2022).

The lubrication ability of the contact lenses is crucial. The sliding friction of silicone-hydrogel-based contact lenses hilaficon-B, lotrafilcon-B, and the effect of various lubricants including distilled water, care solution, and eye drops were explored. Eyedrop and care solution have reduced friction and provided greater lubrication due to tribofilm formation. The care solution also greatly reduces wear debris (Qin et al., 2019). Machines are available for measuring contact lens friction to test their wear properties. Tribometer apparatus can simultaneously apply the normal force, while measuring the friction force response (Angelini et al., 2012). A pendulum-type friction tester measures various friction and wear parameters of contact lenses under physiological conditions (Mabuchi et al., 2021).

1.9 CHALLENGES AND LIMITATIONS

One of the major problems observed after total joint replacement therapy was excessive friction and loosening (Dowson, 2012). Apart from these complications, postoperative dislocation and infection are still most critical problems limiting the long-term success of the joint replacement therapy (Yamamoto et al., 2016). Aseptic loosening following periprosthetic osteolysis is a huge issue that limits clinical success and patient survival post-implantation. Within 10 years of implantation, 20% of the patients developed aseptic loosening, and nearly half of these patients experience severe pain and become disabled (Dumbleton et al., 2002; Ishihara, 2015). The only remedy for this is secondary surgery, which may also increase the economic burden of the treatment (Ishihara, 2015; Kurtz et al., 2007).

Biomaterials have different elastic moduli from those of the natural synovial joints (Katti, 2004). Natural cartilage is made of soft materials compared to the biomaterials that are available to replace them (Seal et al., 2001). Compared to natural materials, biomaterials with a low elastic modulus deform under modest pressure in solid-to-solid contact in artificial joints (Dowson, 2012). Unique materials for the lubrication of these joints that are similar to the natural or biological synovial joints are important. Tribological properties such as cells' potential response to frictional forces, both in vivo and in vitro conditions, are studied in great depth for cartilage and the cornea. However, the transduction signalling pathways of sliding contact forces on cartilage and the cornea has not been studied extensively (Angelini et al., 2012). Studying such molecular regulations will further assist in choosing the right biomaterial and in designing the artificial prosthesis with appropriate tribological properties so that the contact cell fates are not disturbed.

Wear and adverse biochemical reactions to wear debris are the major cause of failure in joint replacement after implantation. The preclinical simulations estimate the wear rates under standard walking conditions leading to failures. Revising the testing procedure systematically with the inclusion of various lifestyles of the patients may assist in predicting and understanding wear-related joint failure and associated tribological performances (Fisher, 2012). When the wear of the polymer liner occurs, small particles are released into the bloodstream. This initiates the foreign body response within various organs, which results in increased taxic effect and organ damage (Urban et al., 2000). Malpositioned joint prosthesis affects every step of the recovery and tribological performance (Fisher, 2012). Once inside the body after the implantation, the bone modulus is affected, and the load gets transferred to the higher modulus value material (Co, Cr, Ti, etc. implant). This results in bone weakness, promoting a stress-shielding effect, which causes brittleness in the bone, and eventually it might face catastrophic failure (Shekhawat et al., 2021). It is difficult to study the tribological characteristics in vivo. It is equally challenging to mathematically model and completely represent the biomechanics in experimental and computational simulators (Mukherjee et al., 2020). The complex tissue architecture involved cannot be mimicked through mathematical modelling. There are no standardized methods for testing biotribological properties since it is an emerging field. However, there is huge potential, and various procedures are being developed.

1.10 SUMMARY

Millions of patients around the globe have benefited from the developments in the field of biomaterials engineering. Restoration of function has improved the quality of life for millions of patients, helping them to regain their normal livelihood. Numerous compatible materials are used for various health care applications. Biomaterials development and artificial prosthesis design are challenging fields that involve multidisciplinary efforts. Tribological studies assist in identifying the materials and surface treatments that minimize friction and wear in medical devices. This can lead to devices that are more durable and have a longer lifespan. Investigating biomaterial interactions within the host tissue environment, along with wear, friction, and lubrication, is necessary for improving the design of existing biomaterials and the development of new biomaterial devices. More biotribological studies and preclinical trials are needed to find the appropriate biomaterials for designing artificial joints with low friction, wear, and better lubrication. Bioengineers, tribologists, and implant designers must also focus on the wide range of kinematic performance of joint prostheses with minimum wear. With the increasing demand for implant materials and joint prostheses in the market, the tribology of biomaterials is a growing field of research with potential applications. The future holds opportunities to design and develop biomaterials and artificial prosthesis that mimic natural biotribology, revolutionizing regenerative medicine.

1.10.1 ACKNOWLEDGEMENTS

The author is grateful for the support and facilities provided by NIT Warangal.

REFERENCES

Abdelgaied, A., Fisher, J., & Jennings, L. M. (2018). A comprehensive combined experimental and computational framework for pre-clinical wear simulation of total knee replacements. *Journal of the Mechanical Behavior of Biomedical Materials*, *78*, 282–291. https://doi.org/10.1016/j.jmbbm.2017.11.022

Adams, M. J., Briscoe, B. J., & Johnson, S. A. (2007). Friction and lubrication of human skin. *Tribology Letters*, *26*(3), 239–253. https://doi.org/10.1007/s11249-007-9206-0

Affatato, S., Ruggiero, A., & Merola, M. (2015). Advanced biomaterials in hip joint arthroplasty. A review on polymer and ceramics composites as alternative bearings. *Composites Part B: Engineering*, *83*, 276–283.

Aghamollaei, H., Pirhadi, S., Shafiee, S., Sehri, M., Goodarzi, V., & Jadidi, K. (2019). Application of polymethylmethacrylate, acrylic, and silicone in ophthalmology. In *Materials for Biomedical Engineering* (pp. 507–554). Elsevier.

Amin, I., Brekel, H. V. D., Nemani, K., Batyrev, E., de Vooys, A., van der Weijde, H., Anasori, B., & Shiju, N. R. (2022). Ti(3)C(2)T(x) MXene polymer composites for anticorrosion: An overview and perspective. *ACS Applied Materials & Interfaces*, *14*(38), 43749–43758. https://doi.org/10.1021/acsami.2c11953

Anderson, J. M. (2001). Biological responses to materials. *Annual Review of Materials Research*, *31*(1), 81–110. https://doi.org/10.1146/annurev.matsci.31.1.81

Angelini, T., Dunn, A., Urueña, J., Dickrell, D., Burris, D., & Sawyer, W. (2012). Cell friction. *Faraday Discussions*, *156*(1), 31–39.

Armentano, I., Dottori, M., Fortunati, E., Mattioli, S., & Kenny, J. (2010). Biodegradable polymer matrix nanocomposites for tissue engineering: A review. *Polymer Degradation and Stability*, *95*(11), 2126–2146.

Bandyopadhyay, A., Mitra, I., Goodman, S. B., Kumar, M., & Bose, S. (2023). Improving biocompatibility for next generation of metallic implants. *Progress in Materials Science*, *133*. https://doi.org/10.1016/j.pmatsci.2022.101053

Bhamra, T. S., Tighe, B. J., & Li, J. (2019). High modulus hydrogels for ophthalmic and related biomedical applications. *Journal of Biomedical Materials Research Part B-Applied Biomaterials*, *107*(5), 1645–1653. https://doi.org/10.1002/jbm.b.34257

Biesiekierski, A., Munir, K., Li, Y., & Wen, C. (2020). 2 — Material selection for medical devices. In C. Wen (Ed.), *Metallic Biomaterials Processing and Medical Device Manufacturing* (pp. 31–94). Woodhead Publishing. https://doi.org/10.1016/B978-0-08-102965-7.00002-3

Brockett, C. (2023). Biomechanics and tribology of total ankle replacement. *Foot and Ankle Clinics*, *28*(1), 1–12. https://doi.org/10.1016/j.fcl.2022.10.002

Dowson, D. (2012). Bio-tribology. *Faraday Discussions*, *156*, 9–30; discussion 87–103. https://doi.org/10.1039/c2fd20103h

Dumbleton, J. H., Manley, M. T., & Edidin, A. A. (2002). A literature review of the association between wear rate and osteolysis in total hip arthroplasty. *The Journal of Arthroplasty*, *17*(5), 649–661. https://doi.org/10.1054/arth.2002.33664

Dunlop, J. W., & Fratzl, P. (2010). Biological composites. *Annual Review of Materials Research*, *40*, 1–24.

Dunn, A. C., Tichy, J. A., Urueña, J. M., & Sawyer, W. G. (2013). Lubrication regimes in contact lens wear during a blink. *Tribology International*, *63*, 45–50. https://doi.org/10.1016/j.triboint.2013.01.008

Dutta, S., Gupta, S., & Roy, M. (2020). Recent developments in magnesium metal–matrix composites for biomedical applications: A review. *ACS Biomaterials Science & Engineering*, *6*(9), 4748–4773.

Fisher, J. (2012). A stratified approach to pre-clinical tribological evaluation of joint replacements representing a wider range of clinical conditions advancing beyond the current standard. *Faraday Discussions*, *156*, 59–68; discussion 87–103. https://doi.org/10.1039/c2fd00001f

Freed, L. E., Engelmayr, G. C., Jr., Borenstein, J. T., Moutos, F. T., & Guilak, F. (2009). Advanced material strategies for tissue engineering scaffolds. *Advanced Materials*, *21*(32–33), 3410–3418. https://doi.org/10.1002/adma.200900303

Georgescu, C., Deleanu, L., Chiper Titire, L., & Ceoromila, A. C. (2021). Tribology of polymer blends PBT + PTFE. *Materials (Basel)*, *14*(4). https://doi.org/10.3390/ma14040997

Habraken, W., Wolke, J., & Jansen, J. (2007). Ceramic composites as matrices and scaffolds for drug delivery in tissue engineering. *Advanced Drug Delivery Reviews*, *59*(4–5), 234–248.

Hasan Basheet, M., Kareem Farhan, F., & Abed, A. N. (2022). Wear and friction analysis of bio-ceramic cordierite system as orthopedic material. *Materials Today: Proceedings*, *60*, 1934–1941. https://doi.org/10.1016/j.matpr.2022.01.031

Ishihara, K. (2015). Highly lubricated polymer interfaces for advanced artificial hip joints through biomimetic design. *Polymer Journal*, *47*(9), 585–597. https://doi.org/10.1038/pj.2015.45

Jesson, D. A., & Watts, J. F. (2012). The interface and interphase in polymer matrix composites: Effect on mechanical properties and methods for identification. *Polymer Reviews*, *52*(3), 321–354.

Jozwik, J., Dziedzic, K., Barszcz, M., & Pashechko, M. (2019). Analysis and comparative assessment of basic tribological properties of selected polymer composites. *Materials (Basel)*, *13*(1). https://doi.org/10.3390/ma13010075

Kamiyama, S., & Khonsari, M. (2000). Hydrodynamics of a soft contact lens during sliding motion. *Journal of Tribology*, *122*(3), 573–577.

Karachalios, T. S., Koutalos, A. A., & Komnos, G. A. (2020). Total hip arthroplasty in patients with osteoporosis. *HIP International*, *30*(4), 370–379. https://doi.org/10.1177/1120700019883244

Katti, K. S. (2004). Biomaterials in total joint replacement. *Colloids and Surfaces B: Biointerfaces*, *39*(3), 133–142.

Kirchhof, S., Goepferich, A. M., & Brandl, F. P. (2015). Hydrogels in ophthalmic applications. *European Journal of Pharmaceutics and Biopharmaceutics*, *95*(Pt B), 227–238. https://doi.org/10.1016/j.ejpb.2015.05.016

Kowalczewski, J. B., Milecki, M., Wielopolski, A., Slosarczyk, A., Marczak, D., & Okon, T. (2010). Zastosowanie HA+beta-tCP w uzupelnianiu ubytkow kostnych w realloplastykach stawu biodrowego i kolanowego [Usefulness of HA+beta-TCP in bone defects repair during revision hip and knee arthroplasty]. *Chirurgia Narządów Ruchu i Ortopedia Polska*, *75*(6), 348–352. www.ncbi.nlm.nih.gov/pubmed/21648152

Krishnakumar, S., & Senthilvelan, T. (2021). Polymer composites in dentistry and orthopedic applications-a review. *Materials Today: Proceedings*, *46*, 9707–9713.

Kurtz, S. M., Ong, K. L., Schmier, J., Mowat, F., Saleh, K., Dybvik, E., Karrholm, J., Garellick, G., Havelin, L. I., Furnes, O., Malchau, H., & Lau, E. (2007). Future clinical and economic impact of revision total hip and knee arthroplasty. *The*

Journal of Bone & Joint Surgery, *89*(Suppl 3), 144–151. https://doi.org/10.2106/JBJS. G.00587

Lakes, R. S. (2003). Composite biomaterials. In *The Biomedical Engineering Handbook* (pp. 79–80). CRC Press.

Learmonth, I. D., Young, C., & Rorabeck, C. (2007). The operation of the century: Total hip replacement. *Lancet*, *370*(9597), 1508–1519. https://doi.org/10.1016/S0140-6736(07)60457-7

Lloyd, A. W., Faragher, R. G., & Denyer, S. P. (2001). Ocular biomaterials and implants. *Biomaterials*, *22*(8), 769–785.

Mabuchi, K., Iwashita, H., Sakai, R., Ujihira, M., & Hori, Y. (2021). Development of a pendulum machine for measuring contact lens friction. *Biosurface and Biotribology*, *7*(3), 154–161.

Mukherjee, S., Nazemi, M., Jonkers, I., & Geris, L. (2020). Use of computational modeling to study joint degeneration: A review. *Frontiers in Bioengineering and Biotechnology*, *8*, 93. https://doi.org/10.3389/fbioe.2020.00093

Neu, C. P., Komvopoulos, K., & Reddi, A. H. (2008). The interface of functional biotribology and regenerative medicine in synovial joints. *Tissue Engineering, Part B: Reviews*, *14*(3), 235–247. https://doi.org/10.1089/ten.teb.2008.0047

Osaheni, A. O., Mather, P. T., & Blum, M. M. (2020). Mechanics and tribology of a zwitterionic polymer blend: Impact of molecular weight. *Materials Science & Engineering C-Materials for Biological Applications*, *111*, 110736. https://doi.org/10.1016/j.msec.2020.110736

Park, S., Krishnan, R., Nicoll, S. B., & Ateshian, G. A. (2003). Cartilage interstitial fluid load support in unconfined compression. *Journal of Biomechanics*, *36*(12), 1785–1796. https://doi.org/10.1016/s0021-9290(03)00231-8

Pramanik, S., Cherusseri, J., Baban, N. S., Sowntharya, L., & Kar, K. K. (2017). Metal matrix composites: Theory, techniques, and applications. *Composite Materials: Processing, Applications, Characterizations*, 369–411.

Qin, D., Zhu, L. T., Zhou, T., Liao, Z. Q., Liang, M., Qin, L., & Cai, Z. B. (2019). Tribological behaviour of two kinds of typical hydrogel contact lenses in different lubricants. *Biosurface and Biotribology*, *5*(4), 110–117.

Ratner, B. D. (2019). Biomaterials: Been there, done that, and evolving into the future. *Annual Review of Biomedical Engineering*, *21*, 171–191. https://doi.org/10.1146/annurev-bioeng-062117-120940

Ratner, B. D., & Bryant, S. J. (2004). Biomaterials: Where we have been and where we are going. *Annual Review of Biomedical Engineering*, *6*, 41–75. https://doi.org/10.1146/annurev.bioeng.6.040803.140027

Ratner, B. E., Hoffman, A. S., Schoen, F. J., & Lemons, J. E. E. (2013). (Third ed.). *Biomaterials Science An Introduction to Materials in Medicine*. Academic Press. https://doi.org/10.1016/C2009-0-02433-7

Rokaya, D., Kritsana, J., Amornvit, P., Dhakal, N., Khurshid, Z., Zafar, M. S., & Saonanon, P. (2022). Magnification of iris through clear acrylic resin in ocular prosthesis. *Journal of Functional Biomaterials*, *13*(1), 29.

Seal, B., Otero, T., & Panitch, A. (2001). Polymeric biomaterials for tissue and organ regeneration. *Materials Science and Engineering: R: Reports*, *34*(4–5), 147–230.

Shekhawat, D., Singh, A., & Patnaik, A. (2021). Tribo-behaviour of biomaterials for hip arthroplasty. *Materials Today: Proceedings*, *44*, 4809–4815. https://doi.org/10.1016/j.matpr.2020.11.420

Urban, R. M., Jacobs, J. J., Tomlinson, M. J., Gavrilovic, J., Black, J., & Peoc'h, M. (2000). Dissemination of wear particles to the liver, spleen, and abdominal lymph nodes of patients with hip or knee replacement. *The Journal of Bone and Joint Surgery*, *82*(4), 457.

Vancso, G. J., Ji, J., Ishihara, K., Martins, M. C. L., & Jiang, S. (2022). Introduction to bioinspired surfaces engineering for biomaterials. *Journal of Materials Chemistry B*, *10*(14), 2277–2279. https://doi.org/10.1039/d2tb90044k

Vroman, I., & Tighzert, L. (2009). Biodegradable polymers. *Materials*, *2*(2), 307–344.

Walczak, M., & Drozd, K. (2016). Tribological characteristics of dental metal biomaterials. *Current Issues in Pharmacy and Medical Sciences*, *29*(4), 158–162.

Wan, Y., Xiong, P., Liu, J., Feng, F., Xun, X., Gama, F. M., Zhang, Q., Yao, F., Yang, Z., Luo, H., & Xu, Y. (2021). Ultrathin, strong, and highly flexible Ti(3)C(2)T(x) MXene/bacterial cellulose composite films for high-performance electromagnetic interference shielding. *ACS Nano*, *15*(5), 8439–8449. https://doi.org/10.1021/acsnano.0c10666

Yamamoto, K., Takagi, M., & Ito, H. (2016). Emerging insights on surgical techniques and biomaterials for total hip and knee arthroplasty. *BioMed Research International*, *2016*, 1496529. https://doi.org/10.1155/2016/1496529

Yin, F., Bedrov, D., Smith, G. D., & Kilbey, S. M. (2007). A Langevin dynamics simulation study of the tribology of polymer loop brushes. *The Journal of Chemical Physics*, *127*(8), 084910. https://doi.org/10.1063/1.2757620

2 Role of Biomaterials in the Health Care System

Momina Shanwaz Mohammad
and Perugu Shyam
National Institute of Technology
Warangal, Telangana, India

2.1 INTRODUCTION

Human health has always been a priority. The development of new biomaterials is increasing daily owing to their extensive application in the health industry. A biomaterial is defined as a substance engineered from biological systems for medical purposes, such as treatment, repair, replacement, and diagnosis (Chintapula et al. 2023; Basu et al. 2022). Biomaterials is an integrative field that deals with biology, medicine, chemistry, tissue engineering, and material science (Ferreira et al. 2020). For ages, the use of biomaterials is common in health care industry, going back nearly 1000 years (Bhat and Kumar 2013). It is known that the Egyptians were the first to use animal biomaterial sinew as sutures (Ige, Umoru, and Aribo 2012). The use of biomaterials has rapidly increased after World War II due to the increased requirement for replacements of the body tissues that were loss in war (El-Husseiny et al. 2011). The US Food and Drug Administration has authorized more than 6000 types of medical devices (FDA). These include US use of biomaterials as prosthetic heart valves, pacemakers, bone-repair plates, and hip and knee replacements.

2.2 CLASSIFICATION OF BIOMATERIALS

Biomaterials can be classified according to their sources and the raw materials used. Biomaterials synthesized from synthetic sources are in daily use. Biomaterials synthesized from natural sources have abundant opportunities for new developments (Joyce et al. 2021). Biomaterials are of four types according to the raw materials used—metals, ceramics, and polymers—and other types are mixtures of these materials as composites. Natural biomaterials are designed to be biocompatible, biodegradable, available, and renewable. Natural biomaterials have a major source of raw material from plants, microorganisms, and animals. Plants, especially flowering plants, are widespread and accumulate many biomaterials (Khrunyk et al. 2020). The discussion begins with natural biomaterials from various sources.

Biomaterials are of three major types according to their sources of raw materials: natural biomaterials, synthetic biomaterials, and hybrid biomaterials, as shown Figure 2.1. Natural biomaterials are extracted from nature, whereas

DOI: 10.1201/9781003384847-2

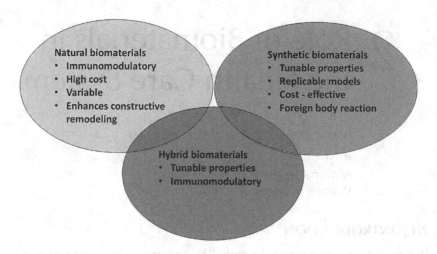

FIGURE 2.1   Classification of biomaterials.

synthetic ones are human-made, such as ceramics, polymers, or composites (Corradetti et al. 2017). Hybrid biomaterials have both the immune modulatory properties of natural sources and the tunable properties of synthetic (Ramakrishna et al. 2001).

2.2.1 Natural Biomaterials

A conserved and regulated utilization of natural habitats can be a great method for biomaterial synthesis. Natural biomaterials from animals are widely used due to their availability and usefulness. Animal kingdom is classified into mammals, birds, insects, reptiles, molluscs, corals, and water animals. Each of the animal species has its own impact on the biomaterials produced in various forms. The biological world has evolved to become a suitable testing ground for materials engineering (Green et al. 2016; Klanrit 2022; Shyngys et al. 2021). The biomaterials from animal sources are illustrated in Figure 2.2.

Natural biomaterials from plants and microorganisms contribute a major portion of natural biomaterials as shown in Figure 2.3. Due to their structural traits and physicochemical properties, their very broad diversity provides an abundance of possibilities for biomaterials from the basic to the interdisciplinary field and applications. The majority of plants are flowering plants. As a result, our expertise with natural biomaterials is still quite restricted, and the identification of novel biomaterials from marine and terrestrial organisms that demonstrate unexpected features may contribute to progress in health care. Yet difficulties with scaling up, purity, and reproducibility persist in the conversion of natural biomaterials into products. Here we illustrate the development of biomaterials derived from plants as well as microorganisms.

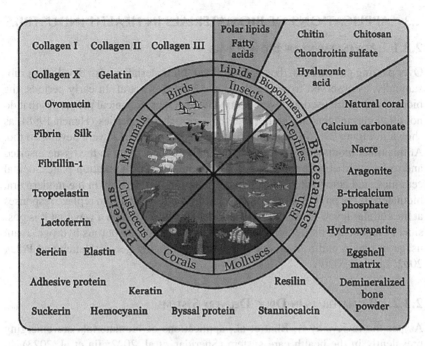

FIGURE 2.2 Animal biosystem and related biomaterials. (Image adapted from Insuasti-Cruz et al., 2022.)

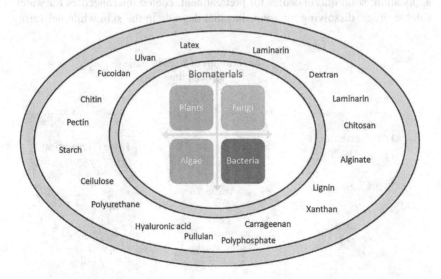

FIGURE 2.3 Biomaterials from plants and microorganisms.

2.3 APPLICATIONS OF BIOMATERIALS IN HEALTH INDUSTRIES

2.3.1 Advancement of Biomaterials

Over passing generations, the applicability of biomaterials is also developing substantially, as observed from the study by Hench L. L et al. In early periods, the biomaterials were used and were seen to have great mechanical properties that do not elicit carcinogenicity and possess anticorrosive properties (Hench 1998), as shown in Figure 2.4. As the generations passed, biomaterials were developed too. At this time, biomaterials were designed to have bioactivity in the tissue inserted and to be resorbable in the tissue, for example, forth orthofixation plates, dental ceramics, and composites (Hench and Thompson 2010). Now in the modern era, biomaterials are paving way to produce artificial tissues that can replace responses at the cellular level. These biomaterials are developed in such a way that it is possible to regenerate tissue, for example, bioactive glass and porous hydrogel foam usage in repair, and to reproduce tissues by activating genes (Hench and Polak 2002; Li et al. 2020).

2.3.2 Biomaterials in Drug Delivery Systems

As per the review by S. Bhat et al., applications of biomaterials are emerging prevalently in the health care system (Sheridan et al. 2022; Jia et al. 2023). In place of traditional needles for drug or vaccines, microneedles are in focus to overcome the limitations of their predecessors. These are made up of silicon, metals, ceramics, glass, and polymers. Microneedles are typed according to the application: solid microneedles for pretreatment, coated microneedles for water-soluble drugs, dissolving microneedles that degrade in the skin while delivering

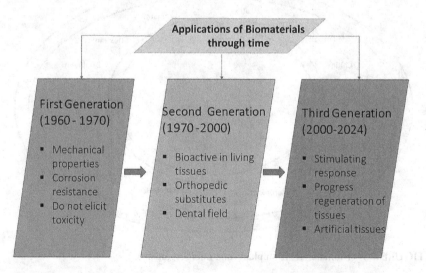

FIGURE 2.4 Developmental applications of biomaterials through the generations.

efficiently across the skin. Drugs with low molecular weight, such as lidocaine, insulin, BCG vaccine, are preferably delivered through this process. In the present cosmetic market, these are meeting with huge demand (Kim, Park, and Prausnitz 2012; Zhang et al. 2022).

To deliver drugs, an advanced biomaterial used is hydrogel. Hydrogels are polymers that can absorb the water or fluid in the tissue without changing its structure; they are replicable as an extra cellular matrix of cells. In tissue engineering, the natural biomaterials from animals, such as collagen and hyaluronic acid, are widely used (Guo et al. 2020). A complex hydrogel developed by Hu et al. has the ability to protect insulin in adverse conditions and release it at neutral pH phases to enhance bioactivity (Hu et al. 2022). They are known for the combined properties of strength, elasticity, and self-healing.

Gene therapy is combined with biomaterials in order to mend injured organs. In this context, a study by Susan Park et al. observed that the terpolymer poly(lysine-g-(lactide-b-ethylene glycol)) protected DNA from nuclease attack by forming a nanoparticulate coating around the DNA (Park and Healy 2003). The research is going on to heal the incision of surgery by inserting DNA into suture materials; one such synthetic polymer that dissolves and that delivers DNA is poly(lactic-co-glycolic acid) (PLGA).

2.3.3 BIOMATERIALS FOR WOMEN

In women, biomaterials are useful in fulfilling various contraceptive purposes as a barrier system included in condoms, diaphragms, hormonal drug delivery devices, and intravaginal rings (Claure et al. 2020). On the other hand, to reduce infertility occurring due to various reasons, biomaterials are useful in a way where hydrogels, such as fibrin, alginate, PEG, and porous gelatin hydrogels, are developed from artificial ovary regeneration to preserve fertility (Lee, Ozkavukcu, and Ku 2021; Morris et al. 2022). Matrigel is a well-known hydrogel used in organoids development and is a natural biomaterial comprised of collagen, PEG, laminin, and glycoproteins (Oefner et al. 2015). As it is derived from nature, there exists some inconsistency of mechanical properties (Zambuto, Clancy, and Harley 2021); for alternate purposes, methacrylated gelatin and porous collagen synthetic matrices are used (Hernandez-Gordillo et al. 2020). Other than these, biomaterials are enjoy many advantages in boosting women's health (Oyen 2022), such as preventing preterm birth by associating cyanoacrylate, fibrin tissues, hydrogels, and membrane patches (Winkler, Harrison, and Messersmith 2019). The research is moving in developing biomaterials in the most vital and sensitive areas like placenta, ovarian organoids, and pelvic floor disorders (Wang et al. 2022).

2.3.4 BIOMATERIALS IN THE MEDICAL FIELD

Biomaterials are widely utilized in the biomedical field. Lignin is used as a nanogel for wound healing and acts as a membrane shield in the treatment of osteoarthritis. Similarly, the plant-extract-mediated biomaterials from various plants like curcumin, citric acid, tannic acid, and grapefruit seed extract are useful in advancing tissue engineering, wound regeneration, wound healing, nanofibers, dressing for wounds, and sunscreen (Gwak, Hong, and Park 2021; Xu et al. 2020).

2.3.5 BIOMATERIALS IN INDUSTRY

In the industrial sector, biomaterials are also used for packaging purposes; mainly in food and pharmaceuticals packaging, polymer-based biomaterials are used that possess antioxidant activity and also improve preserving capacity (Abdalrazeq et al. 2021). Chitosan is the biomaterial most readily available in nature after cellulose; it is mostly used in the packaging of drugs due to its mechanical properties such as film forming ability, nontoxicity, biologically digestive nature, and antimicrobial and antioxidant properties (Istiqomah et al. 2022).

2.3.6 BIOMATERIALS AS BIOSENSORS

Biomaterial development is paving the way in the development of cryogels, a super microporous gel matrix formed at extremely low temperatures of −12°C that facilitate cell proliferation and migration activities. Future research is focusing on the synthesis of cryogels in various feasible structures as sheets, beads, and interconnected networks with enhanced mechanical properties (Tripathi and Kumar 2011). Biosensors are designed in the form of biomaterials to identify diseases in their early stages by detecting changes in the cellular environment. Biosensors, such as quantum dot, graphene-based biosensors, carbon biosensors, carbon nanotubes, and microfluidic biosensors, make use of conventional biomaterials such as chitosan, PEG, and biopolymers (Patel et al. 2016). Some hydrogel sensors are able to sense emergencies and are capable even of intervening in this situation; these are helpful in cardiac emergency conditions (Liu et al. 2019).

2.4 CONCLUSION

So far, biomaterials have emerged as a basic source in fulfilling many needs in diverse fields such as medicine, food, pharmaceuticals, material engineering, textile, and electronic devices. Especially in health care systems, the usage of biomaterials has drastically increased. At each step in the health care system, there are tremendous uses from right at the start in diagnosing a disease to treating it. As discussed, biomaterials are used in medical instruments, orthopedics, ophthalmology in dentistry, wound healing, biosensors, drug delivery systems, tissue engineering, gene therapy, cosmetic implants, first aid, and many more upcoming integrated fields. Even with all these uses, biomaterials still lack the practical advancement in reality due to a few drawbacks such as the inconsistency of mechanical, physical, and chemical properties, lack of clinical study data, immunogenic reactions in tissue, material infection and degradation, and corrosion issues. The exploitation of natural ecosystems for natural biomaterial resources also stands as a prime and major obstacle for the application of biomaterials in health care systems. As biomaterials research is at the budding stage, more innovative implementation and investigations are needed to efficiently employ them in the health care sector. Currently, biomaterials are used in vast and diverse fields that were not expected in the past, and many hidden applications are yet to be revealed through deep investigation and extensive clinical studies.

2.5 FUTURE SCOPE

Biomaterials can have a huge impact in opening the gateway to the future. Especially natural biomaterials have a huge potential for innovation. In the present situation, biomaterials are used for tissue engineering and organ regenerations. For the best outcomes from biomaterials, one has to overcome the accompanying challenges such as unbalanced mechanical properties, biodegradation rate, and clinical studies (Ullah and Chen, 2020). In natural biomaterials, the porous structures can be utilized for better performance in tissue regeneration as they can be transported more easily and allow oxygen, nutrients, and nanoparticles/drugs through them (Tan et al. 2022). In this chapter, we took a broad perspective of biomaterials classification, their applications, the challenges to overcome, and unique solutions for natural ailments. The drawbacks of contemporary biomaterials in the direct application of 3D organ/tissue regeneration can be handled by amalgamation of the basic natural biomaterials with synthetic biomaterials (Galler et al. 2018) for mechanical support. Extensive investigations of the clinical studies of these modern biomaterials will bring effective advantages.

REFERENCES

Abdalrazeq, Manar, Nidal Jaradat, Mohammad Qadi, C Valeria L Giosafatto, Eliana Dell'Olmo, Rosa Gaglione, Angela Arciello, and Raffaele Porta. 2021. "Physico-chemical and Antimicrobial Properties of Whey Protein-Based Films Functionalized with Palestinian Satureja Capitata Essential Oil." Coatings 11 (11): 1364.

Basu, Bikramjit, NH Gowtham, Yang Xiao, Surya R Kalidindi, and Kam W Leong. 2022. "Biomaterialomics: Data Science-Driven Pathways to Develop Fourth-Generation Biomaterials." Acta Biomaterialia 143: 1–25.

Bhat, Sumrita, and Ashok Kumar. 2013. "Biomaterials and Bioengineering Tomorrow's Healthcare." Biomatter 3 (3): e24717.

Chintapula, Uday, Tanmayee Chikate, Deepsundar Sahoo, Amie Kieu, Ingrid D Guerrero Rodriguez, Kytai T Nguyen, and Daniel Trott. 2023. "Immunomodulation in Age-related Disorders and Nanotechnology Interventions." Wiley Interdisciplinary Reviews: Nanomedicine and Nanobiotechnology 15 (1): e1840.

Claure, Isabella, Deborah Anderson, Catherine M Klapperich, Wendy Kuohung, and Joyce Y Wong. 2020. "Biomaterials and Contraception: Promises and Pitfalls." Annals of Biomedical Engineering 48: 2113–31.

Corradetti, Bruna, ME Scarritt, R Londono, SF Badylak, and M Hildebrandt. 2017. The Immune Response to Implanted Materials and Devices. Springer.

El-Husseiny, Inas N, A Ali Marwa, Ayman A Mostafa, and H Elshakankery Mahmoud. 2011. "Surgical Management of Patellar Ligament Rupture in Dogs Using a Prosthetic Woven Fabric: Experimental Study." Journal of American Science 7 (6): 482–90.

Ferreira, Marcel Rodrigues, Renato Milani, Elidiane C Rangel, Maikel Peppelenbosch, and Willian Zambuzzi. 2020. "OsteoBLAST: Computational Routine of Global Molecular Analysis Applied to Biomaterials Development." Frontiers in Bioengineering and Biotechnology 8: 565901.

Galler, KM, FP Brandl, S Kirchhof, M Widbiller, A Eidt, W Buchalla, A Göpferich, and G Schmalz. 2018. "Suitability of Different Natural and Synthetic Biomaterials for Dental Pulp Tissue Engineering." Tissue Engineering Part A 24 (3–4): 234–44.

Green, DW, Gregory S Watson, Jolanta A Watson, D-J Lee, J-M Lee, and H-S Jung. 2016. "Diversification and Enrichment of Clinical Biomaterials Inspired by Darwinian Evolution." Acta Biomaterialia 42: 33–45.

Guo, Youhong, Jiwoong Bae, Zhiwei Fang, Panpan Li, Fei Zhao, and Guihua Yu. 2020. "Hydrogels and Hydrogel-Derived Materials for Energy and Water Sustainability." Chemical Reviews 120 (15): 7642–707.

Gwak, Min A, Bo Min Hong, and Won Ho Park. 2021. "Hyaluronic Acid/Tannic Acid Hydrogel Sunscreen with Excellent Anti-UV, Antioxidant, and Cooling Effects." International Journal of Biological Macromolecules 191: 918–24.

Hench, Larry L. 1998. "Biomaterials: A Forecast for the Future." Biomaterials 19 (16): 1419–23.

Hench, Larry L, and Julia M Polak. 2002. "Third-Generation Biomedical Materials." Science 295 (5557): 1014–17.

Hench, Larry L, and Ian Thompson. 2010. "Twenty-First Century Challenges for Biomaterials." Journal of the Royal Society Interface 7 (suppl_4): S379–91.

Hernandez-Gordillo, Victor, Timothy Kassis, Arinola Lampejo, GiHun Choi, Mario E Gamboa, Juan S Gnecco, Alexander Brown, David T Breault, Rebecca Carrier, and Linda G Griffith. 2020. "Fully Synthetic Matrices for In Vitro Culture of Primary Human Intestinal Enteroids and Endometrial Organoids." Biomaterials 254: 120125.

Hu, Yuwei, Shujun Gao, Hongfang Lu, and Jackie Y Ying. 2022. "Acid-Resistant and Physiological PH-Responsive DNA Hydrogel Composed of A-Motif and i-Motif toward Oral Insulin Delivery." Journal of the American Chemical Society 144 (12): 5461–70.

Ige, Oladeji O, Lasisi E Umoru, and Sunday Aribo. 2012. "Natural Products: A Minefield of Biomaterials." International Scholarly Research Notices 2012: 983062.

Insuasti-Cruz, Erick, Victoria Suárez-Jaramillo, Kevin Andres Mena Urresta, Kevin O Pila-Varela, Xiomira Fiallos-Ayala, Si Amar Dahoumane, and Frank Alexis. 2022. "Natural Biomaterials from Biodiversity for Healthcare Applications." Advanced Healthcare Materials 11 (1): 2101389.

Istiqomah, Annisa, Wahyu Eko Prasetyo, Maulidan Firdaus, and Triana Kusumaningsih. 2022. "Valorisation of Lemongrass Essential Oils onto Chitosan-Starch Film for Sustainable Active Packaging: Greatly Enhanced Antibacterial and Antioxidant Activity." International Journal of Biological Macromolecules 210: 669–81.

Jia, Zhaojun, Xiaoxue Xu, Donghui Zhu, and Yufeng Zheng. 2023. "Design, Printing, and Engineering of Regenerative Biomaterials for Personalized Bone Healthcare." Progress in Materials Science 134: 101072.

Joyce, Kieran, Georgina Targa Fabra, Yagmur Bozkurt, and Abhay Pandit. 2021. "Bioactive Potential of Natural Biomaterials: Identification, Retention and Assessment of Biological Properties." Signal Transduction and Targeted Therapy 6 (1): 122.

Khrunyk, Yuliya, Slawomir Lach, Iaroslav Petrenko, and Hermann Ehrlich. 2020. "Progress in Modern Marine Biomaterials Research." Marine Drugs 18 (12): 589.

Kim, Yeu-Chun, Jung-Hwan Park, and Mark R Prausnitz. 2012. "Microneedles for Drug and Vaccine Delivery." Advanced Drug Delivery Reviews 64 (14): 1547–68.

Klanrit, Poramate. 2022. "Organic Feedstock as Biomaterial for Tissue Engineering." In High-Performance Materials from Bio-based Feedstocks, 247–60. John Wiley & Sons Ltd.

Lee, Sanghoon, Sinan Ozkavukcu, and Seung-Yup Ku. 2021. "Current and Future Perspectives for Improving Ovarian Tissue Cryopreservation and Transplantation Outcomes for Cancer Patients." Reproductive Sciences 28: 1746–58.

Li, Jinhua, Chengtie Wu, Paul K Chu, and Michael Gelinsky. 2020. "3D Printing of Hydrogels: Rational Design Strategies and Emerging Biomedical Applications." Materials Science and Engineering: R: Reports 140: 100543.

Liu, Haoran, Jun Ge, Eugene Ma, and Lei Yang. 2019. "Advanced Biomaterials for Biosensor and Theranostics." In Biomaterials in Translational Medicine, 213–55. Elsevier.

Morris, Mary E, Marie-Charlotte Meinsohn, Maeva Chauvin, Hatice D Saatcioglu, Aki Kashiwagi, Natalie A Sicher, Ngoc Nguyen, Selena Yuan, Rhian Stavely, and Minsuk Hyun. 2022. "A Single-Cell Atlas of the Cycling Murine Ovary." Elife 11: e77239.

Oefner, CM, A Sharkey, L Gardner, H Critchley, M Oyen, and A Moffett. 2015. "Collagen Type IV at the Fetal–Maternal Interface." Placenta 36 (1): 59–68.

Oyen, Michelle L. 2022. "Biomaterials Science and Engineering to Address Unmet Needs in Women's Health." MRS Bulletin 47 (8): 864–71.

Park, Susan, and Kevin E Healy. 2003. "Nanoparticulate DNA Packaging Using Terpolymers of Poly (Lysine-g-(Lactide-b-Ethylene Glycol))." Bioconjugate Chemistry 14 (2): 311–19.

Patel, Suprava, Rachita Nanda, Sibasish Sahoo, and Eli Mohapatra. 2016. "Biosensors in Health Care: The Milestones Achieved in Their Development towards Lab-on-Chip-Analysis." Biochemistry Research International 2016.

Ramakrishna, S, J Mayer, E Wintermantel, and Kam W Leong. 2001. "Biomedical Applications of Polymer-Composite Materials: A Review." Composites Science and Technology 61 (9): 1189–224.

Sheridan, Mark, Caitriona Winters, Fernanda Zamboni, and Maurice N Collins. 2022. "Biomaterials: Antimicrobial Surfaces in Biomedical Engineering and Healthcare." Current Opinion in Biomedical Engineering, 100373.

Shyngys, Moldir, Jia Ren, Xiaoqi Liang, Jiechen Miao, Anna Blocki, and Sebastian Beyer. 2021. "Metal-Organic Framework (MOF)-Based Biomaterials for Tissue Engineering and Regenerative Medicine." Frontiers in Bioengineering and Biotechnology 9: 603608.

Tan, SH, ZH Ngo, D Leavesley, and K Liang. 2022. "Recent Advances in the Design of Three-Dimensional and Bioprinted Scaffolds for Full-Thickness Wound Healing." Tissue Engineering Part B: Reviews 28 (1): 160–81.

Tripathi, Anuj, and Ashok Kumar. 2011. "Multi-featured Macroporous Agarose–Alginate Cryogel: Synthesis and Characterization for Bioengineering Applications." Macromolecular Bioscience 11 (1): 22–35.

Ullah, S and X Chen. 2020. "Fabrication, Applications and Challenges of Natural Biomaterials in Tissue Engineering." Applied Materials Today 20: 100656.

Wang, Bo, Tian Wang, Xiaoran Zhu, Mei Li, Yibao Huang, Liru Xue, Yingying Chen, Qingqing Zhu, and Mingfu Wu. 2022. "Global Burden and Trends of Pelvic Organ Prolapse Associated with Aging Women: An Observational Trend Study from 1990 to 2019." Frontiers in Public Health 10: 975829.

Winkler, Sally M, Michael R Harrison, and Phillip B Messersmith. 2019. "Biomaterials in Fetal Surgery." Biomaterials Science 7 (8): 3092–109.

Xu, Zejun, Shuyan Han, Zhipeng Gu, and Jun Wu. 2020. "Advances and Impact of Anti-
    oxidant Hydrogel in Chronic Wound Healing." Advanced Healthcare Materials 9 (5):
    1901502.
Zambuto, Samantha G, Kathryn BH Clancy, and Brendan AC Harley. 2021. "Tuning Tro-
    phoblast Motility in a Gelatin Hydrogel via Soluble Cues from the Maternal–Fetal
    Interface." Tissue Engineering Part A 27 (15–16): 1064–73.
Zhang, Xiao Peng, Yu Ting He, Wen Xuan Li, Bo Zhi Chen, Can Yang Zhang, Yong Cui,
    and Xin Dong Guo. 2022. "An Update on Biomaterials as the Microneedle Matrixes
    for Biomedical Applications." Journal of Materials Chemistry B 10: 6059–77.

3 Tribology Assessment Methods and Standards on Biomaterials

R Prayer Riju, S Arulvel, D Dsilva Winfred
Rufuss, Jayakrishna Kandasamy,
and Mohanram Murugan
Vellore Institute of Technology
Vellore, Tamil Nadu, India

3.1 INTRODUCTION

Biotribology is a field that focuses on applying tribological concepts like wear, friction, and lubrication to the moving surfaces within the human body. This includes the study of friction and wear in various body parts such as joints, hips, eyelids, and eyeballs (Jin et al. 2016). The term "biotribology" was first coined by Dowson in 1970, relating tribology to living systems. Since then, biotribology has played a crucial role in investigating biological systems, as understanding tribological principles has been useful in this field (Zhou and Jin 2015).

This biotribology plays a major role to assess the wear behavior of implants (metals, ceramics, and polymers) in biomedical engineering. Among the various materials, titanium and stainless steel are the most often used biomaterials for humans (Vallet-Regí, Izquierdo-Barba, and Gil 2003) due to their high strength and biocompatibility. It is commonly used for implants and temporary devices in orthopaedic surgery. But in some cases, these alloys have localized corrosion and release a lot of iron into the tissue around the device, which causes fibrosis (Tracana, Sousa, and Carvalho 1994). In addition to this, the tissue growth, depletion, and osteolysis (Conradi et al. 2011; Hosseinalipour et al. 2010) are some of the main reasons why implants have failed over the past 30 years (Jones, Tsao, and Topoleski 2013).

Wear in the implants is caused by the loading and the interaction of prosthetic parts against one another or the movement of an implant against the host bone. When rubbing against the body tissues, the metal should have a low friction coefficient and strong resistance to wear. This is because the implant may loosen at a high friction coefficient, which substantially increases the wear. Additionally, the debris produced due to wear could be harmful (Sahoo, Das, and Paulo Davim 2019) and reduce the wear life of the implant.

Biotribology plays a key factor in determining the performance and long-term success of the biomaterials in various applications, such as orthopedic implants,

DOI: 10.1201/9781003384847-3

dental implants, and artificial joints. For example, in the case of artificial joints, excessive friction and wear between the joint surfaces can lead to increased wear debris and degradation of the joint, causing pain, inflammation, and ultimately requiring revision surgery. On the other hand, a joint surface with low friction and wear can make it last longer and be more durable, reducing the need for revision surgery and improving patient outcomes. So it is important to have standard validation techniques to recommend the biomaterials for biotribology applications. The standards formulated by organizations like ISO and ASTM are generally used to find the biotribology behavior of the implants and coatings used in recent years. These standards enable the researchers and manufacturers to test and optimize the tribological properties of biomaterials, which are recommended for joint replacements, dental implants, and cardiovascular stents (Stefano, Aliberti, and Ruggiero 2022).

Literally, no chapters or articles are focused on the complete review of standard validation techniques used for the assessment of biotribology properties. Therefore, the present chapter briefly addresses the standards like the International Standard Organization (ISO) and American Society for Testing and Materials (ASTM). In addition, the impacts of wear parameters, lubrication type, and the preparation of biolubricants like simulated body fluids (SBF) in the biotribological test are also elaborated.

3.2   ESSENTIAL STANDARD FOR BIOMATERIALS

Metals like Ti alloy, stainless steels, and Co alloys have been widely used in various medical applications, specifically to support and replace biological tissues such as in the replacements of joints, dental tooth roots, and stents. The biomaterials must meet specific requirements such as corrosion resistance, biocompatibility, and wear resistance, in addition to other mechanical properties. However, the currently available biomaterials do not meet all of these requirements. Importantly, corrosion and wear are the main causes for the failure of implant in dentures, heart valves, bone fracture repair, and artificial heart pump. Among these, wear is a key factor that affects the long-term clinical performance of metallic substances. So it is important for the biomaterials to have the following properties to ensure their long-term survival and safety in human body (Nakano 2010).

3.2.1   MECHANICAL PROPERTIES

To improve an implant's load-bearing capacity and to prevent loosening, mechanical properties are crucial. Specifically, a material with a low modulus of rigidity is ideal for prolonging the implant's service life and avoiding revision surgery due to implant failure and stress shielding effects. Table 3.1 lists the mechanical properties of various biomaterials. Generally, human bones have a lower modulus of elasticity, ranging from 4 to 30 GPa. Therefore, a material intended for use in implants should have a similar or greater modulus of elasticity to be effective.

TABLE 3.1

Mechanical Characteristics of Biomaterials for Implant Applications

Biomaterial	Modulus of Elasticity (GPa)	Tensile Strength (MPa)	Corrosion Resistance	Bioactivity	Reference
Titanium	110–114	880–1000	Excellent	Nonbioactive	(Agha et al. 2016)
Zirconia	200–240	800–1200	Excellent	Nonbioactive	(Pezzotti 2014)
Ceramic	70–300	100–400	Good	Nonbioactive	(Chen et al. 2017)
Stainless Steel	190–220	500–1000	Fair	Nonbioactive	(Marattukalam et al. 2020)
Cobalt-chromium	200–250	900–1300	Good	Nonbioactive	(Muñoz-García et al. 2014)
Polyethylene	0.2–1.2	20–30	N/A	Nonbioactive	(Knight et al. 2017)
Poly (methyl methacrylate)	2.4–3.4	47–78	Poor	Nonbioactive	(Boroujeni et al. 2013)

Compared to bone, metallic materials have a higher modulus, making metals like stainless steel, Co-Cr, and titanium alloys common choices for implants. However, titanium stands out as an excellent candidate due to its high biocompatibility and low modulus of rigidity of 110 GPa (Moghadasi et al. 2022).

3.2.2 BIOCOMPATIBILITY

Biocompatibility refers to a material's ability to coexist with living things without posing a threat to human health. The materials should possess a high resistance toward the detrimental effects of the bone, extracellular tissues, and ionic composition of the blood (Hussain, Saleem, and Ahmad 2019). Also, the implant must not be harmful to cells, i.e., cytotoxic, which can cause changes in the DNA of the genome, i.e., be genotoxic (Buyuksungur et al. 2023). The biocompatibilities of some commonly used biomaterials are tabulated in Table 3.2.

3.2.3 HIGH WEAR RESISTANCE

The material used in contact with body tissues should have a low friction coefficient and be highly resistant to wear when rubbed against the tissues. The reason for requiring low friction and high wear resistance in the material used in contact with body tissues is that higher friction may lead to implant loosening and increased wear rate. Increased wear rate can also result in the release of wear debris into the bloodstream, which can have negative effects on both the implant's longevity and the patient's health (Ramsden et al. 2007).

TABLE 3.2
Biocompatibility of Biomaterials

Material	Advantages	Disadvantages	Biocompatibility Rate (high to low)
Titanium	• Excellent strength • Corrosion resistance • Biocompatibility • Osseointegration	• Expensive • Specialized processes • Allergic reactions	High
Zirconia	• High strength • Biocompatibility • Coloured to natural teeth	• New to market • Long-term safety questionable • Causes wear on counter-face	High
Ceramic	• Biocompatible, • Aesthetic • resistant to wear	• Brittle • Fracture under stress	High
Stainless steel	• Mechanical strength • Inexpensive	• Corrode over time • Causes allergic reactions	Moderate
Cobalt-chromium	• Wear-resistant	• Causes allergic reactions • Corrode over time	Moderate
Polyethylene	• Low sliding friction • Low rate of wear	• High wear rate at high load • Release inflammation particles	Low

Currently, there is a growing trend in the medical field to use implants with high wear-resistant coatings. Popular examples of such coatings include diamond-like carbon coating and titanium nitride coating (Penkov et al. 2016). These coatings are highly biocompatible and possess excellent mechanical strength. Moreover, they provide a protective layer on the implant surface that resists wear and corrosion. Another effective method to enhance the wear properties of implants is micro-arc oxidation with heat treatment. Recent research also indicates that heat treatment can improve the wear and corrosion resistance of magnesium coatings on titanium implants (Muhammad et al. 2023). Further, researchers have extensively studied various coatings to increase the wear resistance of implant coatings, including collagen, chitosan coatings, hydroxyapatite, and tricalcium phosphate (Fabry et al. 2018).

3.2.4 OSSEOINTEGRATION

The concept of osseointegration, which refers to the direct relationship between living bone and load-bearing implants, is a crucial aspect in implantology. The surface properties of the implant, such as roughness, chemistry, and topography, play a vital role in achieving successful osseointegration (Xu et al. 2023). When the implant surface does not integrate with the adjacent bone, the implant may become loose. Some researchers have not recommended osseointegration properties for the temporary implants (Barfeie, Wilson, and Rees 2015) because it is difficult to remove the implant from the human tissues after successful tissue growth. However, in recent years, researchers have demonstrated that the implant can be safely removed after tissue growth (Wang et al. 2019). Therefore, osseointegration was found to be a desirable property for biomaterial applications in order to ensure a proper integration of tissues with the bone.

3.2.5 HIGH CORROSION RESISTANCE

When a biomaterial implant is used in the body, it can release metal ions into the surrounding tissues, when the implant reacts with the blood plasma, which in turn causes harmful responses in humans. So it is important to have a material with better corrosion resistance (Hallab et al. 2005) for biotribological applications. Corrosion of metallic implants can have detrimental effects on the surrounding tissues in multiple ways (Kamachimudali, Sridhar, and Raj 2003). Three different types of corrosion can affect the passivation layer of implants: pitting, crevice, and fretting corrosion. Pitting corrosion occurs when the localized cavities form in the oxide layer around the implant. Crevice corrosion is triggered by differences in the oxygen concentration on different regions of the implant surface. Fretting corrosion occurs when two surfaces rub against each other under load conditions, resulting in the production of wear debris that can further exacerbate the damage (Agarwal et al. 2014). So it is clear that the various corrosions are serious issues in implants and have to be considered before the selection of materials for the implants.

3.2.6 HIGH FATIGUE LIFE

Fatigue properties are among the most important properties of the biomaterials in reducing implant failure and stress shielding effects. Hip prostheses are an example of implants that have failed due to fatigue (Sun et al. 2022). The fatigue life of the implants can be improved through various surface treatments and coatings. Shot blasting is one of the techniques that produces a compressive residual stress and roughness in the surface of the materials that can benefit the fatigue life of dental implants (Pérez et al. 2020). Also, researchers have explored various coating methods to improve the fatigue life of materials. For instance, a study found that a TiN coating has a high fatigue strength compared to steel (Madhukar† et al. 2018). Similarly, the carbon coating on the PEEK composite has exhibited a high fatigue safety factor (12.73%), which is important for hip implants (Teoh 2000).

3.3 OVERVIEW OF STANDARDS AND SPECIFICATIONS OF BIOMATERIAL

The preferred standards and specifications are extremely important to ensure that the applications of biomaterials are safe in operation. These standards and specifications serve as a benchmark for how the materials should be manufactured and tested, as well as for how they perform. Several organizations work on the formulation of standards and specifications for biomaterials. Table 3.3 shows a list of commonly used ASTM guidelines for the application of biomaterials.

TABLE 3.3

ASTM Guidelines for the Application of Biomaterials

ASTM Standard	Description/Title of Standards
ASTM F451–19	Standard Specification for Acetabular Prosthesis
ASTM F2026–19	This standard refers to the guidelines or protocol that have been established for the characterization and testing of biomaterial scaffolds used in tissue-engineered medical products.
ASTM F3039–20	Standard for Design, Manufacture, and Testing of Transcutaneous Oxygen Tension Monitoring Devices
ASTM F2026–19	Standard for Testing of Biomaterial Scaffolds Used in Tissue-Engineered Medical Products
ASTM F3183–20	Standard for Design and Performance of a Stent-Graft for the Treatment of Abdominal Aortic Aneurysms
ASTM F3184–19	Standard Specification for Metallic Bone Plates
ASTM F3187–20	This standard refers to the set of guidelines or specifications that have been established to define the performance of materials used in medical face masks.

The standards and specifications for biomaterials affect different areas, such as material properties, performance expectations, testing methods, labeling, marking requirements, environmental and biocompatibility requirements. For example, a few of the standards specify the minimum level of strength, resistance to fatigue, and biocompatibility for biomaterials. The standards utilized for various biomaterials are depicted in Figure 3.1.

3.3.1 BIOMATERIAL (POLYMER) STANDARDS

Polymer-based biomaterials comprise various materials such as polyethylene glycol (PEG), poly(lactic-co-glycolic acid) (PLGA), polyhydroxyalkanoates (PHA), and poly(caprolactone) (PCL). PEG is frequently utilized in drug delivery systems as it can enhance the solubility and bioavailability of drugs. On the other hand, PLGA and PHA are frequently used in tissue engineering applications because they are biodegradable and can support cell growth.

Despite the advantages, the polymer-based biomaterials have limitations such as low strength and stiffness compared to metallic biomaterials. Also, the use of polymers in the human body can lead to immune responses or inflammation. So it is very important to assess the biocompatibility of the polymers before subjecting them to the applications. The only biopolymer with better mechanical properties that is widely used in biomedical implants (knee and hip replacements) is ultra-high-molecular-weight polyethylene (UHMWPE). UHMWPE has several desirable properties, such as a low friction coefficient, high wear resistance, and biocompatibility. However, there are concerns regarding its

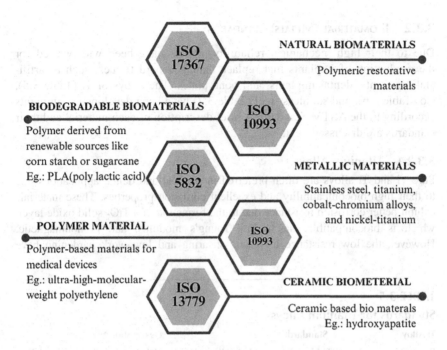

FIGURE 3.1 ISO standards for biomaterials.

TABLE 3.4
Standards for Polymer-Based Biomaterials (Outlined by ASTM and ISO)

Standard (for polymer)	Description
ASTM F2150	Provides guidelines for the testing of synthetic polymer-based biomaterials for use in medical implants.
ASTM F2027	Provides guidelines for the evaluation of the wear properties of polymer-based biomaterials.
ASTM F2024	Provides guidelines for the evaluation of the mechanical properties of polymer-based biomaterials used in medical devices.
ISO 10993	Specifies the biological evaluation polymer-based biomaterials to assess their potential toxicity.
ISO 14630	Provides guidelines for the characterization of polymeric biomaterials used in medical devices.
ISO 5832	Specifies the requirements for metallic and nonmetallic biomaterials for use in orthopedic implants.
ISO 10993–5	Specifies the tests for the in vitro cytotoxicity of polymer-based biomaterials

long-term performance and its potential for wear-debris-induced inflammatory response. Table 3.4 provides a compilation of frequently employed standards for polymer-based biomaterials, as outlined by ASTM and ISO.

3.3.2 Biomaterial (Metals) Standards

Due to their high mechanical reliability, metals have been widely used for the production of implants that replace damaged hard tissues, such as artificial hip joints, dental implants, and bone plates. The alloys of Ti (Table 3.5), Co (Table 3.6), and stainless steel (Table 3.7) have been developed as implants according to the ASTM Standard. A brief description of each material and their standards are discussed next.

3.3.2.1 Titanium Alloys

Pure Ti and Ti alloys are often preferred in medical and dental applications due to their high biocompatibility and excellent corrosion properties. These materials exhibit better corrosion resistance due to the formation of a TiO_2 solid oxide layer, which is biocompatible, has a low Young's modulus, and is nonmagnetic. However, the low resistance to plastic shearing and low work hardening have

TABLE 3.5
Standards for Titanium Alloys

Ti Alloy	Standard	Description
Pure Ti	ASTM F67–89	• Applies to both wrought and cast titanium materials. • Covers the requirements for the microstructure, surface finish, and permissible variations in dimensions.
Pure Ti	ASTM F67–19	• Specifies the mechanical, chemical, and metallurgical requirements for commercially available titanium. • Standards for seamless tubing and rod used for the manufacture of surgical implants.
Ti-6Al-4V	ASTM F620–87, F136–84	• Covers the chemical and mechanical requirements for titanium-6 aluminum-4 vanadium ELI alloy. • Standards for wire, bar, and forging stock.
Ti-6Al-4V	ASTM F1108–88	• Covers the requirements for titanium-6 aluminum-4 vanadium in surgical implants. • Covers chemical composition, mechanical properties, dimensions, and workmanship. • Standard for casting and testing the alloy. high strength, and low density.
Ti-6Al-4V (Extra low interstitial)	ASTM F1295–92	• Covers the chemical composition and mechanical properties, • Covers manufacturing and testing requirements for wrought bars, wire, forgings, and extrusions.
Ti-13Nb-13Zr	ASTM F1713–96	• Covers the requirements for the chemical composition and mechanical properties, • Standards for bars, wires, sheets, and strips.
Ti-12Mo-6Zr-2Fe	ASTM F1813–97	• Covers the requirements for chemical composition, mechanical properties, and biocompatibility. • Standards for bars, wires, and forgings.

TABLE 3.6
Standards for Stainless Steel Alloys

Stainless Steel Alloy	Standards	Description
18Cr-14Ni-2.5Mo alloy	ASTM F138–08	• Covers chemical and mechanical requirements for surgical implants. • Standards for bar and wire.
Stainless steel (UNS S31673)		• Stainless steel bar and wire used in surgical implants or other medical devices. • In the biomedical field, this standard is of paramount importance due to its focus on ensuring the safety, reliability, and quality of materials used in medical applications.
Wrought 18Cr-14Ni-2.5Mo stainless steel strip and sheet for surgical implants (UNS S31673)	ASTM F139–08	• Covers chemical and mechanical requirements for surgical implants. • Standards for sheet and strip.
Wrought stainless steel—implants for surgery	ISO 5832–1:2017	• Covers the chemical composition, mechanical properties, and specific requirements for seven types of stainless steel. • Guidelines for sampling, testing, and marking of the materials.
High nitrogen stainless steel	ISO 5832–9:2017	• Outlines the criteria for wrought high nitrogen stainless steel used in surgical implants. • Covers chemical composition, mechanical properties, and test methods for the material. • Provides information on appropriate cleaning and passivation procedures.

TABLE 3.7
Standards for Cobalt- Chromium Alloys

Cobalt-Chromium and Its Alloys	Standard	Description
Cobalt-chromium casting alloy for surgical implants (UNS R30075)	ASTM F75–12a	• Chemical and mechanical requirements • For cast and wrought Co-Cr alloy
Casting alloy of cobalt-chromium-molybdenum	ISO 5832–4:2014	• Requirements for Co-Cr casting alloy
Cobalt-chromium-molybdenum (wrought) alloys	ISO 5832–12:2016	• Requirements to produce surgical implants

been identified as drawbacks for Ti implants (Lu et al. 2021). Researchers have addressed these issues by exploring various surface modifications and coatings to enhance cell adhesion, proliferation, differentiation, and osteogenic differentiation. Different coatings, such as hydroxyapatite, bioactive glass, microporous coatings with hydroxyapatite and calcium titanate, and antibacterial coatings have been investigated to promote implant fixation, bacterial inhibition, and drug delivery. Table 3.5 outlines the established criteria and standards for titanium alloys (Thukkaram et al. 2020).

ASTM has developed two standards for pure titanium, which is mostly used in surgical implants: ASTM F67 and ASTM F136. ASTM F67 covers the requirements for unalloyed titanium, while ASTM F136 covers requirements for titanium alloy. Both standards recommend the chemical composition, mechanical properties, and testing requirements for titanium used in surgical implants. The use of these standards helps to ensure that titanium implants are safe and effective for use in medical procedures. In addition to these standards, there are also standards for other materials used in surgical implants such as surgical stainless-steel wire and ceramic materials. However, titanium continues to be a popular choice due to its strength, biocompatibility, and the standardization of its manufacturing processes. ASTM F136–84 is a standard that covers the requirements for wrought titanium-6 aluminum-4 vanadium alloy used in surgical implant applications. It also covers the requirements for the manufacture, finishing, and packaging of the material. The standard was revised in 2013 to include additional requirements for biocompatibility testing. Besides the standard discussed earlier, several other standards have been developed by ASTM International for different Ti alloys. These standards include ASTM F1108–88, ASTM F1295–92, ASTM F1713–96, and ASTM F1813–97. Each of these standards provides detailed requirements and specifications for the materials used in surgical implants.

3.3.2.2 Stainless Steel

Among the various alloys, SS316L is widely used in biomedical applications. However, some studies have shown that the presence of nickel in this alloy can lead to allergic reactions. In addition, the reports have indicated problems like pitting, crevice, and stress corrosion in implants made from SS316L. To mitigate the problem of allergic reactions triggered by nickel, stainless steels with elevated nitrogen levels have been formulated. The ongoing research emphasis is on producing nickel-free stainless steels (Fahad et al. 2023). From Table 3.6, it is clear that the standards are generally formulated based on materials, applications, and requirements. The ASTM F138–08 standard details the mechanical properties and chemical composition of wrought stainless steel (wire and bar) required for surgical implants. At the same time, for testing sheet- and strip-type implants (wrought stainless steel), the ASTM F139–08 standard was preferred. ISO 5832 is a collection of international standards that specify the standards for metallic materials used in the manufacture of surgical implants. The series is composed of multiple segments, each concentrating on a particular category of materials, including stainless steel, cobalt-chromium alloys, and titanium alloys. The standards cover the chemical composition, mechanical properties, and other requirements of these materials, as well as guidelines for testing, sampling, and marking them. Adherence to these standards has certainly helped to ensure the safety and effectiveness of surgical implants used in medical procedures.

3.3.2.3 Co-Cr Alloys

Cobalt-chromium (Co-Cr) alloys are more resistant to wear compared to both titanium (Ti) alloys and stainless steel alloys, and Co-Cr-Mo alloys are commonly used in artificial hip joints due to their high strength and ductility. Adding carbide to Co alloys enhances their wear resistance, and transforming the γ phase to the ε martensitic phase can also improve wear resistance. However, the Ni content in Co-Cr alloys can cause allergic reactions (Odaira et al. 2022). The Young's modulus of Co-Cr alloys and stainless steel is about ten times higher than that of bone, which may lead to stress shielding. In contrast, the Young's modulus of Ti and its alloys is about half that of stainless steel, making them less likely to cause stress shielding. Table 3.7 presents the main standards used for the classification of Co-Cr and its alloys, including ASTM F75, which outlines the requirements for Co-Cr-Mo alloy castings for surgical implant applications. This standard specifies the chemical composition, mechanical properties, and testing requirements for Co-Cr-Mo castings used in orthopedic implants, dental implants, and other surgical implants. ISO 5832 is a series of international standards that provide guidelines for metallic materials used in the production of surgical implants, with each guideline focusing on specific types of materials such as stainless steel, cobalt-chromium alloys, and titanium alloys.

3.4 TRIBOLOGY ASSESSMENT METHODS IN BIOMEDICAL IMPLANTS

The prediction of biomedical implant wear is crucial for the longevity and success of the implant in its intended application. The capacity of biomedical implants to endure wear and degradation over time is a crucial consideration in their design, particularly for implants that are intended to remain in the body for prolonged periods, like dental implants or joint replacements. The following are some of the experiments commonly used to predict implant wear.

3.4.1 WEAR SIMULATION TESTS

These tests involve simulating the relative motion between the implant and its surrounding tissues in a controlled laboratory environment. Various tests, such as pin-on-disk, reciprocating sliding, and ball-on-disk tests, can be conducted to evaluate the wear rate and wear mechanism of the implant material (Fu et al. 2022).

3.4.2 IN VITRO WEAR TESTING

This involves exposing the implant to a simulated body fluid, such as a saline solution, to simulate the wear that may occur in the body. The outcome of these tests can offer insights into the implant material's corrosion and wear resistance.

3.4.3 FINITE ELEMENT ANALYSIS (FEA)

Computational methods can be employed to anticipate the wear of the implant through the simulation of the implant's movement relative to the surrounding tissues, as well as the implant's load and motion.

3.4.4 SURFACE ANALYSIS

The evaluation of the surface properties of implant materials, such as their roughness and topography, is important as it can impact the implant's resistance to wear and corrosion.

3.4.5 IN VIVO TESTING

This involves implanting the device into an animal model to monitor the wear and degradation of the implant over time. The testing of implants in simulated physiological environments can help to evaluate their long-term performance and assess the wear and corrosion occurring under realistic conditions. Table 3.8 provides a list of standards related to biotribology, friction, lubrication, and wear in biological systems. These standards elaborate the range of topics related to biotribology, including testing methods, materials selection, and surface characterization.

3.5 TRIBOLOGY ASSESSMENT METHOD: GENERAL TRIBOMETERS USED IN BIOMATERIAL

Sir John Charnley, inventor of modern joint arthroplasty, created the first biomaterials wear tester in 1960. Different wear tester designs were developed for biomaterial testing, including unidirectional disk-on-plate, unidirectional pin-on-disk, bidirectional thrust-washer, reciprocating pin-on-disk, and unidirectional sphere-on-disk, all of which relied on Archard's law. The wear rates measured in these designs were significantly lower than those observed during in vivo wear rate testing. Nevertheless, achieving a wear rate similar to clinical values did not ensure the same wear mechanisms inside the human body. So it is important to have a sophisticated technique to compare the retrieved implants with those from articulating surfaces. Figure 3.2 illustrates the fundamental Biotribology assessment method that is currently in practice.

TABLE 3.8
Standards Related to Biotribology

ASTM Standard Number	Description/Title of Standards
ASTM G99–17	Standard Test Method for wear Testing Using Pin-on-Disk Apparatus
ASTM F2423–18	Method for Evaluating the Wear of Total Joint Prostheses
ASTM F732–19	Method for Evaluating the Wear Properties of Polymer Composite Materials Used in Joint Prostheses
ASTM F732–12	Method for Measuring Wear Properties of Endoprosthetic Materials and Devices
ASTM F746–08(2017)	Test Method for Measuring Abrasion Resistance of Polymer Composite Materials
ASTM F2612–13	Test Method for Wear Testing of Polyethylene against Polyethylene or Metal Counter faces
ASTM F2162–02(2019)	Test Method for Determining the Wear Properties of Polyethylene Used in Joint Replacements
ASTM F1717–13	Test Method for Evaluating the Wear of UHMWPE as a Bearing in Total Joint Replacements
ASTM F1841–16	Test Method for Evaluating Lubrication Properties of Bearings and Joint Simulator Lubricants
ASTM F2538–17	Test Method for Orthopedic Bearing's Friction and Wear Properties.
ASTM F2706–11(2017)	Test Method for Determining the Wear and Frictional Properties of Spinal Implant Motion Segments
ISO 14242–1	Standard for wear testing machines and environmental conditions for wear testing of total hip-joint prostheses.
ISO 14243–1/3	Knee wear test Experiment

3.5.1 PIN-ON-DISK TRIBOMETER FOR BIOMEDICAL DEVICES

A pin-on-disk tribometer (Figure 3.3) is a commonly used biotribology testing device to evaluate the wear and friction properties of biomaterials, particularly in the biomedical field to assess implant devices. It includes a stationary pin and rotating disk with controlled load and speed, with the contacting surface exposed to simulated body fluid. During the test, the frictional force between the pin and the disk is measured, and the wear of the materials is evaluated (Aherwar et al. 2019).

The pin-on-disk tribometer can also be used to evaluate the frictional properties of materials used in implants (ASTM G99 standard) (Borjali, Monson, and

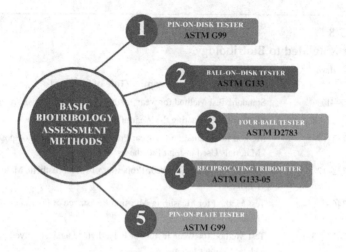

FIGURE 3.2   Basic biotribology assessment method.

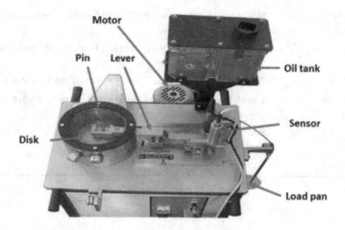

FIGURE 3.3   Pin-on-disk tribometer. (Kumar Kurre et al. 2023.)

Raeymaekers 2019). By evaluating the frictional properties of materials in a pin-on-disk tribometer, researchers can gain valuable insights into the behavior of a biomaterial in real human tissue applications. The attribute of friction is connected to the texture of a surface, and for better biological compatibility, it needs to correspond with the roughness of bone (Salguero et al. 2018).

3.5.2   Ball-on-Disk Tribometer for Biomedical Devices

Ball-on-disk tribometer is the next widely used device for measuring the wear characteristics of materials in various industries, including the biomedical field. There are several ASTM and ISO standards that provide guidelines for the use

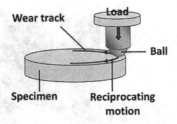

FIGURE 3.4 Ball-on-disk tribometer. (Ajibola et al. 2021.)

of ball-on-disk tribometers in biomedical applications. ASTM F2028 and ISO 14242 are two such standards that specify the testing conditions and parameters for evaluating the wear of orthopedic implants. ASTM F732 and ISO 6474 provide guidelines for testing the wear and frictional properties of hip implants. The use of these standards helps to ensure consistent and accurate testing of materials for biomedical applications.

The device comprises a stationary flat disk, which serves as a test specimen, and a spherical ball that rotates on the disk surface, applying a controlled load to the disk. The disk and ball can be made of different materials to simulate the actual wear conditions in a specific biomedical implant, such as a hip joint or knee prosthesis. The ball-on-disk tribometer (Figure 3.4) is a useful tool in evaluating the tribological performance of biomedical implants. It measures various parameters such as friction coefficient, wear volume, and wear rate, which are indicators of the wear behavior of the implants. Factors like contact pressure, sliding speed, lubrication conditions, and material properties can influence these parameters (Sadowski and Stupkiewicz 2019). During the testing procedure, the ball is rotated at a controlled speed while applying a load to the disk, and wear debris generated is collected and weighed. Tests are performed at a temperature of 37 ±0.1°C using simulated body fluids like Ringer's solution or fluids containing NaCl and PBS (phosphate-buffered solutions). The pin-on-disk, block-on-disk, and ball-on-disk methods are commonly used to study the tribological behavior of metallic biomaterials. Some studies have also conducted tests under dry sliding conditions (Cortes et al. 2019).

3.5.3 Wear and Total Hip Replacement (THR)

Total hip replacement (THR) surgeries are effective for treating degenerative joint diseases, but after 15 years of use, the implants' lifespan decreases significantly, leading to inflammation, loosening, and failure. To prolong their lifespan, researchers are focusing on improving the biotribological performance of orthopedic implants. Hip joint simulators have been developed to evaluate implant wear under body-simulated conditions and provide wear rates and particles similar to those observed in vivo. However, few simulator designs include friction measurement, which is an essential factor in understanding the dynamic performance of

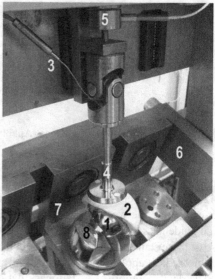

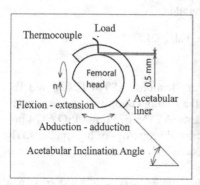

FIGURE 3.5   Hip simulator: (1) femoral module, (2) acetabular module, (3) thermocouple junction wire, (4) load bar, (5) transducer, (6) flexion–extension cradle, (7) abduction–adduction cradle, (8) femoral holder. (Saikko 2023.)

prostheses during wear tests. The wear rates obtained from these tests are crucial, but other properties of the prostheses articulating surfaces are needed to fully understand their dynamic performance. Hip simulator wear tests typically last over 3 months for 5 million cycles (Callaghan et al. 2003). The schematic layout of THR is shown in Figure 3.5.

ASTM F2887–18 provides a guide for evaluating the design and performance of femoral prostheses used in THR. ASTM F1714–08 covers the testing and evaluation of modular connection strength and fatigue performance for hip implants. ISO 7206–4:2021 outlines the testing procedures and criteria for determining the endurance properties of femoral components used in total hip replacement surgeries. ISO 7206–6:2013 provides guidelines for the assessment of the surface finish of metallic hip stems. These standards help to ensure that THR components and procedures meet specific requirements for safety and effectiveness.

3.5.4   KNEE SIMULATORS

A total knee simulator developed by EndoLab® is one of the well-known knee simulators that can be used to determine the wear of total knee endoprostheses and implant kinematics. The simulator allows testing in either force control or displacement control and has excellent machine accuracy due to its servohydraulic actuators (Maag et al. 2021). ASTM F1800 is the standard guide for the selection

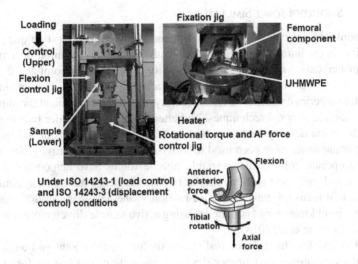

FIGURE 3.6   Knee simulator. (Okazaki et al. 2019.)

of knee simulators for testing knee implants, and it provides guidance on the use, design, and calibration of knee simulators. Another ASTM standard related to knee simulators (Figure 3.6) is ASTM F1714, which provides a method for the mechanical testing of knee implants using a four-station multiaxis simulator. ISO 14243 is an international standard that provides requirements and guidance for the performance of knee joint simulators for the evaluation of knee implants.

3.5.5   ANKLE JOINT SIMULATORS

Ankle joint simulators are utilized to imitate the loading and motion of the ankle joint, commonly for the purpose of examining the mechanics of the ankle joint or evaluating orthopedic implant. These simulators can replicate the complex motions of the ankle joint, including dorsiflexion, plantarflexion, inversion, and eversion, and can apply controlled loads to the joint during testing. They often use a combination of mechanical components, such as motors and sensors, and biological components, such as cadaveric tissue or animal models, to simulate the ankle joint (Wang et al. 2020).

Several ASTM and ISO standards exist for ankle joint simulators. ASTM F2996–13 is a standard guide for evaluating ankle arthroplasty devices using a physiological simulation. This standard provides guidelines for the design and testing of ankle simulators, as well as recommendations for test protocols and data analysis. ISO 22675:2018 is another standard that provides guidance on the mechanical testing of ankle joint prostheses, including the use of simulators. It covers testing methods for evaluating the durability and wear resistance of ankle prostheses, as well as guidelines for interpreting and reporting the results.

3.5.6 SHOULDER JOINT SIMULATORS

The shoulder joint requires both stability and mobility, making it unique among the joints in the human body. Shoulder prostheses are less common than knee or hip replacements, likely due to the complexity of the shoulder joint and the challenges of finding suitable models for replacement. As a result, the outcomes of shoulder surgeries can often be unsatisfactory, highlighting the need for improved prostheses and surgical techniques. To better understand shoulder biomechanics and inform the development of new surgical approaches, experimental shoulder testing apparatuses have been used to analyse motion and sensitivity. Simulators that incorporate continuously variable muscle forces have demonstrated more accurate and consistent motions similar to physiological conditions, as compared to those that focus on static or passive motion. Nonetheless, the studies that have explored joint kinematics and kinetics using active muscle-driven motion are limited (McCracken et al. 2018).

ASTM and ISO have developed standards for shoulder joint and ankle joint simulators to ensure their proper design, construction, and testing for evaluating the performance of joint implants. ASTM F2028–19 and F2346–16 provide standards for the characterization and presentation of the dimensional attributes of osteochondral allografts and the static and dynamic characterization of spinal artificial disks, respectively. ISO 14243–3:2014 is specifically used for wear testing of total ankle joint prostheses, providing loading and displacement parameters for the wear testing machine. These standards aim to ensure the safety, reliability, and effectiveness of shoulder and ankle joint simulators in evaluating the performance of joint implants (Verjans et al. 2016).

3.6 WEAR CHARACTERIZATION TECHNIQUES FOR BIOMATERIAL

3.6.1 WEAR MECHANISM ANALYSIS

The identification of wear mechanisms is crucial in accurately assessing the wear performance of biomaterials. It involves understanding the prevailing mechanisms of wear, including abrasion, adhesion, fatigue, and tribo-chemical reactions that exist in a biomaterial.

3.6.2 WEAR RATE MEASUREMENT

The measurement of wear rate is of utmost importance in evaluating the durability and appropriateness of a biomaterial for various biomedical purposes. For instance, The wear rate of polyethylene-on-metal hip implants is typically in the range of 10–100 mm³/million cycles. Cross-linked polyethylene has lower wear rates, typically in the range of 1–10 mm³/million cycles. Hence finding the appropriate wear rate is very import for effective sustainment of the implant in the host bone or tissue

3.6.3 FRICTIONAL BEHAVIOR

The assessment of the coefficient of friction and the determination of frictional forces encountered by the biomaterial when in contact with opposing surfaces are valuable in comprehending the material's interaction and its propensity for experiencing wear.

3.6.4 TOPOGRAPHY ANALYSIS

Surface analysis involves the examination and evaluation of the topographical and morphological characteristics of a worn biomaterial. This analysis enables the identification and understanding of wear mechanisms and the generation of wear debris. It also denotes whether cell adhesion is possible on the implant surface

3.6.5 WEAR DEBRIS ANALYSIS

The analysis of wear debris by examining the properties of the debris formed during wear tests is a valuable approach for evaluating the biological impact and biocompatibility of biomaterials. If some oxides or any other new substance forms during the wear process, this may cause a hazard to the recipient patient.

3.6.6 SCRATCH TEST

The assessment of a material's wear resistance is of paramount importance in determining its appropriateness for use in load-bearing applications, such as joint replacements.

3.6.7 INFLUENCE OF OPERATING CONDITIONS

The assessment of the impact of different operating conditions, including load, speed, and environmental elements, on wear behavior are crucial for comprehending the material's performance in practical scenarios.

3.6.8 LUBRICATION EFFECTS

The assessment of lubrication effects holds significance in the context of wear behavior analysis, particularly in relation to articulating implants. This evaluation encompasses the examination of both natural bodily fluids and synthetic lubricants.

3.6.9 FATIGUE AND WEAR

The comprehension of the relationship between fatigue and wear is essential in evaluating the performance of biomaterials subjected to repetitive loading.

3.7 LUBRICANTS FOR BIOTRIBOLOGY TESTING OF BIOMATERIALS

In biomaterial tribology testing, lubricants are used to simulate wear and assess the performance of materials in a liquid environment. Biolubricants, such as boric acid (H_3BO_3) and edible vegetable oils, are being explored as natural and environmentally friendly alternatives to traditional lubricants (Trzepieciński 2020). Nowadays, researchers used simulated body fluid for the biotribological testing as they eventually mimic the actual body fluid. Simulated body fluid (SBF) is an in vitro solution that has a similar composition as human plasma and is utilized to evaluate the bioactivity of materials. To determine the bone-bonding ability under in vivo conditions, SBF immersion experiments can be conducted to assess the potential of a material to develop an apatite coating on the implants (Shahabuddin et al. 2022).

Simulated body fluids (SBF) should maintain a comparable ion concentration to human blood plasma while being maintained under mild pH conditions and identical temperature. Simulated body fluids come in various forms, such as simulated gastric fluid (SGF), Hank's balanced salt solution (HBSS), and simulated intestinal fluid (SIF) (Jalota, Bhaduri, and Tas 2008).

3.8 SUMMARY AND FUTURE SCOPE

To sum up, this chapter provides a detailed overview of the different methods and standards used in the field of biomaterials to assess tribology. It explains the fundamental concepts of tribology and emphasizes the significance of wear and friction testing in evaluating the effectiveness of biomaterials. Furthermore, it describes the different testing techniques and standards that are commonly used in this area. Due to the rising demand for biomaterials in medical devices and implants, it is crucial to ensure that they meet the required performance criteria and are safe for use in the human body. This chapter's various tribological tests and standards offer a comprehensive approach to assessing the wear, friction, and corrosion properties of biomaterials.

The ISO and ASTM standards mentioned in this chapter provide guidelines for testing and characterizing biomaterials to ensure that they meet the necessary criteria for clinical use. The use of standardized testing methods and protocols helps to ensure that the results obtained are reliable, accurate, and can be compared across different studies and laboratories. The continued development and improvement of tribology assessment methods and standards will undoubtedly lead to the production of safer and more effective biomaterials in the future, which will have a positive impact on patient outcomes.

The field of tribology assessment methods and standards for biomaterials has made significant progress in ensuring the safety and effectiveness of medical devices and implants. Nevertheless, there is still room for further research and development in this field. One promising future direction is the development of advanced in vitro and in vivo testing methods that can more accurately simulate the complex physiological conditions of the human body. For instance, sophisticated computational models and simulations can be utilized to predict the wear and friction behavior of biomaterials under different loading conditions. Moreover, the use of more advanced testing techniques, such as micro- and nanoscale tribology, can offer more detailed insights into the mechanisms of wear and degradation.

Another important area of future research is the development of new and innovative biomaterials that can offer superior tribological properties. This could involve the use of new types of polymers, metals, ceramics, and composites, as well as the development of surface coatings and modifications that can reduce wear and friction. Furthermore, the use of rapid manufacturing techniques such as 3D printing and additive manufacturing could enable the creation of complex geometries and customized implants with optimized tribological properties.

Finally, there is a need for continued collaboration between researchers, regulatory agencies, and industry stakeholders to ensure that the latest research and best practices are incorporated into regulatory standards and guidelines. Adopting these advanced testing methods can play a significant role in guaranteeing the safety, efficiency, and reliability of novel medical devices and implants. At the same time, it can foster innovation and technological progress in the field.

REFERENCES

Agarwal, Anuja, Amit Tyagi, Anshuman Ahuja, Nishant Kumar, Nayana De, and Himanshu Bhutani. 2014. "Corrosion Aspect of Dental Implants—An Overview and Literature Review." *Open Journal of Stomatology* 4 (2): 56–60. doi:10.4236/ojst.2014.42010.

Agha, Nezha Ahmad, Frank Feyerabend, Boriana Mihailova, Stefanie Heidrich, Ulrich Bismayer, and Regine Willumeit-Römer. 2016. "Magnesium Degradation Influenced by Buffering Salts in Concentrations Typical of In Vitro and In Vivo Models." *Materials Science and Engineering: C* 58 (January): 817–25. doi:10.1016/j.msec.2015.09.067.

Aherwar, Amit, Amar Patnaik, Marjan Bahraminasab, and Amit Singh. 2019. "Preliminary Evaluations on Development of New Materials for Hip Joint Femoral Head." *Proceedings of the Institution of Mechanical Engineers, Part L: Journal of Materials: Design and Applications* 233 (5): 885–99. doi:10.1177/1464420717714495.

Ajibola, Olawale O., Abdullahi O. Adebayo, Sunday G. Borisade, Adebayo F. Owa, and Oladeji O. Ige. 2021. "Characterisation and Tribological Behaviour of Zinc-Aluminium (Zn-Al) Alloy under Dry Sliding Reciprocating Ball on Disk Tribometer." *Materials Today: Proceedings* 38: 1140–46. doi:10.1016/j.matpr.2020.07.135.

Barfeie, A., J. Wilson, and J. Rees. 2015. "Implant Surface Characteristics and Their Effect on Osseointegration." *British Dental Journal* 218 (5): E9. doi:10.1038/sj.bdj.2015.171.

Borjali, A., K. Monson, and B. Raeymaekers. 2019. "Predicting the Polyethylene Wear Rate in Pin-on-Disc Experiments in the Context of Prosthetic Hip Implants: Deriving a Data-Driven Model Using Machine Learning Methods." *Tribology International* 133 (May): 101–10. doi:10.1016/j.triboint.2019.01.014.

Boroujeni, Nariman Mansoori, Huan Zhou, Timothy J.F. Luchini, and Sarit B. Bhaduri. 2013. "Development of Multi-Walled Carbon Nanotubes Reinforced Monetite Bionanocomposite Cements for Orthopedic Applications." *Materials Science and Engineering: C* 33 (7): 4323–30. doi:10.1016/j.msec.2013.06.029.

Buyuksungur, Senem, Pinar Yilgor Huri, Jürgen Schmidt, Iulian Pana, Mihaela Dinu, Catalin Vitelaru, Adrian E. Kiss, et al. 2023. "In Vitro Cytotoxicity, Corrosion and Antibacterial Efficiencies of Zn Doped Hydroxyapatite Coated Ti Based Implant Materials." *Ceramics International* 49 (8): 12570–84. doi:10.1016/j.ceramint.2022.12.119.

Callaghan, John J., Douglas R. Pedersen, Richard C. Johnston, and Thomas D. Brown. 2003. "Clinical Biomechanics of Wear in Total Hip Arthroplasty." *The Iowa Orthopaedic Journal* 23: 1–12. www.ncbi.nlm.nih.gov/pubmed/14575243.

Chen, Lili, Fangling Ji, Yongming Bao, Jing Xia, Lianying Guo, Jingyun Wang, and Yachen Li. 2017. "Biocompatible Cationic Pullulan-g-Desoxycholic Acid-g-PEI Micelles Used to Co-Deliver Drug and Gene for Cancer Therapy." *Materials Science and Engineering: C* 70 (January): 418–29. doi:10.1016/j.msec.2016.09.019.

Conradi, Marjetka, Peter M. Schön, Aleksandra Kocijan, M. Jenko, and G. Julius Vancso. 2011. "Surface Analysis of Localized Corrosion of Austenitic 316L and Duplex 2205 Stainless Steels in Simulated Body Solutions." *Materials Chemistry and Physics* 130 (1–2): 708–13. doi:10.1016/j.matchemphys.2011.07.049.

Cortes, Vicente, Carlos A. Rodriguez Betancourth, Javier A. Ortega, and Hasina Huq. 2019. "Multidirectional Pin-on-Disk Testing Device to Evaluate the Cross-Shear Effect on the Wear of Biocompatible Materials." *Instruments* 3 (3): 35. doi:10.3390/instruments3030035.

Fabry, Christian, Carmen Zietz, Axel Baumann, Reinhard Ehall, and Rainer Bader. 2018. "High Wear Resistance of Femoral Components Coated with Titanium Nitride: A Retrieval Analysis." *Knee Surgery, Sports Traumatology, Arthroscopy* 26 (9): 2630–39. doi:10.1007/s00167-017-4578-7.

Fahad, Nesreen Dakhel, Nabaa Sattar Radhi, Zainab S. Al-Khafaji, and Abass Ali Diwan. 2023. "Surface Modification of Hybrid Composite Multilayers Spin Cold Spraying for Biomedical Duplex Stainless Steel." *Heliyon* 9 (3): e14103. doi:10.1016/j.heliyon.2023.e14103.

Fu, Wenqi, Shuang Liu, Jun Jiao, Zhiwen Xie, Xinfang Huang, Yun Lu, Huiying Liu, et al. 2022. "Wear Resistance and Biocompatibility of Co-Cr Dental Alloys Fabricated with CAST and SLM Techniques." *Materials* 15 (9): 3263. doi:10.3390/ma15093263.

Hallab, Nadim James, Shelley Anderson, Tiffany Stafford, Tibor Glant, and Joshua J. Jacobs. 2005. "Lymphocyte Responses in Patients with Total Hip Arthroplasty." *Journal of Orthopaedic Research* 23 (2): 384–91. doi:10.1016/j.orthres.2004.09.001.

Hosseinalipour, S.M., A. Ershad-langroudi, Amir Nemati Hayati, and A.M. Nabizade-Haghighi. 2010. "Characterization of Sol–Gel Coated 316L Stainless Steel for Biomedical Applications." *Progress in Organic Coatings* 67 (4): 371–74. doi:10.1016/j.porgcoat.2010.01.002.

Hussain, Omar, Shahid Saleem, and Babar Ahmad. 2019. "Implant Materials for Knee and Hip Joint Replacement: A Review from the Tribological Perspective." *IOP Conference Series: Materials Science and Engineering* 561 (1): 012007. doi:10.1088/1757-899X/561/1/012007.

Jalota, Sahil, Sarit B. Bhaduri, and A. Cuneyt Tas. 2008. "Using a Synthetic Body Fluid (SBF) Solution of 27 MM HCO_3- to Make Bone Substitutes More Osteointegrative." *Materials Science and Engineering: C* 28 (1): 129–40. doi:10.1016/j.msec.2007.10.058.

Jin, Z.M., J. Zheng, W. Li, and Z.R. Zhou. 2016. "Tribology of Medical Devices." *Biosurface and Biotribology* 2 (4): 173–92. doi:10.1016/j.bsbt.2016.12.001.

Jones, L.C., A.K. Tsao, and L.D.T. Topoleski. 2013. "Factors Contributing to Orthopaedic Implant Wear." In *Wear of Orthopaedic Implants and Artificial Joints*, 310–50. Elsevier. doi:10.1533/9780857096128.1.310.

Kamachimudali, U., T. M. Sridhar, and Baldev Raj. 2003. "Corrosion of Bio Implants."
    Sadhana 28 (3–4): 601–37. doi:10.1007/BF02706450.
Knight, Spencer J., Christine L. Abraham, Christopher L. Peters, Jeffrey A. Weiss, and
    Andrew E. Anderson. 2017. "Changes in Chondrolabral Mechanics, Coverage,
    and Congruency Following Peri-Acetabular Osteotomy for Treatment of Acetabu-
    lar Retroversion: A Patient-Specific Finite Element Study." *Journal of Orthopaedic
    Research* 35 (11): 2567–76. doi:10.1002/jor.23566.
Kumar Kurre, Santosh, Jitendra Yadav, Ashish Mudgal, Nikhil Malhotra, Akarsh Shukla,
    and V.K. Srivastava. 2023. "Experimental Study of Friction and Wear Characteristics
    of Bio-Based Lubricant on Pin-on-Disk Tribometer." *Materials Today: Proceedings*,
    February. doi:10.1016/j.matpr.2023.02.071.
Lu, Xiaoxuan, Zichen Wu, Kehui Xu, Xiaowei Wang, Shuang Wang, Hua Qiu, Xiangyang
    Li, and Jialong Chen. 2021. "Multifunctional Coatings of Titanium Implants Toward
    Promoting Osseointegration and Preventing Infection: Recent Developments." *Frontiers
    in Bioengineering and Biotechnology* 9 (December). doi:10.3389/fbioe.2021.783816.
Maag, Chase, Amber Metcalfe, Ioan Cracaoanu, Casey Wise, and Daniel D. Auger. 2021.
    "The Development of Simulator Testing for Total Knee Replacements." *Biosurface
    and Biotribology* 7 (2): 70–82. doi:10.1049/bsb2.12001.
Madhukar†, Samatham, Birudala Raga Harshith Reddy, Gyara Ajay Kumar, and Ramawath
    Prashanth Naik†. 2018. "A Study on Improvement of Fatigue Life of Materials by
    Surface Coatings." *International Journal of Current Engineering and Technology* 8
    (1): 5–9. doi:10.14741/ijcet.v8i01.10878.
Marattukalam, Jithin James, Dennis Karlsson, Victor Pacheco, Přemysl Beran, Urban
    Wiklund, Ulf Jansson, Björgvin Hjörvarsson, and Martin Sahlberg. 2020. "The
    Effect of Laser Scanning Strategies on Texture, Mechanical Properties, and Site-
    Specific Grain Orientation in Selective Laser Melted 316L SS." *Materials & Design*
    193 (August): 108852. doi:10.1016/j.matdes.2020.108852.
McCracken, Laura C., Ana Luisa Trejos, Marie-Eve LeBel, Behnaz Poursartip, Abelardo
    Escoto, Rajni V. Patel, and Michael D. Naish. 2018. "Development of a Physical Shoul-
    der Simulator for the Training of Basic Arthroscopic Skills." *The International Journal of
    Medical Robotics and Computer Assisted Surgery* 14 (1): e1868. doi:10.1002/rcs.1868.
Moghadasi, Kaveh, Mohammad Syahid Mohd Isa, Mohammad Ashraf Ariffin, Muhammad
    Zulhiqmi Mohd jamil, Sufian Raja, Bo Wu, Mehrdad Yamani, et al. 2022. "A Review
    on Biomedical Implant Materials and the Effect of Friction Stir Based Techniques on
    Their Mechanical and Tribological Properties." *Journal of Materials Research and
    Technology* 17 (March): 1054–121. doi:10.1016/j.jmrt.2022.01.050.
Muhammad, Ibrahim, Xiaoming Yu, Qingchuan Wang, Yanfang Li, Weirong Li, Lili Tan,
    and Ke Yang. 2023. "Enhancing Corrosion and Wear Resistance of Mg Coating on
    Titanium Implants by Micro-Arc Oxidation and Heat Treatment." *Materials Technol-
    ogy* 38 (1). doi:10.1080/10667857.2023.2176971.
Muñoz-García, Javier, Luis Vázquez, Mario Castro, Raúl Gago, Andrés Redondo-Cubero,
    Ana Moreno-Barrado, and Rodolfo Cuerno. 2014. "Self-Organized Nanopatterning
    of Silicon Surfaces by Ion Beam Sputtering." *Materials Science and Engineering:
    R: Reports* 86 (December): 1–44. doi:10.1016/j.mser.2014.09.001.
Nakano, T. 2010. "Mechanical Properties of Metallic Biomaterials." In *Metals for Bio-
    medical Devices*, 71–98. Elsevier. doi:10.1533/9781845699246.2.71.
Odaira, Takumi, Sheng Xu, Kenji Hirata, Xiao Xu, Toshihiro Omori, Kosuke Ueki,
    Kyosuke Ueda, et al. 2022. "Flexible and Tough Superelastic Co–Cr Alloys for
    Biomedical Applications." *Advanced Materials* 34 (27): 2202305. doi:10.1002/
    adma.202202305.

Okazaki, Yoshimitsu, Minako Hosoba, Syuichi Miura, and Tadashi Mochizuki. 2019. "Effects of Knee Simulator Control Method and Radiation Dose on UHMWPE Wear Rate, and Relationship between Wear Rate and Clinical Revision Rate in National Joint Registry." *Journal of the Mechanical Behavior of Biomedical Materials* 90 (February): 182–90. doi:10.1016/j.jmbbm.2018.09.034.

Penkov, Oleksiy V., Vladimir E. Pukha, Svetlana L. Starikova, Mahdi Khadem, Vadym V. Starikov, Maxim V. Maleev, and Dae-Eun Kim. 2016. "Highly Wear-Resistant and Biocompatible Carbon Nanocomposite Coatings for Dental Implants." *Biomaterials* 102 (September): 130–36. doi:10.1016/j.biomaterials.2016.06.029.

Pérez, R.A., J. Gargallo, P. Altuna, M. Herrero-Climent, and F.J. Gil. 2020. "Fatigue of Narrow Dental Implants: Influence of the Hardening Method." *Materials* 13 (6): 1429. doi:10.3390/ma13061429.

Pezzotti, Giuseppe. 2014. "Bioceramics for Hip Joints: The Physical Chemistry Viewpoint." *Materials* 7 (6): 4367–4410. doi:10.3390/ma7064367.

Ramsden, J.J., D.M. Allen, D.J. Stephenson, J.R. Alcock, G.N. Peggs, G. Fuller, and G. Goch. 2007. "The Design and Manufacture of Biomedical Surfaces." *CIRP Annals* 56 (2): 687–711. doi:10.1016/j.cirp.2007.10.001.

Sadowski, Przemysław, and Stanisław Stupkiewicz. 2019. "Friction in Lubricated Soft-on-Hard, Hard-on-Soft and Soft-on-Soft Sliding Contacts." *Tribology International* 129 (January): 246–56. doi:10.1016/j.triboint.2018.08.025.

Sahoo, Prasanta, Suman Kalyan Das, and J. Paulo Davim. 2019. "Tribology of Materials for Biomedical Applications." In *Mechanical Behaviour of Biomaterials*, 1–45. Elsevier. doi:10.1016/B978-0-08-102174-3.00001-2.

Saikko, Vesa. 2023. "VEXLPE Friction Studied with a Multidirectional Hip Joint Simulator Using Contact Temperature Control." *Tribology International* 187 (September): 108707. doi:10.1016/j.triboint.2023.108707.

Salguero, Jorge, Juan Vazquez-Martinez, Irene Sol, and Moises Batista. 2018. "Application of Pin-On-Disc Techniques for the Study of Tribological Interferences in the Dry Machining of A92024-T3 (Al–Cu) Alloys." *Materials* 11 (7): 1236. doi:10.3390/ma11071236.

Shahabuddin, M., M. Mofijur, I.M. Rizwanul Fattah, M.A. Kalam, H.H. Masjuki, M.A. Chowdhury, and Nayem Hossain. 2022. "Study on the Tribological Characteristics of Plant Oil-Based Bio-Lubricant with Automotive Liner-Piston Ring Materials." *Current Research in Green and Sustainable Chemistry* 5: 100262. doi:10.1016/j.crgsc.2022.100262.

Stefano, Marco De, Silvana Mirella Aliberti, and Alessandro Ruggiero. 2022. "(Bio)Tribocorrosion in Dental Implants: Principles and Techniques of Investigation." *Applied Sciences* 12 (15): 7421. doi:10.3390/app12157421.

Sun, Fei, Wei Cheng, Baohong Zhao, and Zeng Lin. 2022. "Fatigue Properties of Plasma Nitriding for Dental Implant Application." *The Journal of Prosthetic Dentistry* 131 (2): 329.e1–e8. doi:10.1016/j.prosdent.2022.01.019.

Teoh, S. 2000. "Fatigue of Biomaterials: A Review." *International Journal of Fatigue* 22 (10): 825–37. doi:10.1016/S0142-1123(00)00052-9.

Thukkaram, Monica, Renee Coryn, Mahtab Asadian, Parinaz Saadat Esbah Tabaei, Petra Rigole, Naveenkumar Rajendhran, Anton Nikiforov, et al. 2020. "Fabrication of Microporous Coatings on Titanium Implants with Improved Mechanical, Antibacterial, and Cell-Interactive Properties." *ACS Applied Materials & Interfaces* 12 (27): 30155–69. doi:10.1021/acsami.0c07234.

Tracana, R. B., J. P. Sousa, and G. S. Carvalho. 1994. "Mouse Inflammatory Response to Stainless Steel Corrosion Products." *Journal of Materials Science: Materials in Medicine* 5 (9–10): 596–600. doi:10.1007/BF00120337.

Trzepieciński, Tomasz. 2020. "Tribological Performance of Environmentally Friendly Bio-Degradable Lubricants Based on a Combination of Boric Acid and Bio-Based Oils." *Materials* 13 (17): 3892. doi:10.3390/ma13173892.

Vallet-Regí, M., I. Izquierdo-Barba, and F. J. Gil. 2003. "Localized Corrosion of 316L Stainless Steel with SiO 2-CaO Films Obtained by Means of Sol-Gel Treatment." *Journal of Biomedical Materials Research Part A* 67A (2): 674–78. doi:10.1002/jbm.a.10159.

Verjans, Mark, Nad Siroros, Jörg Eschweiler, and Klaus Radermacher. 2016. "Technical Concept and Evaluation of a Novel Shoulder Simulator with Adaptive Muscle Force Generation and Free Motion." *Current Directions in Biomedical Engineering* 2 (1): 61–5. doi:10.1515/cdbme-2016-0017.

Wang, Chenchen, Hongxing Hu, Zhipeng Li, Yifan Shen, Yong Xu, Gangqiang Zhang, Xiangqiong Zeng, et al. 2019. "Enhanced Osseointegration of Titanium Alloy Implants with Laser Microgrooved Surfaces and Graphene Oxide Coating." *ACS Applied Materials & Interfaces* 11 (43): 39470–83. doi:10.1021/acsami.9b12733.

Wang, Dongmei, Wei Wang, Qinyang Guo, Guanglin Shi, Genrui Zhu, Xu Wang, and Anmin Liu. 2020. "Design and Validation of a Foot–Ankle Dynamic Simulator with a 6-Degree-of-Freedom Parallel Mechanism." *Proceedings of the Institution of Mechanical Engineers, Part H: Journal of Engineering in Medicine* 234 (10): 1070–82. doi:10.1177/0954411920938902.

Xu, Xianxing, Hailun Xu, Qihao Chai, Ziyang Li, Zhentao Man, and Wei Li. 2023. "Novel Functionalized Ti6Al4V Scaffold for Preventing Infection and Promoting Rapid Osseointegration." *Materials & Design* 226 (February): 111612. doi:10.1016/j.matdes.2023.111612.

Zhou, Z.R., and Z.M. Jin. 2015. "Biotribology: Recent Progresses and Future Perspectives." *Biosurface and Biotribology* 1 (1): 3–24. doi:10.1016/j.bsbt.2015.03.001.

4 Tribological Behaviors of Implants

Ravivarman R
National Institute of Technology
Agartala, Tripura, India

4.1 INTRODUCTION TO TRIBOLOGY IN IMPLANTS

Tribology in biomedical implants refers to the study of material surface interaction regarding friction, wear, and lubrication, as well as the ways in which these factors interact within the body [1] and the implants. The tribological principles are used to study the moving mechanisms in artificial biological systems. The moving mechanism includes the articulating joints like the hip, knee, shoulder, and ankle in the biological systems. According to recent studies, approximately 2 million joint replacements have been executed in the last decade, and this figure is expected to increase significantly in the years to come [2,3]. In the last two years, COVID-19 has also caused a sharp rise in implant transplantation, especially hip implantation [4]. In the investigations done, the hip implant mortality was greater for the COVID-19-positive group. A steady rise in joint problems is also noted because of COVID-19 postoperative complications. This necessitates a prolonged study on the aftereffects of implantation, including the study of tribological characteristics with bone surfaces. Accessing the tribological characteristics involves comprehending and managing the wear mechanisms that happen in the implant materials inside the body with respect to the tissues and fluids. The successful use of biomaterials in a variety of replacement operations has been enhanced by the recent growth of biotribology [5] research in the medical field. Nowadays, a variety of material combinations—including metals, carbon ceramics, and polymers—are employed in biological applications. Among the materials used, polymers showed predominant results [6,7] with tribological characteristics like minimum friction coefficient, enhanced wear strength, and biocompatibility within the body [7]. The functionality of the implants is affected due to improper selection of friction coefficient between the articulating surfaces, which demands the proper choice of friction coefficient. High-wear-resistant material with proper durability is anticipated to ensure appropriate function for a prolonged period in the lifetime of the implants. Biocompatibility also must be considered as the tissues and fluids present in the human body come into direct interaction with the implants. All these tribological characteristics were found to be enhanced in the recently developed polyethylene material [8], compared to the existing materials. In the realm of medical implants, tribology is concerned in maximising devices' functionality and design to guarantee their robustness, safety, and biocompatibility. It also entails analysing the wear resistance of materials, examining the frictional behavior between

DOI: 10.1201/9781003384847-4

implant components and creating lubrication strategies to lessen wear and friction inside the body. Biomedical implants such as orthopedic joint replacements, dental prosthetics, and cardiovascular implants like stents and artificial heart valves require an understanding of commitment to enhance longevity and its efficacy through tribological qualities. The capacity of these implants to survive the intricate and dynamic mechanical conditions found within the human body determines both their effectiveness and lifespan.

The importance of understanding tribology in the background of biomedical sciences is crucial for reasons like biocompatibility, durability, functionality, and reduction of complications. A deeper exploration of the various tribological aspects and challenges related to biomedical implants is necessary for understanding and optimizing the tribological behaviors of implant materials. A crucial forecast is also needed to evaluate the success of implants in individual patients and to advance in the domain of medical device engineering and health care. In this chapter, research studies focusing on these parameters like wear mechanism, surface coatings, friction coefficient, and lubrication are deliberated to attain elementary and stable knowledge.

4.2 SIGNIFICANCE OF TRIBOLOGY STUDY IN IMPLANTS

The design of implants largely relies on the tribology of interacting surfaces in relative motion [9]. Implants frequently have surfaces in contact during regular activities. Debris and particles are produced due to the wear and friction between these surfaces, potentially resulting in implant failure, tissue injury, and inflammation [10]. Tribology and surface treatments aid in designing materials with reduced wear and friction in order to prolong the life and improve the functionality of implants.

In the hip and knee joint replacements portrayed in Figure 4.1, anthropological factors turn out to be vital to replicating the joints' natural movements. Because the articulating surface contacts in these joints [11] need to be carefully developed to minimise wear and friction. The success of joint replacements is a significant milestone in the

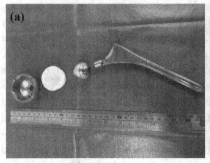
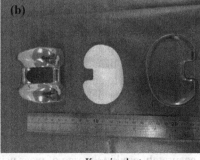

Hip implant Knee implant

FIGURE 4.1 Joints contacts: (a) hip implant, (b) knee implant.

history of orthopaedics during the 20th century. Even though the success rate is high, the material science community is quite concerned about the number of revision procedures that are needed because of implant wear. Patients, doctors, and health care systems [12] also bear a significant burden because of revision surgeries. Problems like osteolysis [13] or the loss of bone around an implant because of wear debris necessitate revision surgeries, which can be prevented by enhancing tribological features. The stability of implants is also influenced by tribological variables. For instance, in orthopedic implants osseointegration [14], the implant fuses with the surrounding bone that is impacted by the contacts between the implant and the bone.

The demand for dental implant is increasing each year globally as the number of accidental tooth loss cases rises and population aging becomes a global problem [15]. Dental implants must have great strength, superior corrosion resistance, and outstanding biocompatibility to fulfil the demanding biological criteria [16,17]. Dental implant [18] materials must be strong enough to endure the mechanical stresses of biting and chewing without putting undue strain on neighbouring teeth or adjacent tissues. Additionally, tribological factors also help in the design of surfaces that inhibit bacterial bonding [19], thereby reducing the risk of infection.

Thus, improving tribological characteristics can help the implant integrate more fully with the host tissue and be more stable. Decreased wear and friction improve patient comfort while extending the life of implants. Patients who have implants with little wear and seamless functioning are likely to have a higher quality of life. From these discussions, it is concluded that tribology plays a vital role in the development, design, and functionality of implants. It guarantees that implants are biologically compatible and mechanically sound, which enhances the stability, lifespan, and general success of the implantation in the long term. The goal of improved durability of the implant has kept the research going owing to these restraints.

4.3 TRIBOLOGICAL ASPECTS OF IMPLANTS

4.3.1 WEAR MECHANISM

When implant materials are subjected to mechanical stresses, they deteriorate and lose material in different ways. Understanding the wear mechanisms is essential for designing and selecting materials for biomedical implants. Several primary wear mechanisms like adhesive, abrasive, fatigue, pitting, erosive, and creep wear are observed in implant materials. When two surfaces come in contact and adhere owing to friction, then the wear developed is called adhesive wear. Material slides from one surface to another due to this wear. Adhesive wear in implant materials may result in wear debris [20,21] production and surface degradation. Implant wear rate prediction has been carried out using both experimental and numerical methods. Recently developed advanced finite element techniques [22,23], conducted on the ultra-high-molecular-weight polyethylene (UHMWPE), proposed to accurately predict the rate of wear using the most cited Archard law [24].

$$V = kF_N s \tag{1}$$

where V = wear volume, k = wear coefficient, F_{N-} = normal force in contact, and s = sliding distance.

Compared to the wear tests conducted experimentally as depicted in Figure 4.2, wear predictive models of implants are becoming more widespread for the preclinical evaluation. This is because they enable fast and inexpensive acquisition of information on the long-term functioning of these devices. Adhesive wear is reduced with the proper combination of surface treatments and lubrication in orthopedic [25] and dental implants [26].

Another type of wear mechanism in implants is called abrasive wear, which is the result of material being removed due to asperities or abrasive particles on one or both surfaces. Abrasive wear can happen when hard particles, such as bone fragments or debris from implants, encounter the surface. The totally conformal reciprocating sliding contact against UHMWPE [27] and the three-body abrasive wear behavior using the titanium debris was deliberated in the study conducted in the orthopedic implant surface. Titanium alloy microabrasion wear behavior was [28] investigated for various friction pairs using the abrasion tester shown in Figure 4.3. The abrasive wear loss on different friction pairings varied with varying sliding distance, and the mode progressively transitioned from two-body to mixed and finally three-body abrasion. This kind of wear entails the release of minuscule wear debris or particles that may discover their way into the surrounding tissues or bloodstream. Implant materials biocompatibility can be significantly impacted by microscopic wear.

An implant material experiences fatigue wear because of repeated loading and unloading due to the patient's activities, which can cause cracks to start and propagate. Owing to cyclic loading during daily activities, several implants are vulnerable to cyclic loads and wear, which is a concern for the fretting of orthopedic implants [29]. Fretting wear develops when there is constant and oscillatory relative motion between the surfaces. Particularly at the implant–bone interface in orthopedic implants, this wear may cause material loss and surface degradation [30]. Fatigue failure is also considered to be one of the most common types

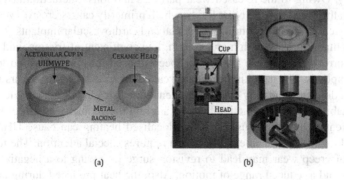

(a) (b)

FIGURE 4.2 Hip implant: (a) UHMWPE acetabular cup and ceramic head, (b) KUPA E-Sim hip joint simulator.

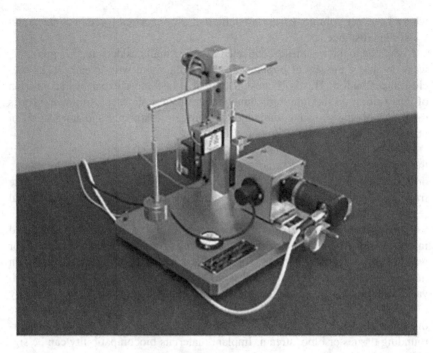

FIGURE 4.3　Abrasion tester at microscale level.

of failure in dental implants [31], which adds regular investigation to recognize the variables influencing the fatigue life of dental implants. High-fatigue-resistant materials with a proper surface coating are used in these implants to enhance the fatigue strength and reduce pitting, which leads to crater formation.

When a material is exposed to corrosive conditions (such as bodily fluids) due to mechanical activity, its results in a mix of wear and corrosion. This is a serious concern in implants, which predominantly occurs in the event of metal components. This may also release wear particles and ions that could be harmful to the body. Owing to the released wear particles and ions, interaction takes place between the blood and the other fluids, which primarily causes erosive wear. This erosive wear is more predominant in dental and cardiovascular implants. To counter this, titanium alloy with high strength, low coefficient of friction, and exceptional corrosion resistance [32,33] has been utilised most as compared to other metal implants. The next kind of wear is called creep wear, and it occurs when a material deforms gradually over time when loaded steadily. It may result in wear and instability in orthopedic implants by altering the geometry and fit of implant components. One study suggested that localised heating can cause UHMWPE material to oxidise and creep [34], which requires special attention. The intricate nature of creep wear may lead to revision surgeries owing to a negative tissue reaction and a reduced range of motion. Also, the heat produced during articulation must be considered in forecasting the femoral implant surfaces' articulating systems to achieve long-term performance. It is clear from such various wear mechanisms that ongoing research and development needs to be conducted to create mutually biocompatible and long-lasting implant materials.

4.3.1.1 Wear Characterization and Testing Methods

From the previous section it is understood that, to guarantee the effectiveness and durability of biomedical implants, the wear and tribological characteristics of implant materials must be accessed intensely. These features are assessed using a variety of techniques and testing procedures. The following are a few standard techniques for assessing the tribological characteristics and wear of implant materials:

4.3.1.1.1 Pin-on-Disk Testing

In this technique, a pin—which stands in for the implant material—is rotated in controlled circumstances against a flat disk, which stands in for a counter surface [35]. Frictional force and wear rate measurements are made to get information on the materials' tribological behavior. Pin-on-disk testing is a useful technique for evaluating the impact of material interactions, lubrication, and environmental factors. Many studies [36] have evaluated the suitability of utilising a multidirectional pin-on-disk tribometer for various combinations of materials. Compared to joint simulators that replicate clinical circumstances, which can be costly to set up and maintain, this device is straightforward to use and reasonably priced. Widespread wear for various material combinations in prosthetic hip implants is quantified using pin-on-disk experiment results [37]. The most recent work on titanium alloys [38] examined the tribological properties in dry conditions with ASTM G99–95a standards, considering input factors such as normal load, sliding distance, and speed. This was done using the pin-on-disk tribometers shown in Figure 4.4. The results of the trial presented the interaction of sliding speed and sliding distance, wear mass loss, and friction coefficient.

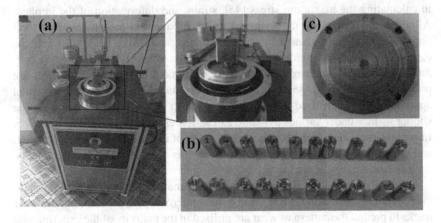

FIGURE 4.4   (a) Pin on disc—triobometer, (b) titanium alloy pins, (c) counterpart surface steel disk.

4.3.1.1.2   Linear Reciprocating Sliding Testing
Using this technique, an implant sample, typically a pin or flat specimen material, moves linearly back and forth across a stationary counter surface. Investigation of continuous wear monitoring was performed in the titanium alloy [39] against the alumina using the linear reciprocating sliding mechanism at different normal loads and sliding velocities. The factors obtained from the test are the penetration depth and wear rate. This test was used to simulate the sliding motion [40,41] found in some implant applications such as prosthetic joints.

4.3.1.1.3   Block-on-Ring Testing
To simulate the behavior of materials in rolling or sliding contact, a block specimen is slid on a rotating ring in this test setup. Few research [42–44] utilised the block on ring tester in their study to assess the wear and friction characteristics of orthopedic implant materials.

4.3.1.1.4   Hip Simulator Testing
The most recently designed hip simulators (Figure 4.2) are specifically made to replicate the intricate hip joint motion and load circumstances to evaluate the wear behavior of hip joint replacements. This simulator monitors the wear of components in the femoral head and the acetabular cup using a lubricating fluid.

4.3.1.1.5   Structural Finite Element Analysis (FEA)
FEA is also widely performed to understand and predict the wear behavior and performance of prostheses. FEA plays a crucial part in assessing static and dynamic loading scenarios, evaluating the influence of fatigue and cyclic loading, understanding failure mechanisms, and optimising implant geometry and material properties. Static loading is the most performed type of analysis in implants as it helps to assess the mechanical response and stability of the implant under normal physiological conditions. The geometry of the prostheses plays an influential role in calculating the maximum stress [45], strain, and deformation of the implant. Although the design and dimensions vary from patient to patient based on their physical condition, a standard design is chosen, and, using FEA software, the essential boundary conditions are specified based on the ASTM and loading conditions as per ISO standards to predict the outcome. The models of implants are prepared using 3D CAD application. A finite element modelling and experimental approach [46] was carried out in a hip implant to examine the wear against the sliding surface under various dynamic gait activities, as represented in Figure 4.5. In recent times, FEA helped to decrease the risk of implant failure, wear, fracture, and infection. It also used to explore novel designs and materials for hip implants, such as functionally graded lattice or bioinspired structures [47].

A microhardness tester like Vickers for estimating the hardness [48], scanning electron microscopy (SEM), and optical microscopy for examining the wear tracks to predict the pattern of wear are utilised in the majority of the experimental works conducted in the tribological characterisation of implants in biomedical sciences. The real-world data from in vivo and retrieval studies offer important

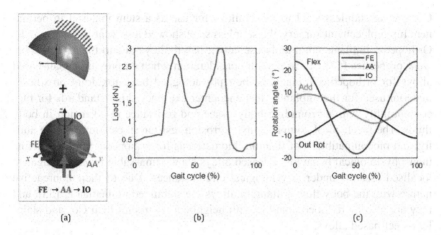

(a)   (b)   (c)

FIGURE 4.5 Dynamic gait activities: (a) normal load, (b) and rotation angle, and (c) curves trailed ISO 14242.

insights about how the implant materials function [49] in the human body, even though laboratory testing is still necessary. To comprehend long-term wear and performance, these investigations analyse the tissues and implants that have been taken out from the body. Combining multiple testing methods can provide a comprehensive assessment of an implant's overall performance in terms of tribological characteristics.

4.3.2 MATERIALS AND SURFACE PROPERTIES IMPACT ON TRIBOLOGICAL BEHAVIORS

The tribological behavior of implant materials is largely determined by their surface characteristics. The properties of friction and wear can be influenced by surface roughness and chemical topography. To minimise friction and encourage tissue integration, engineers frequently create smooth bioactive implant surfaces. Enhancing wear resistance in bioimplants requires careful material selection and alterations in surfaces using some surface treatment operations. The application and implant type determine the materials and surface treatments to be used. Metals are divided into numerous groups: stainless steel, Co-based alloys, Ti-based alloys, Mg-based alloys, Fe-based alloys, and Zn-based alloy [50]. Due to their adequate strength, ductility, corrosion resistance, biocompatibility, and fracture toughness, metallic materials are frequently utilized in orthopedic implants

As the properties of stainless steel are long-lasting and resistant to corrosion, it is widely utilised in a variety of implants, such as screws, pins, fracture plates and hip nails [50]. The iron- (Fe-) based alloys that make up stainless steel often include some percentage of Cr and Ni. Significant levels of the alloying metals like molybdenum and manganese, as well as trace quantities of carbon, nitrogen, phosphorus, sulphur, and silicon, are also present in medical-grade stainless steel.

Comparing stainless steel to other alloys for use as a stem material in permanent hip replacement surgery, the stainless steel showed less wear resistance [51]. Orthopedic implants commonly use cobalt-based alloys due to their remarkable wear properties [52]. An important consideration when employing cobalt-based alloys for orthopedic implants is their physiological behavior. Joint prostheses material used for the implants must encounter extremely high standards for biocompatibility with surrounding body tissue and resistance to corrosion in body fluids. The mechanical compatibility, corrosion resistance, osteointegration ability, and biocompatibility of titanium biomaterials for orthopedic implants define their physiological behavior. Ti-based alloys show remarkable resistance against localised assaults under physiological circumstances. Due to their nonreactive nature with the body fluids, titanium alloys are stabilized immediately [53], and they are also more biocompatible with neighbouring tissues than Co- and stainless-steel-based alloys.

The main categories of orthopedic ceramics are bioinert and bioactive ceramics. In the human body, bioinert ceramics undergo physical or chemical alterations over an extended duration and stimulate minimal response in living tissues. For these reasons, bioinert ceramic materials are not conventionally used in fracture repair applications, although they are used in articular components of total joint replacements [50]. Al_2O_3 (alumina), ZrO_2 (zirconia), and Si_3N_4 (silicon nitride) are a few bioinert ceramics that are widely in use for the following reasons. Alumina is employed in knee and hip replacements because of its wear resistance and biocompatibility [54,55]. Another ceramic material utilised in orthopedic implants is zirconia [56], which is selected for its high hardness and the inert nature of the debris created due to low wear rate. For the last four years, silicon nitride has been widely used in spinal surgeries without causing any problems. Few ceramics that are bioactive can develop direct interactions with the surrounding biological bone tissues [57] due to the biological affinity.

Polymers are long-chain molecules made up of numerous tiny repeating monomers, or composer units. Polymers can be attained from synthetic organic sources or from natural sources. In recent joint replacements surgeries, cross-linked [58] ultra-high-molecular-weight polyethylene (UHMWPE) is utilised for enhanced wear resistance at the articulating surface. Numerous orthopedic implants are made of polyetheretherketone (PEEK) [59–61], which can be reinforced with carbon fibres to increase its resistance to wear. Table 4.1 lists the tribological properties of materials with their applications in biomedical sciences.

4.3.2.1 Surface Treatments

The biomechanical circumstances of the body and the anticipated endurance of implant functionality are the unique requirements of the implant that should be considered when choosing materials and surface treatments to enhance wear resistance. To ensure that the chosen materials and treatments fulfil the requisite wear resistance criteria and biocompatibility requirements, extensive techniques and assessment are required. Hydroxyapatite (HA) coating are the most prevalent techniques carried out with titanium alloys to improve the inertness and stability

TABLE 4.1
Materials Used as Implants with Applications (50–61)

Materials	Characteristics	Applications
Metals		
Stainless steel	Excellent corrosion resistance Good biocompatibility High strength	Pins, screws, fracture plates, and hip nails
Ti-based alloys	Excellent corrosion resistance Good biocompatibility	Prostheses stems Dental implant
Co-based alloys	Excellent corrosion resistance Good biocompatibility High strength High wear resistance	Femoral head Hip and knee prostheses Prostheses stems
Mg-based alloys	Excellent corrosion resistance Good high temperature mechanical properties Light weight	Hip joints Cardiovascular stents Dental implants
Ceramics		
Alumina	Excellent biocompatibility Moderate tensile strength High melting point Low friction coefficient	Hip and knee replacement
Zirconia	Excellent biocompatibility Good fracture toughness Wear resistance	Dental implants Hip replacement
Polymers		
Poly(methylmethacrylate)	Good mechanical properties Light weight	Hip prostheses Acrylic bone cements Vertebroplasty
Polyetheretherketone	Good chemical resistance Good wear and abrasion resistance Stable at high temperature	Spinal implant Hip prostheses Knee prostheses Orbital prostheses
Ultra-high-molecular weight-polyethylene	High impact strength Good chemical resistance Low moisture absorption Excellent abrasion resistance Low friction	Liner of acetabulum cups in total hip prosthesis. Tibia insert and patellar component in total knee arthroplasty

of the implant. The functionality of the implant is also improved by introducing ions at the HA coatings [62] for enhancing surface properties. Ion implantation is a process by which ions are shot onto the implant material surface to form a hardened coating. Through this procedure, the materials bulk properties can be preserved while enhancing the wear resistance. Diamond-like carbon (DLC) coatings are also performed over the stainless steel through a saddle field source deposition system to improve their hardness and wear strength and to reduce friction. The coated implant displayed improved wear strength compared to the uncoated implants in the femoral head of hip implants [63,64]. Plasma-spray-coated metallic and ceramic implants also displayed improved wear strength related to one uncoated in various implant applications [65]. The cross-linking method in polyethylene to improve abrasion resistance is a novel technique used to strengthen the UHMWPE [66] most recently created material in implantation. Implant longevity can also be increased, and wear can be decreased by adding antiwear particles, like ceramic particles, to the polymer components of implants through surface treatment methods. The quality of the surface roughness and wear-induced surface topography variations are measured using profilometry techniques.

4.3.3 LUBRICATION AND BIOMIMETIC APPROACHES

For bioimplants, like joint replacements and other moving implant components, lubrication with biomimetic techniques is crucial in minimising wear and friction. To improve the functionality and durability of implants, these techniques try to imitate the lubrication and mechanics found naturally in the human body. Synovial fluid (SF) is one such lubricant present at the articular cartilage, which can be useful in the treatment of joint implants, such as prosthetic knees and hips. The rheological features of the natural SF existing in the body joints are replicated by artificial lubricating [67] solutions to lessen wear and friction. Shear rate is predicted to calculate the viscosity of these artificial lubricants. Researchers are focused on creating implant materials that match the mechanical and lubricating qualities of articular cartilage. Biopolymer blends of artificial SF [68] was found to lessen wear between implant component parts and offer a low-friction condition. Another technique of adding a lubricating layer with the implant material surfaces is coating with antimicrobial hydrogel [69]. Because of their ability to absorb and release water, these hydrogels have good cell adhesion with respect to bone growth, and hydrophilicity, proper cushioning, and friction-reducing effect are also absorbed. Antimicrobial hydrogel may find usage in joint implants due to the rapid fixation property with the interface of the bone.

Other alternate methods of adding natural lubrication are conducted through biomimetic approaches. By using this approach, surfaces will be able to release lubricating molecules in response to pressure or shear forces. Researchers are trying to create materials and coatings with [70] long-lasting artificial hip joint implants that can imitate lubrication by increasing surface hydrophilicity. To enhance lubrication in artificial joints, biomimetic techniques seek to cover implant surfaces with lubricin (glycoprotein) molecules [71] or to develop materials that may act as boundary lubricin lines at the joint interfaces during sliding.

The surface modification techniques discussed in the previous section can also influence in lowering friction by reducing irregularity through superhydrophilic coatings [72] in implants. Multiscale micro-/nanotextured surfaces coatings with patterns are made with titanium alloy [73] implants to improve tribological characteristics. Biopolymer coatings [74] that contain antibiotic-loaded polyhydroxyalkanoates (PHAs) on titanium implants helped bioimplants lubricate better. These coatings can imitate the lubricating qualities of natural tissues and have good biocompatible qualities. Certain implants use sophisticated lubricating techniques, like ferrofluid-based and magnetorheological systems [75] in implants. The lubrication level is adjusted in response to changing conditions which can further reduce wear and friction. By minimising direct surface contact and creating a lubricating layer on the implant surface, all these techniques can lower friction between the moving elements of implants. These biomimetic and lubrication techniques hope to prolong the life and improve the functionality of bioimplants by trying to replicate the natural lubrication. Engineers and researchers are still investigating and creating novel ways to lessen wear and friction in bioimplants, thereby improving the patient comfort and the longevity of these implants.

4.4 FUTURE DIRECTIONS OF IMPLANT TRIBOLOGY

Emerging materials and technologies in implant tribology are at the forefront of research and development in the field of biomedical implants. The performance, biocompatibility, and wear resistance of implants are the goals of these advancements. To improve the mechanical characteristics and wear strength in current implant materials, researchers are looking into newest materials and technologies that include the usage of nanocomposites like ceramic nanoparticles and carbon nanotubes of combined metals or polymers alloys [76], as shown in the surface morphology of Figure 4.6.

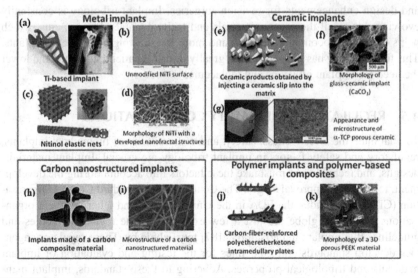

FIGURE 4.6 Surface morphology of different metal implant alloys.

The unique properties of advanced coating processes, such as multilayer coatings, antimicrobial coatings, and bioactive glass, are drawing interest in the recent years. Biologically active chemicals are released via multilayer coatings [77] with customised characteristics. Research is being done on implants with antimicrobial coatings [78] to lower the risk of infections, which can be a major worry during implant surgery. Bioactive glasses [79] have the potential to enhance implant tissue integration by releasing bioactive ions and thereby encouraging bone regeneration. More recently developed, additive manufacturing [80] and surface texturing techniques allow precise control of material composition while creating biomimicry in implant structures. Innovative surface patterns are created for patient-specific implants with surface texturing [81] technology for improving tribological characteristics in the UHMWPE surfaces of orthopedic bearings. Nowadays, actuators and sensors are also included with implants to provide real-time mechanical and wear status monitoring. With the use of this smart implants [82], wear-related problems can be identified early, and implant properties can be changed as desired.

Recent innovations also include development of hybrid and biodegradable materials. Hybrid materials combine the biocompatibility of polymers with the strength of metals to become functionally graded materials [83] by attaining problem-specific characteristics such as wear strength with reduced friction coefficient. The development of biodegradable materials [84] is underway for use in applications where implants are intended to serve a temporary purpose. In this case, the body absorbs and progressively breaks down these components, which lessens the need to remove the implant. Implant behavior is predicted in several patients through the application of well-trained deep-learning algorithm [85,86] with artificial intelligence. By simulating the intricate tribological interactions seen in the body over a period, these technologies can cost-effectively help with material selection and design enhancements for revision surgeries. Implant tribology is constantly evolving due to all these new materials and technological advancements, which helps to create biocompatible, safer, and more long-lasting biomedical implants. This field of study has the potential to greatly improve patient outcomes and lower the need for implant revisions and replacements.

4.5 REGULATORY AND SAFETY CONSIDERATIONS

To guarantee the effectiveness, safety, and compatibility of biomedical implants, regulatory and safety factors in implant tribology are crucial. Implant materials, designs, and technologies must take these factors into account during the development, testing, and approval stages. The Central Drugs Standard Control Organisation (CDSCO) in India, the FDA in the United States, and other pertinent organisations across the globe are just a few examples of the regulatory bodies and guidelines that implant manufacturers [87] must abide by. These regulatory agencies develop standards and guidelines for the testing and evaluation of implant materials and tribological properties. Adhering to these standards, implant manufacturers must prepare complete documentation and data submission attesting to safety and effectiveness. These groups also monitor the efficacy and quality of medical implants. To guarantee constant product quality and safety, implant material and device producers are frequently obliged to put quality management systems (like ISO 13485) into place. Numerous tribology and medical device standards are published by the International Organization for Standardization (ISO). For example, ISO 6474 deals with dental implant systems, and ISO 14243 addresses the wear of total hip joint prostheses. For guaranteeing quality and safety in India, medical implants might need to meet the applicable requirements of the Bureau of Indian Standards (BIS).

Using procedures like preclinical testing, clinical trials, postmarket surveillance, risk assessment, material traceability, and implant labelling, long-term and follow-up studies are carried out to track implant tribological performance and patient outcomes. Both the regulatory approval of new implants and the continued monitoring for enhancement of current implants depend on manufacturers' adherence to these factors. In the field of implant tribology, cooperation among regulatory bodies, implant producers, medical practitioners, and researchers is essential for upholding high standards of performance and safety.

4.6 SUMMARY

The improvement of patient health and well-being is the main objective of biomedical implants. Comprehending and refining tribological behaviors guarantees the efficient operation of implants, mitigating discomfort, restoring mobility, and augmenting the standard of living for patients suffering with different ailments as discussed. The advancement of patient care, medical technology, and the general quality of life for people with a range of medical disorders are all greatly aided by this multidisciplinary area of research and development. Excessive wear and friction can cause tissue damage, infections, discomfort, loosening of the implant, implant failure, and decreased patient satisfaction. From this chapter, it is concluded that, the tribological research will prolong the lifespan of implants by minimising wear and the production of wear debris, lowering the risk of complications, enhancing the functionality of implants, and delaying the need for revision surgeries. This results in substantial cost savings for health care systems and patients by lessening medical procedures. Future patients will benefit from the development of better implant materials, designs, and manufacturing methods due to the continuous ongoing research in biomedical devices.

REFERENCES

1. Fellah M, Labaïz M, Assala O, Dekhil L, Zerniz N, Iost A. Tribological behavior of biomaterial for total hip prosthesis. Matériaux & Techniques. 2014; 102(6–7):601.
2. Urban MK, Wolfe SW, Sanghavi NM, Fields K, Magid SK. The incidence of perioperative cardiac events after orthopedic surgery: a single institutional experience of cases performed over one year. HSS Journal®. 2017 Oct;13(3):248–54.
3. Abdelbary A. 19 Tribological aspects. Tribology and Sustainability. 2021 Aug 26:333.

4. Forlenza EM, Higgins JD, Burnett RA, Serino J, Della Valle CJ. COVID-19 infection after total joint arthroplasty is associated with increased complications. The Journal of Arthroplasty. 2022 Jul 1;37(7):S457–64.

5. Zhou ZR, Jin ZM. Biotribology: recent progresses and future perspectives. Biosurface and Biotribology. 2015 Mar 1;1(1):3–24.

6. Zhang L, Sawae Y, Yamaguchi T, Murakami T, Yang H. Effect of radiation dose on depth-dependent oxidation and wear of shelf-aged gamma-irradiated ultra-high molecular weight polyethylene (UHMWPE). Tribology International. 2015 Sep 1;89:78–85.

7. Bian YY, Zhou L, Zhou G, Jin ZM, Xin SX, Hua ZK, Weng XS. Study on bio-compatibility, tribological property and wear debris characterization of ultra-low-wear polyethylene as artificial joint materials. Journal of the Mechanical Behavior of Biomedical Materials. 2018 Jun 1;82:87–94.

8. Chang BP, Akil HM, Nasir RM. Mechanical and tribological properties of zeolite-reinforced UHMWPE composite for implant application. Procedia Engineering. 2013 Jan 1;68:88–94.

9. Di Puccio F, Mattei L. Biotribology of artificial hip joints. World Journal of Orthopedics. 2015 Jan 1;6(1):77.

10. Goodman SB, Gallo J, Gibon E, Takagi M. Diagnosis and management of implant debris-associated inflammation. Expert Review of Medical Devices. 2020 Jan 2;17(1):41–56.

11. Jin ZM, Zheng J, Li W, Zhou ZR. Tribology of medical devices. Biosurface and Biotribology. 2016 Dec 1;2(4):173–92.

12. Ackerman IN, Ayton D. Orthopaedic surgeons' perceptions of the changing burden of revision joint replacement surgery in Australia: a qualitative study. Musculoskeletal Care. 2022 Mar;20(1):200–8.

13. Goodman SB, Gallo J. Periprosthetic osteolysis: mechanisms, prevention and treatment. Journal of Clinical Medicine. 2019 Dec 1;8(12):2091.

14. Guglielmotti MB, Olmedo DG, Cabrini RL. Research on implants and osseointegration. Periodontology 2000. 2019 Feb;79(1):178–89.

15. Thomas C. Dental care in older adults. British Journal of Community Nursing. 2019 May 2;24(5):233–5.

16. Penkov OV, Pukha VE, Starikova SL, Khadem M, Starikov VV, Maleev MV, Kim DE. Highly wear-resistant and biocompatible carbon nanocomposite coatings for dental implants. Biomaterials. 2016 Sep 1;102:130–6.

17. De Stefano M, Aliberti SM, Ruggiero A. (Bio)Tribocorrosion in dental implants: principles and techniques of investigation. Applied Sciences. 2022 Jul 24;12(15):7421.

18. Zheng Y, Bashandeh K, Shakil A, Jha S, Polycarpou AA. Review of dental tribology: current status and challenges. Tribology International. 2022 Feb 1;166:107354.

19. Yu J, Zhou M, Zhang L, Wei H. Antibacterial adhesion strategy for dental titanium implant surfaces: from mechanisms to application. Journal of Functional Biomaterials. 2022 Sep 29;13(4):169.

20. Dearnaley G. Adhesive, abrasive and oxidative wear in ion-implanted metals. Materials Science and Engineering. 1985 Feb 1;69(1):139–47.

21. Rodrıguez RJ, Sanz A, Medrano A, Garcia-Lorente JA. Tribological properties of ion implanted aluminum alloys. Vacuum. 1999 Jan 1;52(1–2):187–92.

22. Wang A. A unified theory of wear for ultra-high molecular weight polyethylene in multi-directional sliding. Wear. 2001 Mar 1;248(1–2):38–47.

23. Mattei L, Di Puccio F. How accurate is the Archard law to predict wear of UHMWPE in hard-on-soft hip implants? A numerical and experimental investigation. Tribology International. 2023 Sep 1;187:108768.

24. Archard J. Contact and rubbing of flat surfaces. Journal of Applied Physics. 1953 Aug 1;24(8):981–8.
25. Ching HA, Choudhury D, Nine MJ, Osman NA. Effects of surface coating on reducing friction and wear of orthopaedic implants. Science and Technology of Advanced Materials. 2014 Jan 7;15(1):014402.
26. Le Guéhennec L, Soueidan A, Layrolle P, Amouriq Y. Surface treatments of titanium dental implants for rapid osseointegration. Dental Materials. 2007 Jul 1;23(7):844–54.
27. Poggie RA, Mishra AK, Davidson JA. Three-body abrasive wear behaviour of orthopaedic implant bearing surfaces from titanium debris. Journal of Materials Science: Materials in Medicine. 1994 Jun;5:387–92.
28. Wang Z, Huang W, Ma Y. Micro-scale abrasive wear behavior of medical implant material Ti–25Nb–3Mo–3Zr–2Sn alloy on various friction pairs. Materials Science and Engineering: C. 2014 Sep 1;42:211–8.
29. Hoeppner DW, Chandrasekaran V. Fretting in orthopaedic implants: a review. Wear. 1994 Apr 1;173(1–2):189–97.
30. Feyzi M, Fallahnezhad K, Taylor M, Hashemi R. A review on the finite element simulation of fretting wear and corrosion in the taper junction of hip replacement implants. Computers in Biology and Medicine. 2021 Mar 1;130:104196.
31. Gherde C, Dhatrak P, Nimbalkar S, Joshi S. A comprehensive review of factors affecting fatigue life of dental implants. Materials Today: Proceedings. 2021 Jan 1;43:1117–23.
32. Niinomi M, Kuroda D, Fukunaga KI, Morinaga M, Kato Y, Yashiro T, Suzuki A. Corrosion wear fracture of new β type biomedical titanium alloys. Materials Science and Engineering: A. 1999 May 15;263(2):193–9.
33. Kamachimudali U, Sridhar TM, Raj B. Corrosion of bio implants. Sadhana. 2003 Jun;28:601–37.
34. Davidson JA, Schwartz G. Wear, creep, and frictional heat of femoral implant articulating surfaces and the effect on long-term performance—Part I, a review. Journal of Biomedical Materials Research. 1987 Dec 1;21(A3 Suppl):261–85.
35. Kurtz SM, MacDonald DW, Kocagöz S, Tohfafarosh M, Baykal D. Can pin-on-disk testing be used to assess the wear performance of retrieved UHMWPE components for total joint arthroplasty?. BioMed Research International. 2014 Sep 11;2014:581812.
36. Zdero R, Guenther LE, Gascoyne TC. Pin-on-disk wear testing of biomaterials used for total joint replacements. In Experimental Methods in Orthopaedic Biomechanics 2017 Jan 1 (pp. 299–311). Academic Press.
37. Borjali A, Monson K, Raeymaekers B. Predicting the polyethylene wear rate in pin-on-disc experiments in the context of prosthetic hip implants: deriving a data-driven model using machine learning methods. Tribology International. 2019 May 1;133:101–10.
38. Sivaprakasam P, Hailu T, Elias G. Experimental investigation on wear behavior of titanium alloy (Grade 23) by pin on disc tribometer. Results in Materials. 2023 Sep 1;19:100422.
39. Zivic F, Babic M, Mitrovic S, Vencl A. Continuous control as alternative route for wear monitoring by measuring penetration depth during linear reciprocating sliding of Ti6Al4V alloy. Journal of Alloys and Compounds. 2011 May 12;509(19):5748–54.
40. Vilhena L, Oppong G, Ramalho A. Tribocorrosion of different biomaterials under reciprocating sliding conditions in artificial saliva. Lubrication Science. 2019 Dec;31(8):364–80.
41. Kapps V, Almeida CM, Trommer RM, Senna CA, Maru MM. Scatter in delamination wear tests of tribopair materials used in articulated implants. Tribology International. 2019 May 1;133:172–81.

42. Lee CK. Fabrication, characterization and wear corrosion testing of bioactive hydroxy-apatite/nano-TiO2 composite coatings on anodic Ti–6Al–4V substrate for biomedical applications. Materials Science and Engineering: B. 2012 Jun 25;177(11):810–8.

43. Hussin MS, Fernandez J, Ramezani M, Kumar P, Kelly PA. Analytical and computational sliding wear prediction in a novel knee implant: a case study. Computer Methods in Biomechanics and Biomedical Engineering. 2020 Mar 11;23(4):143–54.

44. VV AT, Chukwuike VI, Shtansky DV, Subramanian B. Biocompatibility study of nanocomposite titanium boron nitride (TiBN) thin films for orthopedic implant applications. Surface and Coatings Technology. 2021 Mar 25;410:126968.

45. Chethan KN, Zuber M, Shenoy S. Finite element analysis of different hip implant designs along with femur under static loading conditions. Journal of Biomedical Physics & Engineering. 2019 Oct;9(5):507.

46. Shankar S, Nithyaprakash R, Sugunesh AP, Selvamani KA, Uddin MS. Experimental and finite element wear study of silicon nitride against alumina for hip implants with bio-lubricant for various gait activities. Silicon. 2021 Mar;13:633–44.

47. Kladovasilakis N, Tsongas K, Tzetzis D. Finite element analysis of orthopedic hip implant with functionally graded bioinspired lattice structures. Biomimetics. 2020 Sep 12;5(3):44.

48. Correa DR, Kuroda PA, Lourenço ML, Buzalaf MA, Mendoza ME, Archanjo BS, Achete CA, Rocha LA, Grandini CR. Microstructure and selected mechanical properties of aged Ti-15Zr-based alloys for biomedical applications. Materials Science and Engineering: C. 2018 Oct 1;91:762–71.

49. Makkar P, Sarkar SK, Padalhin AR, Moon BG, Lee YS, Lee BT. In vitro and in vivo assessment of biomedical Mg–Ca alloys for bone implant applications. Journal of Applied Biomaterials & Functional Materials. 2018 Jul;16(3):126–36.

50. Navarro M, Michiardi A, Castano O, Planell JA. Biomaterials in orthopaedics. Journal of the Royal Society Interface. 2008 Oct 6;5(27):1137–58.

51. Derbyshire B, Fisher J, Dowson D, Hardaker C, Brummitt K. Comparative study of the wear of UHMWPE with zirconia ceramic and stainless-steel femoral heads in artificial hip joints. Medical Engineering & Physics. 1994 May 1;16(3):229–36.

52. Jin W, Chu PK. Orthopedic implants. Encyclopedia of Biomedical Engineering. 2019 Jan 1;1(3):425–39.

53. Hanawa T. Biocompatibility of titanium from the viewpoint of its surface. Science and Technology of Advanced Materials. 2022 Dec 31;23(1):457–72.

54. Sathishkumar S, Paulraj J, Chakraborti P, Muthuraj M. Comprehensive review on biomaterials and their inherent behaviors for hip repair applications. ACS Applied Bio Materials. 2023 Oct 23;6(11):4439–64.

55. Hu CY, Yoon TR. Recent updates for biomaterials used in total hip arthroplasty. Biomaterials Research. 2018 Dec;22(1):1–2.

56. Merola M, Affatato S. Materials for hip prostheses: a review of wear and loading considerations. Materials. 2019 Feb 5;12(3):495.

57. Ohtsuki C, Kamitakahara M, Miyazaki T. Bioactive ceramic-based materials with designed reactivity for bone tissue regeneration. Journal of the Royal Society Interface. 2009 Jun 6;6(suppl_3):S349–60.

58. Kayandan S, Doshi BN, Oral E, Muratoglu OK. Surface cross-linked ultra high molecular weight polyethylene by emulsified diffusion of dicumyl peroxide. Journal of Biomedical Materials Research Part B: Applied Biomaterials. 2018 May;106(4):1517–23.

59. Sankar S, Paulraj J, Chakraborti P. Fused filament fabricated PEEK based polymer composites for orthopaedic implants: a review. International Journal of Materials Research. 2023 Oct 23;114(10–11):980–8.

60. Sathishkumar S, Jawahar P, Chakraborti P. Influence of carbonaceous reinforcements on mechanical and tribological properties of PEEK composites–a review. Polymer-Plastics Technology and Materials. 2022 Aug 13;61(12):1367–84.

61. Sathishkumar S, Jawahar P, Chakraborti P. Synthesis, properties, and applications of PEEK-based biomaterials. In Advanced Materials for Biomedical Applications 2022 Dec 13 (pp. 81–107). CRC Press.

62. Li J, Zhang T, Liao Z, Wei Y, Hang R, Huang D. Engineered functional doped hydroxyapatite coating on titanium implants for osseointegration. Journal of Materials Research and Technology. 2023 Sep 27;27:122–52.

63. Hauert R. A review of modified DLC coatings for biological applications. Diamond and Related Materials. 2003 Mar 1;12(3–7):583–9.

64. Love CA, Cook RB, Harvey TJ, Dearnley PA, Wood RJ. Diamond like carbon coatings for potential application in biological implants—a review. Tribology International. 2013 Jul 1;63:141–50.

65. Ganapathy P, Manivasagam G, Rajamanickam A, Natarajan A. Wear studies on plasma-sprayed Al2O3 and 8mole% of Yttrium-stabilized ZrO2 composite coating on biomedical Ti-6Al-4V alloy for orthopedic joint application. International Journal of Nanomedicine. 2015 Oct 1;10(sup2):213–22.

66. Kurtz SM, Muratoglu OK, Evans M, Edidin AA. Advances in the processing, sterilization, and crosslinking of ultra-high molecular weight polyethylene for total joint arthroplasty. Biomaterials. 1999 Sep 1;20(18):1659–88.

67. Yoshioka H, Stevens K, Genovese M, Dillingham MF, Lang P. Articular cartilage of knee: normal patterns at MR imaging that mimic disease in healthy subjects and patients with osteoarthritis. Radiology. 2004 Apr;231(1):31–8.

68. Smith AM, Fleming L, Wudebwe U, Bowen J, Grover LM. Development of a synovial fluid analogue with bio-relevant rheology for wear testing of orthopaedic implants. Journal of the Mechanical Behavior of Biomedical Materials. 2014 Apr 1;32:177–84.

69. Wu X, Liu S, Chen K, Wang F, Feng C, Xu L, Zhang D. 3D printed chitosan-gelatine hydrogel coating on titanium alloy surface as biological fixation interface of artificial joint prosthesis. International Journal of Biological Macromolecules. 2021 Jul 1;182:669–79.

70. Ishihara K. Highly lubricated polymer interfaces for advanced artificial hip joints through biomimetic design. Polymer Journal. 2015 Sep;47(9):585–97.

71. Lawrence A, Xu X, Bible MD, Calve S, Neu CP, Panitch A. Synthesis and characterization of a lubricin mimic (mLub) to reduce friction and adhesion on the articular cartilage surface. Biomaterials. 2015 Dec 1;73:42–50.

72. Kumar R, Sahani AK. Role of superhydrophobic coatings in biomedical applications. Materials Today: Proceedings. 2021 Jan 1;45:5655–9.

73. Zhang M, Zhou B, Gao J, Hei H, Ma Y, Huang X, Liu Z, Xue Y, Yu S, Wu Y. A scalelike micro/nano-textured structure on Ti-based implants with enhanced cytocompatibility and osteogenic activities. Surface and Coatings Technology. 2021 Sep 25;422:127497.

74. Rodríguez-Contreras A, García Y, Manero JM, Rupérez E. Antibacterial PHAs coating for titanium implants. European Polymer Journal. 2017 May 1;90:66–78.

75. Arteaga O, Terán HC, Morales H, Argüello E, Erazo MI, Ortiz M, Morales JJ. Design of human knee smart prosthesis with active torque control. International Journal of Mechanical Engineering and Robotics Research. 2020 Mar;9(3):347–52.

76. Basova TV, Vikulova ES, Dorovskikh SI, Hassan A, Morozova NB. The use of noble metal coatings and nanoparticles for the modification of medical implant materials. Materials & Design. 2021 Jun 1;204:109672.

77. Macdonald ML, Samuel RE, Shah NJ, Padera RF, Beben YM, Hammond PT. Tissue integration of growth factor-eluting layer-by-layer polyelectrolyte multilayer coated implants. Biomaterials. 2011 Feb 1;32(5):1446–53.

78. Shahid A, Aslam B, Muzammil S, Aslam N, Shahid M, Almatroudi A, Allemailem KS, Saqalein M, Nisar MA, Rasool MH, Khurshid M. The prospects of antimicrobial coated medical implants. Journal of Applied Biomaterials & Functional Materials. 2021 Aug;19:22808000211040304.

79. Brauer DS. Bioactive glasses—structure and properties. Angewandte Chemie International Edition. 2015 Mar 27;54(14):4160–81.

80. Vignesh M, Ranjith Kumar G, Sathishkumar M, Manikandan M, Rajyalakshmi G, Ramanujam R, Arivazhagan N. Development of biomedical implants through additive manufacturing: a review. Journal of Materials Engineering and Performance. 2021 Jul;30:4735–44.

81. Rahman MM, Biswas MA, Hoque KN. Recent development on micro-texturing of UHMWPE surfaces for orthopedic bearings: a review. Biotribology. 2022 Jun 30:100216.

82. Ledet EH, Liddle B, Kradinova K, Harper S. Smart implants in orthopedic surgery, improving patient outcomes: a review. Innovation and Entrepreneurship in Health. 2018 Aug 29;5:41–51.

83. Bahraminasab M, Farahmand F. State of the art review on design and manufacture of hybrid biomedical materials: hip and knee prostheses. Proceedings of the Institution of Mechanical Engineers, Part H: Journal of Engineering in Medicine. 2017 Sep;231(9):785–813.

84. Godavitarne C, Robertson A, Peters J, Rogers B. Biodegradable materials. Orthopaedics and Trauma. 2017 Oct 1;31(5):316–20.

85. Karnuta JM, Haeberle HS, Luu BC, Roth AL, Molloy RM, Nystrom LM, Piuzzi NS, Schaffer JL, Chen AF, Iorio R, Krebs VE. Artificial intelligence to identify arthroplasty implants from radiographs of the hip. The Journal of Arthroplasty. 2021 Jul 1;36(7):S290–4.

86. Karnuta JM, Luu BC, Roth AL, Haeberle HS, Chen AF, Iorio R, Schaffer JL, Mont MA, Patterson BM, Krebs VE, Ramkumar PN. Artificial intelligence to identify arthroplasty implants from radiographs of the knee. The Journal of Arthroplasty. 2021 Mar 1;36(3):935–40.

87. Wadhwa A, Talegaonkar S, Popli H. A regulatory overview of hip and knee joint replacement devices. Applied Clinical Research, Clinical Trials and Regulatory Affairs. 2019 Dec 1;6(3):212–30.

5 Tribo-Corrosion Behavior of Implants

Mohanram Murugan, Jayakrishna Kandasamy,
S Arulvel, and R Prayer Riju
Vellore Institute of Technology
Vellore, Tamil Nadu, India

5.1 INTRODUCTION

Tribo-corrosion refers to the occurrence of corrosion and tribological processes (wear and friction) in a material. It is a multidisciplinary field that brings together aspects of electrochemistry, mechanical engineering, and materials science (Mathew et al., 2009). The term "tribo-corrosion" is derived from the Greek words "tribos" meaning "rubbing" and "corrosion" signifying the degradation of a material through chemical reactions with its surroundings (Budinski, 2007). Tribo-corrosion is a prevalent problem affecting several industries, such as aerospace, biomedicine, energy, and transportation, and it can impact materials like metals, ceramics, polymers, and composites. When these materials are subjected to mechanical and environmental stress in various applications, they experience wear and corrosion simultaneously (Zagho et al., 2018).

The tribo-corrosion process can be divided into two stages: initiation and propagation. The initiation stage takes place when a material is first subjected to mechanical and environmental loads, resulting in small cracks, scratches, and other surface defects. These defects serve as initiation sites for corrosion, allowing corrosive agents to penetrate the material and react with the substrate. The propagation stage occurs as the corrosion reactions persist at the surface defects, leading to further material degradation. The rate of degradation depends on various factors including the material type, environment, mechanical loads, and surface roughness (Williams & Campbell, 2006).

Tribo-corrosion is a complex field of study that requires the use of various techniques for evaluating the behavior of materials. Electrochemical methods such as potentiodynamic polarization and electrochemical impedance spectroscopy help in understanding corrosion behavior while mechanical tests such as scratch testing and wear testing examine tribological behavior. Scanning electron microscopy and X-ray diffraction provide insight into the microstructural alterations that occurs during tribo-corrosion.

5.1.1 IMPORTANCE OF TRIBO-CORROSION BEHAVIOR IN IMPLANT MATERIALS

Tribo-corrosion is a significant problem in the field of implant materials, as it can cause implant devices to fail and result in the need for additional surgeries. These

DOI: 10.1201/9781003384847-5

materials are utilised in various biomedical applications, including orthopedic, dental, and cardiovascular treatments. Due to the exposure to both mechanical and environmental stresses, the materials experience simultaneous wear and corrosion (Manivasagam et al., 2010). Dental implants, such as crowns and bridges, are also vulnerable to tribo-corrosion. The materials used in these devices are exposed to a variety of environmental factors, including corrosive substances in the mouth, like saliva and bacteria, as well as mechanical stress caused by regular wear and tear and the patient's chewing and biting habits. The combination of these factors can lead to tribo-corrosion of the material, potentially resulting in device failure (Gaur et al., 2022).

Joint replacement devices and other orthopedic implants are exposed to a combination of mechanical and environmental stresses. The mechanical stresses include normal wear and tear and physical activity, while the environmental stresses include exposure to corrosive substances like body fluids and enzymes. This tribo-corrosion can lead to implant failure. The same holds true for cardiovascular implants such as stents and pacemakers, which are subjected to tribo-corrosion due to the combination of environmental loads from corrosive substances like blood and body fluids, and mechanical loads like normal wear and tear and changes in heart rate and blood pressure. This can result in the potential failure of the device (Mathew et al., 2023).

Tribo-corrosion-induced failure of implant materials can have severe impacts on patients. If an orthopedic implant fails, it can necessitate revision surgeries, which can pose financial and health hazards for the patient. In the event of a failed dental implant, the patient may require a replacement, incurring monetary expense and time consumption. Furthermore, a failure of cardiovascular implants can result in life-threatening complications such as blood clots, heart attack, and stroke. Several strategies have been proposed to tackle the tribo-corrosion issue in implant materials. One such solution is the adoption of more corrosion-resistant materials, like pure titanium and titanium alloys, which have demonstrated their ability to resist corrosion in biological surroundings and are commonly utilised in implantation (Revathi et al., 2016). Another way to address the challenge is to cover the implant materials with protective coatings that boost their tribo-corrosion resistance. Studies have revealed that coatings such as diamond-like carbon can effectively enhance the tribo-corrosion performance of implant materials by serving as a shield between the material and its environment, thus decreasing the rate of corrosion (Rafiq et al., 2022).

5.2   IMPLANT MATERIALS

5.2.1   OVERVIEW OF COMMONLY USED IMPLANT MATERIALS

The selection of materials for implant applications is based on several important factors such as the intended usage, exposure to mechanical and environmental stress, and the desired performance. Among the available options, stainless steel is a popular choice due to its excellent mechanical properties, biocompatibility, and resistance to corrosion. This type of steel contains a minimum of 10.5% chromium, which creates a protective oxide layer that safeguards it from corrosion. Stainless steel is utilised in various implant applications including orthopaedics, dentistry, and cardiovascular medicine (Nouri & Wen, 2021).

Titanium and its alloys are frequently utilised as implant materials due to their biocompatibility, light weight, and strength. These alloys, made by blending titanium with other elements such as aluminium and vanadium, also offer good mechanical properties and resistance to corrosion. They are commonly used in orthopedic and dental implant procedures (Hoque et al., 2022). Another material often used in implant applications is cobalt-chromium alloys, which has good mechanical properties and resistance to corrosion. These alloys are also widely used in orthopedic and dental implant procedures (Al Jabbari, 2014).

Ceramics, a group of inorganic nonmetallic materials, are also a popular implant material. Known for their good wear resistance and biocompatibility, ceramics also resist corrosion, making them ideal for use in orthopedic, dental, and spinal implant procedures (Navarro et al., 2008). Polymers are a popular choice in the field of implant applications due to their advantageous properties such as flexibility, bio-compatibility, and cost-effectiveness. Monomers, which are repeating units, make up these materials. Polymers are frequently utilised in spinal and soft tissue implant applications (Premkumar et al., 2021). In addition to these conventional materials, researchers are investigating the potential of using innovative materials like carbon nanotubes and graphene in implant applications. These materials have exceptional characteristics, including high strength, flexibility, and biocompatibility, that could make them ideal for implant applications (Munir et al., 2019).

5.2.2 PROPERTIES OF IMPLANT MATERIALS THAT AFFECT TRIBO-CORROSION BEHAVIOR

The tribo-corrosion behavior of implant materials can be impacted by a variety of properties. To ensure the creation of long-lasting and durable implant devices, it is crucial to comprehend the properties that affect tribo-corrosion behavior. Among these properties, corrosion resistance holds significant importance. This is the capability of a material to withstand degradation when exposed to corrosive conditions. The level of corrosion resistance varies depending on various factors like the composition, microstructure, and surface finish of the material. For instance, materials with high chromium levels such as stainless steel are known for their excellent corrosion resistance. Furthermore, materials with a smooth and uniform surface finish are less prone to corrosion compared to those with rough and irregular surface finishes (Olugbade, 2022).

The tribo-corrosion behavior of a material is also impacted by its mechanical properties. These properties pertain to a material's resistance to deformation and breaking under mechanical stress and are determined by factors like composition, microstructure, and heat treatment. For instance, materials with superior strength and durability like titanium alloys are less likely to experience mechanical failure compared to those with low strength and durability (Hammood et al., 2019, Feyzi et al., 2022). Additionally, the surface chemistry of the material plays a crucial role in tribo-corrosion behavior. Surface chemistry involves the chemical composition and structure of a material's surface. It can impact the material's resistance to corrosion as well as its ability to form a shielding oxide layer. For example, titanium, which has a high oxygen content, is capable of forming a protective oxide layer on its surface that protects it from corrosion (Liu & Zhang, 2015).

The surface roughness of the material is another important property that affects tribo-corrosion behavior. Surface roughness refers to the texture or irregularity of the surface of a material. The surface roughness of a material can affect its corrosion resistance, as well as its ability to form a protective oxide layer. For example, materials with a smooth and uniform surface finish are less susceptible to corrosion than materials with a rough and irregular surface finish (Toloei et al., 2013). The load and stress applied to the implant material is another important property that affects tribo-corrosion behavior. Load and stress can affect the corrosion rate of the material, as well as its ability to form a protective oxide layer. For example, materials that are subjected to high loads and stresses are more susceptible to corrosion than materials that are subjected to low loads and stresses (Patel, 2019).

5.3 TYPES OF TRIBO-CORROSION IN IMPLANTS

5.3.1 Mechanical Tribo-Corrosion

In Figure 5.1, the mechanical tribo-corrosive behavior of a cardiovascular stent is represented. Mechanical tribo-corrosion is a complex process that involves both tribology (friction and wear) and corrosion, triggered by mechanical factors. This phenomenon occurs at the interface between a material and its surroundings and is impacted by various elements such as material properties, the environment, and the applied stress and loads (Costa & de Brito, 2015). The mechanical tribo-corrosion process can be divided into three phases: initiation, propagation, and stabilization. The initiation phase occurs when the material is exposed to mechanical and environmental loads, leading to the formation of small cracks,

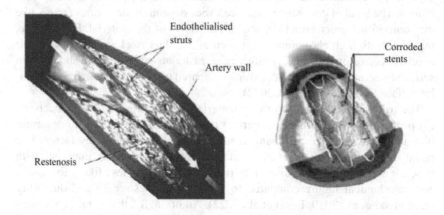

FIGURE 5.1   Mechanical tribo-corrosion. (Manam et al., 2017.)

scratches, and other surface imperfections. These imperfections can act as initiation sites for corrosion, allowing corrosive agents to penetrate the material and react with the substrate (Wang & Chen, 2018). The propagation phase happens when corrosion reactions continue to occur at the defects, leading to further degradation of the material. The rate of degradation depends on various factors such as the material type, environment, mechanical loads, and surface roughness (Smith, 2021). Finally, the stabilization phase occurs when the material reaches a state of balance where the corrosion rate is matched by the rate of material regeneration. This stage is characterised by a constant rate of corrosion and wear, with little change in material properties over time (Smith, 2020).

5.3.2 GALVANIC CORROSION

Galvanic corrosion is a form of corrosion that takes place when two metals or alloys of different compositions come into contact with an electrolyte. It is a result of an electrochemical reaction caused by the difference in electrical potential between the two materials. This type of corrosion can cause faster deterioration of one of the metals, making it particularly relevant in implant technology where close proximity of dissimilar materials is a factor (Lee & Kim, 2010). When two dissimilar metals or alloys are in close proximity, an electrical current will flow between them, forming a galvanic cell. The metal or alloy with a higher electrical potential acts as the cathode, while the one with a lower potential becomes the anode. The anode corrodes at a quicker pace as it loses electrons to the cathode, resulting in what is known as galvanic corrosion (Narayan, 2017). The rate of galvanic corrosion depends on various factors such as the type of metals or alloys involved, the size of their surface area, their distance from each other, and the nature of the electrolyte. The corrosion rate is higher if the anodic material has a larger surface area in contact with the cathodic material, or if the distance between the metals or alloys is greater (Bockris & O'Connell, 1988).

Minimizing galvanic corrosion is possible by using materials with similar electrical potentials. However, in implant applications, this may not always be an option due to specific requirements. Alternative methods can be employed to reduce the effects of galvanic corrosion (Smith & Jones, 2010). One solution is to use coatings on the implant materials to separate them from each other. For instance, a Teflon coating can be applied to the implant materials, preventing any contact between them and thus eliminating galvanic corrosion (Koray & Hasirci, 2005). Another strategy is the use of sacrificial anodes. A sacrificial anode is a metal or alloy with a lower electrical potential than the other materials, and it is intentionally used to corrode first, protecting the more noble materials from galvanic corrosion in implant applications.

5.4 FACTORS AFFECTING TRIBO-CORROSION BEHAVIOR IN IMPLANTS

The phenomenon of tribo-corrosion involves the interaction between an implant material and its surroundings and is influenced by various factors. To enhance the durability and longevity of implant devices, it is crucial to comprehend the elements that shape tribo-corrosion behavior in implants. One of the most significant factors that impact tribo-corrosion behavior is the implant's material properties, such as its composition, microstructure, and surface finish. These properties can determine the implant's corrosion resistance, mechanical strength, and capability of forming a defensive oxide layer. Generally, stainless steel is the most widely used biometallic material in implant applications like orthopedic implants, artificial heart valves, bone fixation, curettes, precision stainless steel tubing, otolaryngology ear scope nozzles, catheters, sensor probes, screws prostheses, and orthopedic plates (Resnik et al., 2020). It offers numerous advantages, including a high modulus of elasticity, biocompatibility, and cost-effectiveness in manufacturing. Despite these advantages, tribo-corrosion plays a major role in affecting the passive film that protects the stainless steel surfaces, leading to increased debris generation. The amount of tribo-corrosion depends on multiple factors like the selection of stainless steel type, corrosive medium, contact stress, and sliding speed. Particularly, stainless steel 316L is the most prominent type as compared to other stainless steels due to its high chromium and low carbon content (Abreu et al., 2021, Parker et al., 2022, Tan et al., 2021, Gassner et al., 2021). For example, the authors of this study (see Figure 5.2) analysed the tribo-corrosion performance of laser-cladded 2-layer coating using Fe-based amorphous powder on stainless steel 316L. They concluded that the tribological performance of two-layer coating using Ringer's solution results in the lowest coefficient of friction and volume loss under all loads from 5 to 20 N. Especially at 5 N load, the volume reduction rate of 316L SS decreased by more than three times due to the two-layer coating (Ji et al., 2022).

Another factor that affects tribo-corrosion behavior is the presence of lubricants or wear debris. The presence of these substances can alter the implant's corrosion rate

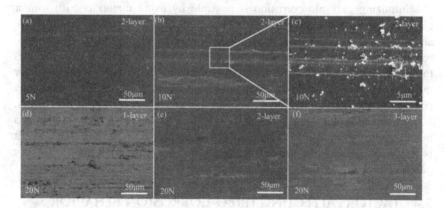

FIGURE 5.2 SEM micrographs of the worn surfaces after tribo-corrosion tests in Ringer's solution at open circuit: (a) 2-layer coating at 5 N load; (b) 2-layer coating at 10 N load; (c) enlarged view of 2-layer coating at 10 N load; (d) 1-layer coating at 20 N load; (e) 2-layer coating at 20 N load; (f) 3-layer coating at 20 N load. (Ji et al., 2022.)

and its ability to form a protective oxide layer. For instance, a lubricant may act as a barrier, reducing the corrosion rate of the implant. However, if the lubricant contains corrosive agents, it may also increase the corrosion rate of the implant (Branco et al., 2019). Finally, the design of the implant is another crucial factor that affects tribo-corrosion behavior. The design of an implant can impact the loads and stresses it experiences and the environment in which it is placed. For example, an implant that is designed to move against another implant or natural tissue will undergo different loads and stresses than one designed to be stationary (Kligman et al., 2021).

5.5 METHODS FOR EVALUATING TRIBO-CORROSION BEHAVIOR OF IMPLANTS

5.5.1 ELECTROCHEMICAL TECHNIQUES

The tribo-corrosion behavior of implant materials is commonly studied through electrochemical methods. These methods enable researchers to assess the corrosion resistance and the formation of a protective oxide layer of the materials, as well as the impact of mechanical loads on the corrosion process. One of the most frequently used electrochemical techniques is the potentiodynamic polarization method, which involves measuring the current–potential relationship of a material based on applied potential. The results of the test reveal the material's corrosion rate and mechanism (Munir et al., 2016).

Electrochemical impedance spectroscopy (EIS) is another popular method, where the electrical impedance of the material is measured as a function of frequency to evaluate its corrosion resistance and oxide layer formation (Magar et al., 2021). Cyclic voltammetry (CV) is a crucial electrochemical technique that measures the current–potential relationship of a material as a function of applied potential in a cyclic manner. The results of the CV test give insight into the material's corrosion rate, mechanism, and the effect of mechanical loads on the corrosion process (Elgrishi et al., 2018). Another technique, scanning electrochemical microscopy (SECM), is used to study the tribo-corrosion behavior of implant materials at the microscale level by measuring the current–potential relationship of the material while scanning a microelectrode tip over its surface (Caniglia & Kranz, 2020).

5.5.2 MECHANICAL TESTING

Mechanical testing plays a crucial role in determining the tribo-corrosion performance of implant materials. These tests allow experts to analyse the mechanical characteristics of the materials, such as their strength, toughness, and wear resistance, as well as how mechanical loads impact the corrosion process. One of the most frequently used mechanical tests for assessing tribo-corrosion in implants is the corrosion fatigue test. This test involves exposing the material to cyclic loads while in a corrosive environment. The results of the corrosion fatigue test offer insights into the fatigue life of the material and the impact of the corrosive environment on the material's fatigue behavior (Antunes & Oliveira, 2012).

The wear test is another commonly used mechanical test. This test involves exposing the material to sliding or rolling contact against another material while in a corrosive environment. The results of the wear test offer insights into the wear resistance of the material and the impact of the corrosive environment on the materials wear behavior (Goudarzi & Rezvanian, 2017). The corrosion creep test is another significant mechanical test. This test involves exposing the material to a constant load while in a corrosive environment. The results of the corrosion creep test offer insights into the creep behavior of the material and the impact of the corrosive environment on the material's creep behavior (Gutman et al., 2001).

Other tests such as tensile, compressive, and bend testing can also be included in mechanical testing to provide information about the mechanical properties of the material, including the ultimate tensile strength, yield strength, and ductility.

5.5.3 MICROSCOPY AND SURFACE ANALYSIS

The assessment of tribo-corrosion behavior in implant materials can be achieved through the use of microscopy and surface analysis techniques. These methods enable the examination of the microstructure and surface features of the materials, as well as the impact of the corrosive environment on the material's surface. One of the most commonly employed microscopy techniques for this purpose is scanning electron microscopy (SEM), which allows for the analysis of the microstructure and surface characteristics at high magnification. SEM results can provide insight into the corrosion rate and the formation and appearance of corrosion products on the surface (Mano et al., 2019).

Transmission electron microscopy (TEM) is another widely used microscopy technique that allows for high-resolution microstructure analysis. TEM results can reveal the corrosion rate and the formation and appearance of corrosion products on the surface (Han et al., 2015). Atomic force microscopy (AFM) is another important microscopy technique that enables the analysis of surface morphology at high resolution. AFM results can offer information on the surface roughness and the formation and appearance of corrosion products on the surface (Duan, 2017). In addition to microscopy techniques, X-ray photoelectron spectroscopy (XPS), Auger electron spectroscopy (AES), and time-of-flight secondary ion mass spectrometry (TOF-SIMS) are surface analysis techniques commonly utilised to evaluate the tribo-corrosion behavior in implants. These techniques allow for the analysis of the chemical composition of the implant material's surface, as well as the formation and distribution of corrosion products (Kim et al., 2019).

5.6 EXPLANATION OF HOW TRIBO-CORROSION PLAYS A MAJOR ROLE IN SURFACE COATING TECHNIQUES

Tribo-corrosion refers to the exposure of a material to mechanical wear and corrosion, which can significantly impact the performance and safety of implants. To address this issue, various surface coating techniques have been implemented to provide protection from tribo-corrosion (Kheder et al., 2021). One such technique is electroplating, where a thin layer of biocompatible and corrosion-resistant material, such as titanium or stainless steel, is deposited onto the implant's surface to act as a barrier against corrosive agents and minimise mechanical wear (Priyadarshini et al., 2019).

Another popular surface coating method is the application of ceramic coatings, like alumina or zirconia, through physical vapor deposition. These ceramic coatings are biocompatible and corrosion-resistant, making them effective in protecting implants from tribo-corrosion (Amirtharaj et al., 2022). Finally, polymeric coatings, such as polyethylene or PTFE, are often used for implants as well. These biocompatible coatings can be applied through dip coating or spray-coating and offer excellent wear resistance properties (Tripathi et al., 2017).

In conclusion, tribo-corrosion is a major concern for implants and can lead to rapid degradation of the implant's surface, leading to failure and potential harm to the patient. To combat this, various surface coating techniques have been developed to protect implants from tribo-corrosion, including the application of biocompatible and corrosion-resistant materials, ceramic coatings, and polymeric coatings. Additionally, surface modification techniques can also be used to improve the tribo-corrosion resistance of implants. These techniques have been shown to be effective in prolonging the lifespan of implants and reducing the risk of failure (Figure 5.3).

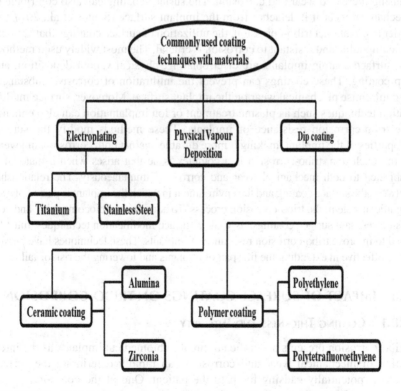

FIGURE 5.3 Flowchart of commonly used coating techniques with materials.

5.7 INTERACTION BETWEEN THE SURFACE COATING AND THE ENVIRONMENT: MECHANISMS OF TRIBO-CORROSION

In the case of implants, interaction between the surface coating and the environment can result in a rapid degradation of the surface, leading to potential failure and harm to the patient. To comprehend tribo-corrosion, it is crucial to examine the relationship between the surface coating and the environment the implant is situated in (Cruz et al., 2011). One significant aspect of tribo-corrosion is the formation of a thin film of corrosion produced on the implant's surface, made of oxides, hydroxides, or other corrosion products due to interaction with the environment. These corrosion products can serve as a barrier and reduce mechanical wear on the implant. However, they can also become detached and contribute to further wear on the implant (Borges et al., 2017).

Another factor is the development of microcracks on the implant surface, caused by the combination of mechanical wear and corrosion, which can lead to a rapid degradation of the surface. These microcracks can also provide a route for corrosive agents to penetrate the implant, hastening the rate of corrosion (Saha & Roy, 2023). The surface coating on an implant plays a crucial part in tribo-corrosion as it acts as a barrier against corrosive agents. However, it can also be a source of tribo-corrosion if it becomes damaged or detached from the implant surface, causing increased wear and corrosion. The surface coating can also contribute to mechanical wear if it detaches from the implant surface (Santos et al., 2017). In order to counteract tribo-corrosion, the utilization of surface coatings that are both biocompatible and resistant to corrosion is crucial. The most widely used methods for surface coating implants are electroplating, physical vapour deposition, and dip coating. These coatings can prevent the infiltration of corrosive substances and minimise mechanical wear on the implant surface. Moreover, surface modification techniques such as plasma treatment or ion implantation can also enhance the tribo-corrosion resistance of implants. These methods modify the surface properties of the implant, making it more durable against both corrosion and wear.

In conclusion, tribo-corrosion is a complex issue that arises when a material is subjected to both mechanical wear and corrosion simultaneously. The relationship between the surface coating and the environment in which the implant is placed plays a significant role in the tribo-corrosion process. To address this, biocompatible and corrosion-resistant surface coatings, as well as surface modification techniques, must be used to improve tribo-corrosion resistance of implants. These techniques have proven to be effective in extending the lifespan of implants and lowering the risk of failure.

5.8 IMPACT OF SURFACE COATINGS ON TRIBO-CORROSION

5.8.1 COATING THICKNESS AND INTEGRITY

Tribo-corrosion presents a significant threat to biomedical implants as the interaction of mechanical wear and corrosion can rapidly deteriorate the surface coating, potentially causing harm to the patient. One of the consequences of tribo-corrosion on biomedical implants is a decline in coating thickness and stability. The thickness of the coating plays a crucial role in the tribo-corrosion resistance of an implant, as a thicker coating offers better protection against both corrosive agents and mechanical wear. However, tribo-corrosion can erode the coating thickness, as the mechanical wear and corrosion can cause the coating to detach from the implant surface. This leads to a decrease in the protective qualities of the coating, increasing the likelihood of failure (Lu et al., 2011).

The state of the coating is a crucial aspect in determining the tribo-corrosion resistance of biomedical implants. An intact coating without any cracks or defects provides better protection against corrosive agents and wear. However, tribo-corrosion can reduce the coating integrity by causing cracks or defects through the combination of mechanical wear and corrosion. These cracks or defects can facilitate the penetration of corrosive agents into the implant surface, leading to accelerated corrosion (Wang et al., 2018). Furthermore, tribo-corrosion can lead to the formation of corrosion products on the implant surface. These products can protect the implant from mechanical wear but can also contribute to wear as they may detach from the surface. Additionally, the corrosion products can also act as a catalyst for the corrosion process (Lin et al., 2005).

In conclusion, tribo-corrosion is a major concern for biomedical implants, as the combination of mechanical wear and corrosion can lead to a rapid degradation of the implant's surface coating. One of the main impacts of tribo-corrosion on surface coatings in biomedical implants is the reduction of coating thickness and integrity, which can lead to an increased risk of failure. To prevent these negative impacts, it is important to use surface coatings that are biocompatible and corrosion-resistant, as well as surface modification techniques that can be used to improve the tribo-corrosion resistance of implants.

5.8.2 Coating Adhesion and Mechanical Properties

Tribo-corrosion can have a profound effect on surface coatings by reducing their adhesion and mechanical properties. This is due to the corrosive and abrasive effects of tribo-corrosion that can cause the formation of microcracks, delamination, and roughness on the surface of the coating, thus impacting its bonding ability and strength (Wood, 2007). Adhesion is a critical aspect of a coating, as it determines its ability to stick to the substrate and offer protection. This property can be influenced by factors such as the chemical composition of the coating and substrate, surface preparation, and application method (Petrovic et al., 2012). The processes of corrosion and wear during tribo-corrosion can result in the creation of microcracks and a roughened surface on the coating. These imperfections act as stress points, potentially causing the separation of the coating from the substrate, known as delamination. This weakens the adhesion between the coating and substrate and increases the likelihood of failure (Shen et al., 2018).

The mechanical properties of a coating refer to its ability to handle stress and deformation, including hardness, elasticity, and ductility. These properties are influenced by factors such as the thickness, composition, microstructure, and porosity of the coating (Guo et al., 2018). The consequences of tribo-corrosion can include material removal from the surface and a reduction in coating thickness, affecting its mechanical properties. The microcracks and roughened surface can also have a negative impact on the mechanical properties by acting as stress concentrators and reducing the coating's ductility and elasticity. The decline in adhesion and mechanical properties can negatively impact the performance and lifespan of the coating. Delamination and the formation of flake-like structures may further increase the risk of failure, and a reduction in mechanical properties can make the coating more vulnerable to deformation and failure under stress (Mischler, 2008).

5.8.3 Corrosion Rate and Susceptibility to Failure

The occurrence of tribological processes (friction and wear) and corrosion on a surface, known as tribo-corrosion, has a major impact on surface coatings. This can result in an increased rate of corrosion and a heightened vulnerability to failure. Factors that can influence the corrosion rate include the coating's chemical composition, microstructure, porosity, and the presence of corrosive agents in the environment. The relative motion between the surface and the environment can also lead to microcracks and surface roughening, contributing to the formation of corrosion products and reducing the coating thickness. A thin liquid film, caused by the relative motion, may act as a lubricant and reduce friction but can also alter the surface's electrochemical properties and contribute to corrosion. In addition, mechanical wear can occur due to the relative motion, leading to material loss from the surface (Jafari & Islam, 2014).

The synergistic effect between corrosion and wear processes can speed up the corrosion rate through tribo-corrosion. This is because the corrosion process can cause the formation of microcracks that increase stress and hasten the wear process. Additionally, the wear process can lead to material removal from the surface, exposing it to the environment and intensifying the corrosion process. This increase in corrosion rate can reduce the lifespan of the coating and increase its chances of failure, which can occur in various forms such as cracking, delamination, and complete breakdown. Furthermore, the corrosion rate can also weaken the mechanical properties of the coating, making it more susceptible to deformation and failure when subjected to load (Wahab et al., 2014).

5.9 PREVENTION AND MITIGATION OF TRIBO-CORROSION

5.9.1 Selection of Appropriate Coating Materials and Methods

The degradation of biomedical implant surfaces due to the combination of mechanical wear and corrosion, known as tribo-corrosion, is a major issue in the field of biomedical engineering. To avoid harm to patients, it is crucial to implement preventative measures through the selection of appropriate coating materials and methods. The first step of preventing and mitigating tribo-corrosion is to choose a biocompatible and corrosion-resistant coating material, such as titanium, gold, stainless steel, or alumina. These materials are well-suited for use in biomedical implants as they do not trigger adverse reactions within the body and provide protection against corrosive agents (Saini et al., 2015).

The next step to prevent and mitigate the tribo-corrosion was to determine suitable coating techniques. Figure 5.4 shows the common methods, including electroplating, physical vapor deposition, and dip coating. Electroplating is a common surface coating technique employed to apply a layer of powdered metal particles onto a metal substrate by using an electrical current (Figure 5.5a). Electroplating technique can be mainly used for corrosion protection and improving the mechani-

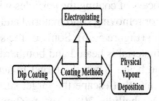

FIGURE 5.4   Commonly used coating method to coat biocompatible materials.

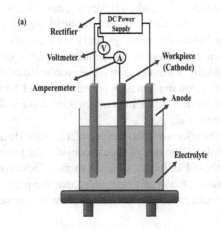

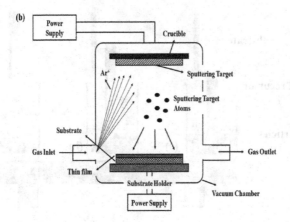

FIGURE 5.5   Schematic images of (a) electroplating coating and (b) PVD coating process.

cal or surface properties of the coating (Augustyn et al., 2021). The electroplating procedure is as follows: (1) The object to be coated (cathode) and the metal to be deposited (anode) are immersed in a solution containing metal ions (electrolyte). (2) When a direct current is passed through the solution, metal ions move toward the cathode and deposit on the surface of the cathode. (3) The anode gradually dissolves and replenishes the metal ions in solution. (4) Continue this process until the desired thickness of the coating is obtained. (Leiden et al., 2020). Physical vapour deposition (PVD) is the process of coating the particles with thin film on a substrate by evaporating, sputtering, or removing solid material and condensing onto the substrate in a vacuum condition (Figure 5.5b). Some of the steps included in the PVD are as follows: The target material is heated and bombarded with an energy source such as an arc, laser, or ion beam. Then the target material evaporates or ionises into atoms, molecules, or ions that escape the target surface and migrate towards the substrate (Bouzakis & Michailidis, 2019, Yap & Zhang, 2015). Dip coating is a process in which a liquid film is applied to the surface of a substrate by immersing it in a solution containing metal ions (Figure 5.6). Some of the steps in dip coating include immersion, dwelling, withdrawal, drying, and curing (Javidi & Hrymak, 2015). Dip coatings can be used for various applications, such as protective coatings, optical coatings, biomedical coatings, and nanomaterials (Tang & Yan, 2017).

The tribo-corrosion resistance of biomedical implants can be improved by utilising different coating methods as well as surface modification techniques like plasma treatment or ion implantation (Figures 5.7 and 5.8). These techniques change the surface properties of the implant, making it more durable against corrosion and wear (Izman et al., 2012).

To further mitigate the effects of tribo-corrosion, it is crucial to have a well-designed and manufactured implant. The design should consider the potential tribo-corrosion and aim to minimise the risk of failure. Cleanroom manufacturing and quality control procedures should also be followed to guarantee that the implant is free of defects or contaminants that could cause tribo-corrosion (Shaw & Sánchez-Herencia, 2017).

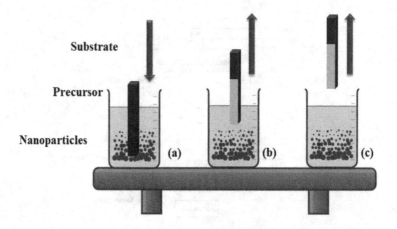

FIGURE 5.6　Dip coating process: (a) dipping, (b) deposition, (c) evaporation.

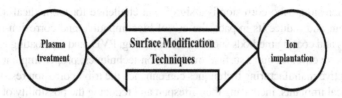

FIGURE 5.7 Commonly used surface modification methods to treat the coated metals.

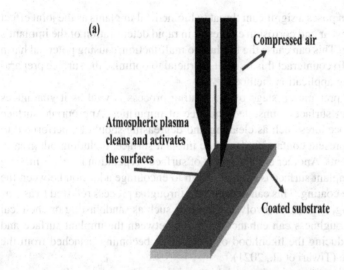

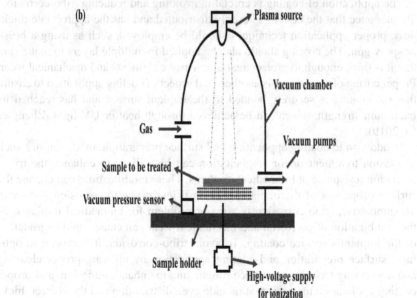

FIGURE 5.8 Schematic images of (a) plasma treatment and (b) ion implantation processes.

In conclusion, tribo-corrosion is a significant challenge for biomedical implants. To prevent and reduce its impact, the use of biocompatible and corrosion-resistant materials and coating methods such as electroplating, PVD, and dip coating is important. Moreover, combining surface modification techniques, proper implant design, and effective manufacturing techniques can enhance the tribo-corrosion resistance of biomedical implants, increasing their lifespan and reducing the possibility of failure.

5.9.2 OPTIMIZATION OF SURFACE PREPARATION AND COATING APPLICATION

Tribo-corrosion poses a significant threat to biomedical implants as the joint effect of mechanical wear and corrosion can result in rapid deterioration of the implant's surface coating. This can cause the implant to malfunction, causing potential harm to the patient. To counteract this issue, it is crucial to optimise the surface preparation and coating application methods.

The surface preparation stage of the coating process is vital as it guarantees that the implant surface is unsoiled and free of impurities. Appropriate surface preparation procedures such as cleaning and degreasing should be performed to eliminate any present contaminants on the implant surface, including oil, grease, or other pollutants. Another crucial aspect of surface preparation involves making sure that the implant surface is rough enough to encourage adhesion between the surface and the coating. This can be achieved through a process referred to as surface roughening, which can involve techniques such as sandblasting or chemical etching. This roughness can enhance the bond between the implant surface and the coating, reducing the likelihood of the coating becoming detached from the implant surface (Tiwari et al., 2021).

The application of coating is crucial in avoiding and reducing tribo-corrosion. To guarantee that the coating is evenly distributed and has the appropriate thickness, proper application techniques should be employed, such as using a brush or spray gun. The coating should also be applied in multiple layers to make sure that it is thick enough to protect against corrosive elements and mechanical wear. Proper curing of the coating is another vital aspect of coating application to ensure that the coating is securely bonded to the implant surface and has reached its maximum strength, which can be achieved through heat or UV light (Zheng & Li, 2019).

In addition to coating application and surface preparation, modifications such as plasma treatment or ion implantation can be utilised to enhance the tribo-corrosion resistance of biomedical implants. These modifications can change the surface properties of the implant, making it less prone to corrosion and wear. To summarise, tribo-corrosion is a major problem for biomedical implants, as the combination of corrosion and mechanical wear can cause rapid degradation of the implant's surface coating. To avoid tribo-corrosion, it is crucial to optimise surface preparation and coating application by utilising proper cleaning and degreasing techniques, surface roughening to enhance adhesion, and proper coating application methods that include even distribution and the correct thickness. These steps extend the lifespan of biomedical implants and reduce the likelihood of failure.

5.9.3 REGULAR MONITORING AND MAINTENANCE OF COATED SURFACES

It is crucial to keep a close eye on the coated surfaces to detect any indications of tribo-corrosion as soon as possible. This can involve visual assessments, such as searching for changes in colour or cracks, or more sophisticated methods like electrochemical impedance spectroscopy (EIS) or scanning electron microscopy (SEM). Regular monitoring helps to pinpoint problems with the coating before they escalate, allowing for prompt fixes or replacements. Maintaining the coated surfaces is another essential step in avoiding and managing tribo-corrosion, which involves regular cleaning to eliminate any contaminants and repairing or reapplying the coating for any faults or cracks (Merten, 2015).

Additionally, it is crucial to make sure that the implant is properly lubricated to minimise mechanical wear on the implant surface and reduce the risk of tribo-corrosion. Proper lubrication also minimises friction between the implant and surrounding tissue, decreasing the likelihood of implant failure (Siddaiah & Menezes, 2016). Finally, to enhance the tribo-corrosion resistance of biomedical implants, regular monitoring and maintenance can include surface modification techniques like plasma treatment or ion implantation. These procedures modify the surface properties of the implant, making it more resistant to corrosion and wear.

5.10 CONCLUSION

Tribo-corrosion is the simultaneous occurrence of tribological factors, such as friction, wear, and corrosion. The tribo-corrosion behavior of an implant material is impacted by several elements, including the material's properties, the environment it is located in, the pressure and stress exerted on it, the presence of lubricants or wear debris, and the design of the implant. The comprehension of tribo-corrosion behavior in implant materials is established through a blend of experimental and theoretical research. The experimental research involves using various methods, such as electrochemical methods, mechanical testing, microscopy, and surface analysis, to examine the tribo-corrosion behavior of implant materials. Theoretical research, on the other hand, involves utilizing mathematical models to forecast the tribo-corrosion behavior of implant materials.

Experiments have demonstrated that the properties of an implant material, such as its composition, microstructure, and surface finish, play a crucial role in determining its tribo-corrosion behavior. For instance, materials with high chromium concentrations, such as stainless steel, exhibit good resistance to corrosion. Meanwhile, materials with a smooth and uniform surface finish are less prone to corrosion than those with a rough and irregular surface finish. The location where the implant is situated has a significant impact on its tribo-corrosion behavior. For instance, implants located in an environment with high oxygen levels, such as air, are more prone to corrosion compared to those in an environment with low oxygen levels, such as oil. In the same way, implants located in a humid environment are more susceptible to corrosion than those placed in a dry environment.

Further, the pressure and stress applied to the implant also influence its tribo-corrosion behavior. The pressure and stress can impact the rate of corrosion and the formation of a protective oxide layer. Implant subjected to high pressure and stress are more susceptible to corrosion than those subjected to low pressure and stress. The tribo-corrosion behavior of an implant can also be influenced by the presence of a lubricant or wear debris. A lubricant can act as a barrier, reducing the rate of corrosion, but if it contains corrosive substances, it can hasten the corrosion rate. Finally, the design of the implant is a critical factor that affects tribo-corrosion behavior. The design can affect the stress and pressure on the implant, as well as the environment it is located in.

Tribo-corrosion is a complicated process that involves the manifestation of tribological and corrosive actions on a surface. This process can significantly affect the performance and lifespan of surface coatings, especially in the realm of biomedical implants, where tribo-corrosion can compromise the effectiveness and longevity of the implant. Consequently, it is crucial to comprehend and manage tribo-corrosion in order to ensure the longevity and reliability of surface coatings in implants.

The consequences of a decrease in coating thickness and integrity (a reduction in adhesion and mechanical properties and an increase in corrosion rate) can result in implant failure, which can harm the patient and require additional cost for the replacement surgeries. To counteract these effects, various strategies are implemented, including choosing the right coating materials and methods, optimizing surface preparation and coating application, and monitoring and maintaining coated surfaces regularly. Opting for appropriate coating materials and methods can guarantee that the coating is appropriate for the specific environment and application, providing the desired properties. For instance, biocompatible and biodegradable materials such as ceramics, polymers, and composites can be considered potential coating materials. These materials can be engineered to have specific properties like improved biocompatibility, corrosion resistance, and mechanical properties. Techniques such as visual inspections, NDT, and electrochemical measurements can be used for monitoring, while maintenance techniques such as cleaning, painting, and repair can be used to address specific issues.

In conclusion, tribo-corrosion is a crucial factor that can greatly affect the performance and lifespan of surface coatings on biomedical implants. Managing tribo-corrosion is vital to maintaining the longevity and efficiency of these coatings. By choosing the right coating materials and methods, optimising surface preparation and application, and regularly monitoring and maintaining the coated surfaces, tribo-corrosion can be effectively managed, enhancing the safety and efficacy of biomedical implants for patients.

5.11   FUTURE RESEARCH DIRECTIONS AND CHALLENGES FOR TRIBO-CORROSION

- In the future, tribo-corrosion research in implant materials needs to overcome several crucial challenges.
- Initially, tribo-corrosion mechanisms need to be developed for the use of advanced analysis methods to examine the microstructure and surface

properties of implant materials, as well as mathematical models to anticipate tribo-corrosion behavior.

- To improve the tribo-corrosion behavior, the selection of long-lasting implant materials is necessary because they react heavily with body tissues in the human body. It can be accomplished by implementing the manufacturing process of implants with biometallic materials and post-treatment techniques.
- To improve the performance and lifespan of these implants, future research should also focus on developing new coating materials specifically designed for biomedical implants and on exploring biocompatible and biodegradable options such as ceramics, polymers, and composites.

REFERENCES

Abreu, D., Silva Jr, W. M., Ardila, M. A. N., & de Mello, J. D. B. (2021). Tribocorrosion in ferritic stainless steels: an improved methodological approach. Materials Research, 25, e20210179.

Al Jabbari, Y. S. (2014). Physico-mechanical properties and prosthodontic applications of Co-Cr dental alloys: a review of the literature. The Journal of Advanced Prosthodontics, 6(2), 138–145.

Amirtharaj Mosas, K. K., Chandrasekar, A. R., Dasan, A., Pakseresht, A., & Galusek, D. (2022). Recent advancements in materials and coatings for biomedical implants. Gels, 8(5), 323.

Antunes, R. A., & de Oliveira, M. C. L. (2012). Corrosion fatigue of biomedical metallic alloys: mechanisms and mitigation. Acta Biomaterialia, 8(3), 937–962.

Augustyn, P., Rytlewski, P., Moraczewski, K., & Mazurkiewicz, A. (2021). A review on the direct electroplating of polymeric materials. Journal of Materials Science, 56(27), 14881–14899.

Bockris, J. F., & O'Connell, D. (1988). Galvanic corrosion of metals: understanding the basics. Journal of Applied Electrochemistry, 18(3), 361–371.

Borges, J. S., Castells, P., & Nóbrega, J. A. (2017). Tribocorrosion behaviour of titanium implants in physiological solutions. Corrosion Science, 120, 360–368.

Bouzakis, K. D., Michailidis, N. (2019). Physical vapor deposition (PVD). In: Chatti, S., Laperrière, L., Reinhart, G., & Tolio, T. (eds) CIRP Encyclopedia of Production Engineering. Springer.

Branco, A. C., Moreira, V., Reis, J. A., Colaço, R., Figueiredo-Pina, C. G., & Serro, A. P. (2019). Influence of contact configuration and lubricating conditions on the microtriboactivity of the Zirconia-Ti6Al4V pair used in dental applications. Journal of the Mechanical Behaviour of Biomedical Materials, 91, 164–173.

Budinski, K. G. (2007). Guide to Friction, Wear, and Erosion Testing. ASTM International.

Caniglia, G., & Kranz, C. (2020). Scanning electrochemical microscopy and its potential for studying biofilms and antimicrobial coatings. Analytical and Bioanalytical Chemistry, 412, 6133–6148.

Costa, J. M., & de Brito, A. A. (2015). Mechanical tribocorrosion: a review of the interaction between friction, wear and corrosion. Wear, 338–339, 183–199.

Cruz, H. V., Souza, J. C. M., Henriques, M., & Rocha, L. A. (2011). Tribocorrosion and bio-tribocorrosion in the oral environment: the case of dental implants. Biomedical Tribology, 1–33.

Duan, X. (2017). Atomic force microscopy (AFM) in corrosion science. Corrosion Science, 123, 78–87.

Elgrishi, N., Rountree, K. J., McCarthy, B. D., Rountree, E. S., Eisenhart, T. T., & Dempsey, J. L. (2018). A practical beginner's guide to cyclic voltammetry. Journal of Chemical Education, 95(2), 197–206.

Feyzi, M., Fallahnezhad, K., Taylor, M., & Hashemi, R. (2022). The tribocorrosion behaviour of Ti-6Al-4 V alloy: the role of both normal force and electrochemical potential. Tribology Letters, 70(3), 83.

Gassner, A., Waidelich, L., Palkowski, H., Wilde, J., & Mozaffari-Jovein, H. (2021). Tribocorrosion mechanisms of martensitic stainless steels. HTM Journal of Heat Treatment and Materials, 76(3), 205–218.

Gaur, S., Agnihotri, R., & Albin, S. (2022). Bio-tribocorrosion of titanium dental implants and its toxicological implications: a scoping review. The Scientific World Journal, 2022, 7371594.

Goudarzi, V., & Rezvanian, A. R. (2017). Effect of surface treatment on the wear and corrosion behaviour of Co-Cr-Mo alloy used for biomedical applications. Journal of Bio- and Tribo-Corrosion, 3(3), 55.

Guo, Y., Ma, J., Zhang, S., & Wang, Y. (2018). Study on mechanical properties of TiN coatings deposited by magnetron sputtering. Journal of Materials Science & Technology, 34(12), 1603–1608.

Gutman, E. M., Eliezer, A., Unigovski, Y., & Abramov, E. (2001). Mechanoelectrochemical behaviour and creep corrosion of magnesium alloys. Materials Science and Engineering: A, 302(1), 63–67.

Hammood, A. S., Thair, L., Altawaly, H. D., & Parvin, N. (2019). Tribocorrosion behaviour of Ti–6Al–4V alloy in biomedical implants: effects of applied load and surface roughness on material degradation. Journal of Bio-and Tribo-Corrosion, 5, 1–12.

Han, Y., Li, Z., & Zhang, Y. (2015). Transmission electron microscopy investigation of corrosion products formed on stainless steel. Journal of Materials Science and Technology, 31, 709–715.

Hoque, M. E., Showva, N. N., Ahmed, M., Rashid, A. B., Sadique, S. E., El-Bialy, T., & Xu, H. (2022). Titanium and titanium alloys in dentistry: current trends, recent developments, and future prospects. Heliyon, 8, e11300.

Izman, S., Abdul-Kadir, M. R., Anwar, M., Nazim, E. M., Rosliza, R., Shah, A., & Hassan, M. A. (2012). Surface modification techniques for biomedical grade of titanium alloys: oxidation, carburization and ion implantation processes. In: Mahmod, R. M., Noor, Z., & Hassan, M. A. (eds.) Titanium Alloys-Towards Achieving Enhanced Properties for Diversified Applications (pp. 201–228). InTech.

Jafari, M. A., & Islam, M. R. (2014). Corrosion rate and its controlling factors in coatings: a review. Progress in Organic Coatings, 84(1–2), 1–9.

Javidi, M., & Hrymak, A. N. (2015). Numerical simulation of the dip-coating process with wall effects on the coating film thickness. Journal of Coatings Technology and Research, 12, 843–853.

Ji, X., Luo, C., Jin, J., Zhang, Y., Sun, Y., & Fu, L. (2022). Tribocorrosion performance of 316L stainless steel enhanced by laser clad 2-layer coating using Fe-based amorphous powder. Journal of Materials Research and Technology, 17, 612–621.

Kheder, W., Al Kawas, S., Khalaf, K., & Samsudin, A. R. (2021). Impact of tribocorrosion and titanium particles release on dental implant complications—a narrative review. Japanese Dental Science Review, 57, 182–189.

Kim, K. S., Lee, Y. K., & Kim, S. H. (2019). Characterization of tribocorrosion behaviour of implant materials using X-ray photoelectron spectroscopy. Journal of Materials Science and Technology, 35, 665–676.

Kligman, S., Ren, Z., Chung, C. H., Perillo, M. A., Chang, Y. C., Koo, H., et al. (2021). The impact of dental implant surface modifications on osseointegration and biofilm formation. Journal of Clinical Medicine, 10(8), 1641.

Koray, A., & Hasirci, V. (2005). Biomedical applications of polymer blends. Progress in Polymer Science, 30(7), 969–1004.

Lee, J. K., & Kim, Y. Y. (2010). Galvanic corrosion of implant materials: a review. Journal of Biomedical Materials Research Part B: Applied Biomaterials, 1(5), 36–57.

Leiden, A., Kölle, S., Thiede, S., Schmid, K., Metzner, M., & Herrmann, C. (2020). Model-based analysis, control and dosing of electroplating electrolytes. The International Journal of Advanced Manufacturing Technology, 111(5–6), 1751–1766.

Lin, J., Gu, Z., Wang, J., & Zhang, D. (2005). The impact of tribocorrosion on surface coatings in biomedical implants. Wear, 259, 87–97.

Liu, Y., & Zhang, X. The role of surface chemistry in tribocorrosion behaviour. Journal of the Electrochemical Society, 162(5), C175–C185.

Lu, J., Kim, H. J., Gao, M., Lu, L., & Kim, Y.G. (2011). Tribocorrosion behaviour and microstructure of TiO2 nanotube arrays as a candidate for biomedical applications. Journal of the Mechanical Behaviour of Biomedical Materials, 3(2), 256.

Magar, H. S., Hassan, R. Y., & Mulchandani, A. (2021). Electrochemical impedance spectroscopy (EIS): principles, construction, and biosensing applications. Sensors, 21(19), 6578.

Manam, N. S., Harun, W. S. W., Shri, D. N. A., Ghani, S. A. C., Kurniawan, T., Ismail, M. H., & Ibrahim, M. H. I. (2017). Study of corrosion in biocompatible metals for implants: a review. Journal of Alloys and Compounds, 701, 698–715.

Manivasagam, G., Dhinasekaran, D., & Rajamanickam, A. (2010). Biomedical implants: corrosion and its prevention—a review. Recent Patents on Corrosion Science, 2(1), 31–40.

Mano, J. F., Martins, A. M. P. S., & de Lemos, M. S. C. (2019). Tribocorrosion studies of biomedical implants by SEM and EDS. Materials Science and Engineering: C, 99, 949–957.

Mathew, M. T., Cheng, K. Y., Sun, Y., & Barao, V. A. (2023). The progress in tribocorrosion research (2010–21): focused on the orthopedics and dental implants. Journal of Bio-and Tribo-Corrosion, 9(3), 48.

Mathew, M. T., Srinivasa Pai, P., Pourzal, R., Fischer, A., & Wimmer, M.A. (2009). Significance of tribocorrosion in biomedical applications: overview and current status. Advances in Tribology, 2009, 250986.

Merten, B. J. (2015). Coating evaluation by electrochemical impedance spectroscopy (EIS): Report ST-2016-7673-1.

Mischler, S. (2008). Triboelectrochemical techniques and interpretation methods in tribocorrosion: a comparative evaluation. Tribology International, 41(7), 573–583.

Munir, K. S., Wen, C., & Li, Y. (2019). Carbon nanotubes and graphene as nanoreinforcements in metallic biomaterials: a review. Advanced Biosystems, 3(3), 1800212.

Munir, S., Pelletier, M. H., & Walsh, W. R. (2016). Potentiodynamic corrosion testing. Journal of Visualized Experiments, 115, e54351.

Narayan, J. M. R. (2017). Galvanic corrosion in dissimilar metal systems. Journal of Electrochemical Science and Technology, 8(2), 61–68.

Navarro, M., Michiardi, A., Castano, O., & Planell, J. A. (2008). Biomaterials in orthopaedics. Journal of the Royal Society Interface, 5(27), 1137–1158.

Nouri, A., & Wen, C. (2021). Stainless steels in orthopedics. In: Sacks, M. S., Yoo, J. J., & Mikos, A. G. (eds) Structural Biomaterials (pp. 67–101). Woodhead Publishing.

Olugbade, T. O. (2022). Corrosion resistance, evaluation methods, and surface treatments of stainless steels. In: Lashin, A. H. A. (ed.) Stainless Steels (pp. 1–31). IntechOpen.

Parker, M. E., Horton, D. J., & Wahl, K. J. (2022). Tribocorrosion behavior of 2205 duplex stainless steel in sodium chloride and sodium sulfate environments. Tribology Letters, 70(3), 70.

Patel, M. (2019). Tribocorrosion behaviour of metallic implants a comparative study of CoCrMo and Ti6AL4V under the effect of normal load. PhD diss.

Petrovic, N., Ugljesic, V., & Nikolic, J. (2012). Adhesion of coatings: a review of fundamental mechanisms and practical considerations. Progress in Organic Coatings, 74, 1–15.

Premkumar, J., SonicaSree, K., & Sudhakar, T. (2021). Polymers in biomedical use. In: Hussain, C. M., & Thomas, S. (eds) Handbook of Polymer and Ceramic Nanotechnology (pp. 1–29). Springer.

Priyadarshini, B., Rama, M., Chetan, & Vijayalakshmi, U. (2019). Bioactive coating as a surface modification technique for biocompatible metallic implants: a review. Journal of Asian Ceramic Societies, 7(4), 397–406.

Rafiq, N. M., Wang, W., Liew, S. L., Chua, C. S., & Wang, S. A review on multifunctional bioceramic coatings in hip implants for osteointegration enhancement. Applied Surface Science Advances, 13, 100353.

Resnik, M., Benčina, M., Levičnik, E., Rawat, N., Iglič, A., & Junkar, I. (2020). Strategies for improving antimicrobial properties of stainless steel. Materials, 13(13), 2944.

Revathi, A., Magesh, S., Balla, V. K., Das, M., & Manivasagam, G. (2016). Current advances in enhancement of wear and corrosion resistance of titanium alloys-a review. Materials Technology, 31(12), 696–704.

Saha, S., & Roy, S. (2023). Metallic dental implants wear mechanisms, materials, and manufacturing processes: a literature review. Materials, 16(1), 161.

Saini, M., Singh, Y., Arora, P., Arora, V., & Jain, K. (2015). Implant biomaterials: a comprehensive review. World Journal of Clinical Cases, 3(1), 52–57.

Santos, C. R., Paiva, A. L., & Oliveira, J. L. (2017). Tribocorrosion in orthopedic implants: a review. Materials Science and Engineering: C, 75, 200–214.

Shaw, J. C., & Sánchez-Herencia, A. J. (2017). Mitigation of tribocorrosion in implantable devices. Journal of Biomedical Materials Research Part A, 105(7), 1751–1760.

Shen, G., Fang, F., & Kang, C. (2018). Tribological performance of bioimplants: a comprehensive review. Nanotechnology and Precision Engineering, 1(2), 107–122.

Siddaiah, A., & Menezes, P. L. (2016). Advances in bio-inspired tribology for engineering applications. Journal of Bio- and Tribo-Corrosion, 2, 1–19.

Smith, J. (2020). Corrosion and wear in materials: understanding the stabilization stage. Materials Science and Engineering Journal, 56(3), 212–219.

Smith, J. (2021). The propagation stage of corrosion: factors affecting degradation rate. Journal of Materials Science, 56(1), 78–87.

Smith, J., & Jones, R. (2010). Galvanic corrosion in implant applications: strategies for mitigation. Journal of Biomedical Materials Research, 42(3), 235–242.

Tan, L., Wang, Z., & Ma, Y. (2021). Tribocorrosion behavior and degradation mechanism of 316L stainless steel in typical corrosive media. Acta Metallurgica Sinica (English Letters), 34, 813–824.

Tang, X., & Yan, X. (2017). Dip-coating for fibrous materials: mechanism, methods and applications. Journal of Sol-Gel Science and Technology, 81, 378–404.

Tiwari, A., Sharma, P., Vishwamitra, B., & Singh, G. (2021). Review on surface treatment for implant infection via gentamicin and antibiotic releasing coatings. Coatings, 11(8), 1006.

Toloei, A., Stoilov, V., & Northwood, D. (2013). The relationship between surface roughness and corrosion. Paper presented at ASME International Mechanical Engineering

Congress and Exposition, San Diego, CA, November 15–21. ASME Digital Collection, V02BT02A054.

Tripathi, V., Singh, A., Bhatnagar, A., & Bhargava, R. K. (2017). Polyethylene coating for improved biocompatibility and wear resistance of orthopedic implants. Journal of Materials Science & Technology, 33(2), 97–104.

Wahab, N. M., Tan, K. K., & Mohamed, A. R. (2014). Tribocorrosion behaviour of electrodeposited Zn-Ni coatings on steel substrates. Corrosion Science, 78, 253–261.

Wang, L., Zhou, X., Wang, J., & Zhang, L. (2018). Tribocorrosion behaviour of Ti-6Al-4V implants with different coating integrity. Surface and Coatings Technology, 347, 1–11.

Wang, Y., & Chen, L. (2018). Mechanical tribocorrosion: a review. Materials and Corrosion, 69(3), 225–240.

Williams, J. A., & Campbell, S. A. (2006). Tribocorrosion: an overview. Journal of Materials Science 41(1), 1–14.

Wood, R. J. (2007). Tribo-corrosion of coatings: a review. Journal of Physics D: Applied Physics, 40(18), 5502.

Yap, Y. K., & Zhang, D. (2015). Physical vapor deposition. In: Bhushan, B. (eds) Encyclopedia of Nanotechnology. Springer.

Zagho, M. M., Hussein, E. A., & Elzatahry, A. A. (2018). Recent overviews in functional polymer composites for biomedical applications. Polymers, 10(7), 739.

Zheng, J., & Li, H. (2019). Prevention and mitigation of tribocorrosion by coating application: a review. Surface and Coatings Technology, 365, 131–144.

6 Tribo-Surface Characteristics of Bioimplant Materials

Sathish S[1], Anandakrishnan V[2], Baskaran M[3], Kumaravel A[3], and Ananthakumar K[4]
[1] Madras Institute of Technology, Anna University Chennai, Tamil Nadu, India
[2] National Institute of Technology Tiruchirappalli, Tamil Nadu, India
[3] K.S. Rangasamy College of Technology Tiruchengode, Tamil Nadu, India
[4] Karpagam college of Engineering Coimbatore, Tamil Nadu, India

6.1 INTRODUCTION

The use of biomedical implants has become increasingly important in the handling of cardiac problems, bone fractures, and other medical issues. Owing to the ever increasing complexity of medical issues, implants are becoming more and more necessary. The modern generation of biomedical implants imitate the natural bone and tissues for improved biocompatibility. The properties of the newer implant materials need to be examined to show the effective employment of implants in view of physical, chemical, mechanical, biological, and tribological properties. Biomedical implants must be reactive free, biocompatible, and functionally equivalent to natural tissues [1]. Metals, ceramics, and polymers are just a few of the materials used to make biomedical implants.

The main causes of diseases like arthritis or joint discomfort, which call for implants to exchange the defective bones and rigid tissues, are getting older, being overweight, accidents, and genetics. Extreme discomfort, inflammation, and functional loss result from the deterioration of bones and knee joints. In addition, conditions like osteoporosis and osteoarthritis gradually deteriorate the mechanical qualities of bones. Reduced bone density, hormonal imbalance, stress, accidents, and changes in the shape of bones all contribute to osteoarthritis. Knee replacements, dental implants, bone implants, vascular stents, and tissue engineering all use biomaterials and implants. Though the materials are found to be good in material strength and biocompatible, the implant materials fail to meet the tribological behavior when it is subjected to relative motions. Further, the worn debris released from the implant

DOI: 10.1201/9781003384847-6

materials gives rise to the risk of chronic inflammation, the release of metal ions, and other issues [2]. Therefore it is mandated to examine the tribological performance of the bioimplant materials to explore their longevity and safeness in the implantation.

Due to better compatibility, increased corrosion resistance, and superior mechanical properties, first-generation metallic implants cobalt, chromium, titanium, and stainless steel are frequently employed in biomaterials. Stainless steel has been used since the early 1900s [1]. Chromium is alloyed with steel implants to combat the issue of rusting and corrosion. Implants made of stainless steel are susceptible to stress cracking because of corrosion brought on by bodily fluids and tensile stress. Because of this cracking, cobalt, chromium, and nickel are released into the body, producing various allergic reactions and diseases. Chromium can lead to problems with the liver, blood, and kidneys. Stainless steel implants are dangerous and unsuitable for long-term use as medical implants. The body responses to an external object are among the most crucial factors in developing and choosing an implant.

When the implant and surrounding tissues come into contact, several reactions happen, and these responses affect the implant's triumph and biocompatibility. Titanium, tantalum, zirconium, molybdenum, niobium, and gold are biocompatible materials, but nickel, vanadium, aluminium, and chromium are deemed harmful to the body [3]. Properties including elongation, Young's modulus, tensile strength, and fatigue strength are taken into consideration while developing implants for load-bearing applications. The protecting effect and prevention of pressure transmission to the surrounding bone can result from the higher bone strength, which can prevent bone restoration and harm to the bone tissues. To prevent any concerns with load and stress management, the implant should have characteristics similar to those of the natural tissues.

The term "bioactive materials" is also used to describe modern biomaterials since the host tissues respond well to the implant. Osseointegration happens when an implant's bioactive components pierce the host tissue. Over time, the host tissues completely replace the implant material due to the release of soluble by-products [4]. The development of host tissues, nutrition availability, pore size, and surface roughness all influence a substance's bioactivity. Polylactic acid-loaded bioglass and porous sol-gel foam are examples of bioactive ceramic materials. To achieve a similar bioactive response, bioactive proteins, such as bone morphogenic protein (BMP) [3], can also be coated on the surface of the porous ceramic implant. Modern biomaterials are also referred to as "bioactive materials" since the host tissues react favourably to the implant. Osseointegration occurs when the host tissue is penetrated by bioactive components in an implant. In time, the release of soluble by-products causes the host tissues to entirely swap the implant material [4]. Pore size, surface roughness, the development of host tissues, and the availability of nutrients all affect how bioactive a substance is. Bioactive ceramic materials include porous sol-gel foam and bioglass that is loaded with polylactic acid. The surface of the porous ceramic implant can also be coated with bioactive proteins, such as bone morph genic protein (BMP) [3], to provide a comparable bioactive response. The chapter highlights the essential mechanical properties required for biomaterials by comparing the elastic modulus, biocompatibility, corrosion resistance, and wear resistance of different biomaterials. The elastic modulus of biomaterials needs to be near the elastic modulus of natural bone in order to avoid serious problems and the stress shielding effect. Different metallic, ceramic, and polymeric implant materials—both degradable and nondegradable—are discussed. Additionally, design factors and materials used in stents and for medication delivery are examined. Similarly, a thorough study of materials utilized in tissue engineering and scaffolds is offered.

6.2 TYPES OF BIOIMPLANT MATERIALS

The biomaterials used for implants are classified into three categories: bio inert materials, bioactive materials, and bioresorbable materials. The material that is suitable for the implant and that does not induce any harm to the body is called bioinert material. Stainless steel, magnesium, titanium, zirconia, and alumina are some of the most common bioinert materials [5,6]. The material that undergoes the process of ion exchange with the surrounding body fluid is a bioactive material. The material that is dissolved and replaced with the generation of a new layer of tissue is bioresorbable material. In addition, implant materials are classified as metals, polymers, and ceramics.

6.2.1 METALLIC MATERIALS

Due to their superior mechanical qualities, ease of availability, and affordable production, metallic implants are favoured. Ancient times saw the first use of Au and Ag in dental and bone implants. [7,8]. The implant material must be toxic-free, have

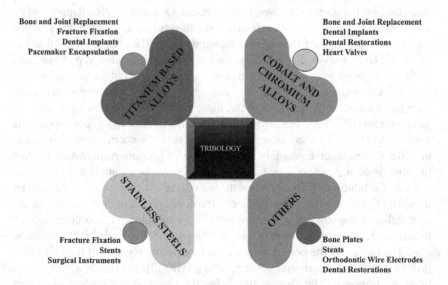

FIGURE 6.1   Bioimplant material and its applications.

nontoxic mechanical qualities that are comparable to those of hard tissues, and have strong corrosion resistance. It is rate based on how well the metallic implant works with the body and how hazardous it is. Depending on requirements, the selection of implant materials is made; a typical application is illustrated in Figure 6.1.

6.2.1.1 Stainless Steel (SS) Implants

The most common SS implant is the clinical grade 316LSS. The mechanical, physical, and chemical properties of 316LSS are diverse. This grade of implant materials is easily accessible and affordable. Numerous alloying components, including molybdenum, chromium, manganese, copper, nickel, silicon, and carbon are present in stainless steel. The coating of chromium oxide in the stainless steel prevents oxidation that results in a strong resistance to corrosion. Stainless steel has the propensity to leach toxic metallic ions including Cr, Ni, and Fe, which can result in major health problems. To counteract the drawbacks of stainless steel, various surface modification techniques are done. In addition, the implants are covered with ceramic, polymer, and composite coatings to stop metallic leaching. SS is often cast off in trauma operations and biomedical implants. Knee, hip, and ankle replacement implants are made of 316LSS. Implants made of stainless steel offer superior mechanical and tribological characteristics and are biocompatible with living things. The implants are typically utilized for temporary purposes because of the problems with metallic leaching in stainless steel. Implant loading conditions can be of static or dynamic, where the dynamic loading ends on the failure of implants through fatigue.

6.2.1.2 Titanium Alloy Implants

Because of its reduced density, better strength, inertness, improved corrosion resistance, increased biocompatibility, and low modulus, alloys related to titanium are favoured for implantations. The metal is suitable for implantation because of its great biocompatibility with the biological environment. Titanium is a better option for implants because its modulus is significantly lower than that of steel- and cobalt-based implants. Despite having a far lower density, titanium-based alloys are just as strong as stainless steel alloys. Heart valves, pacemakers, bone screws, knee and hip replacements, dental implants, and other medical equipment are made of alloys based on titanium. Due to their disadvantages, such as their reduced shear strength, Ti-based alloys are not appropriate for many medical applications. Ti-based alloys' high coefficient of friction can also release wear particles and debris, which in turn can aggravate the body's inflammatory response and cause pain.

6.2.1.3 Magnesium-Based Alloy Implants

Among the minerals that the human body requires the most is magnesium. The traditional implants are need to be removed through a secondary operation that can be quite painful and result in difficulties after the treatment. This issue can be overcome with implants made of a biodegradable Mg-based alloy. Implants made with magnesium can deteriorate over time without producing any hazardous byproducts. Furthermore, magnesium-based alloys have improved castability, machinability, and strength-to-weight ratios. Because of their higher yield strength and lower Young's modulus, implants made of magnesium are more akin to natural bone. Because the implant material and native bone have different Young's moduli, the implant material may be able to support a greater weight, leading to stress shielding. Additional problems that could arise from the stress shielding include inflammation, implant loosening, and thickening of the bone. The mechanical properties of magnesium-based implants prevent them from lowering stress in bone implants.

6.2.1.4 Co Alloy Implants

Cobalt-centred alloys have outstanding mechanical characteristics, increased wear resistance, and greater oxidization resistance at elevated temperatures. Co-based alloys were originally utilized for dental implants in the early 1940s, and further enhancement in Co-based alloys made it the choice in a variety of medical procedures, including knee and orthopedic implants. In comparison to natural bone, Co-based alloys have greater modulus values, which might result in stress shielding and bone resorption. Further, the properties of cobalt-based material are enhanced with the addition of molybdenum, carbon, nickel, and chromium alloying elements.

6.2.1.5 Shape Memory Alloys

The form memory alloys are stronger, have a lower elastic modulus, and have a larger recovery strain. Due to their distinct mechanical properties, titanium-based shape memory alloys, including TiNi, TiZr, TiNiAg, and TiNbSn, are employed in medical implants. Reverse martensitic transition is the basis for the properties of shape memory alloys. TiNi alloys exhibit significantly greater corrosion resistance than cobalt-based alloys and are very biocompatible. TiNi stents had less thrombi than stainless steel stents, and they have superior biocompatibility in both ex vivo and in vivo experiments. Shape memory alloys are appropriate for bone implants, joint replacement, stents, and tissue engineering due to their low stiffness and high strength. The tissue can grow into or along the porous implant thanks to the shape memory result. The creation of various phases with varied ultimate properties and transformation hysteresis behavior can result from even a little change in composition.

6.2.2 Polymer-Based Materials

The demand for biomedical implants is rising daily, and the research accomplishments on polymer-based implant materials are focused in parallel with metal and ceramics to meet the constantly growing demands. To prevent the negative effects of metallic implantations, many revision operations are necessary. In addition, metallic implants can weaken, corrode, produce harmful ions, loosen the implant, trigger allergic reactions, and stress protect. Different organic and synthetic polymer materials are employed in implants and medication delivery systems to address these problems. An additional advantage of natural polymer-based implants is its degradability. For plates, rods, pacemakers, tissue engineering, stents, and dental and bone implants, polymers are employed. Greater strength, inertness, good compatibility, greater chemical resistance, lesser density, good elasticity, greater thermal stability, great durability, and toughness are just a few of the characteristics that polymeric materials possess. The characteristics and flaws of polymer implants can be considerably improved by combining two or more polymers. To enhance the interface qualities and compatibility with the biological surroundings and to address implant material drawbacks, several polymers are employed in the covering of metallic implants. Polymeric implants are now more reasonably priced and biologically compatible thanks to modern production methods like 3D printing. These methods can be utilized to create flexible implants for a variety of uses, including tissue repairs and medication delivery.

6.2.3 CERAMIC-BASED MATERIALS

Ceramic-based implants are used in a variety of orthopedic and dental implant applications. Ceramic implants have an impact on the biological environment in a number of ways, such as through physical attachment to tissues, implant fixation, and the development of bone tissue inside the porous ceramic implant. Calcium phosphate, also referred to as hydroxyapatite (HA), is one of the most widely used bioactive ceramic materials for implants. Ceramic materials based on calcium are further classified into different groups according to the ratio of calcium to phosphate. The ratio is essential for hydroxyapatite to be bioactive for implants. Another biodegradable material that can be used in a variety of non-load-bearing implants is hydroxyapatite. When water and a particular temperature are applied to degradable ceramic implants, like calcium phosphate, the HA phase is created.

The production of these degradable implants is problematic because they are temperature sensitive. Additionally, HA is applied via plasma spraying and laser coating to a variety of metallic implants. These coatings enhance the interfacial characteristics, increase biocompatibility, and guard against deterioration of the underlying substance. HA is used in prosthetic joints as bone cement. SiO_2, P_2O_5, CaO, and Na_2O are examples of additional ceramic materials that are utilized for similar applications. For load-bearing applications like orthopedic and dental implants, alumina (Al_2O_3) is frequently employed owing to its bioinert, biocompatible, greater wear and corrosion resistance. Because Al_2O_3-based implants are so much more biocompatible, they don't need cementing materials to be fixed.

6.3 NEED FOR TRIBOLOGICAL ANALYSIS

The materials implanted in the human body are subjected to micromotion even though it is a fixed implant [9,10]. In some cases, like the implants in dentistry and orthopedics, it is deliberately involved in relative motion with the contact surface. Such relative motion between contact surfaces ends in the synergic wear of material, which leads to the reduced life of the implant materials. In addition, the wear debris ends up in the discharge of metal ions by the corrosive action with the surrounding fluids and induces inflammation [2]. Material with higher wear resistance increases the longevity of the implant material and reduces risk. Therefore it is essential to explore the tribological behavior of the implant material to find its suitability, stability, and lifespan [11].

6.4 WEAR MECHANISMS

6.4.1 ABRASIVE WEAR

When harder particles have a relative motion with the contact surface, the wear loss is abrasive wear. The mechanisms of cutting, fracture, fatigue, and grain pull-out are closely related to abrasive wear. The mechanisms that reveal abrasive wear are ploughing and microcutting. The mechanism of fracture is evident with the generation of subsurface cracks by brittle failure. The crack is observed in three modes: crack propagation at 30° to surface, deep median crack, and localized fragmentations. The material displacement along the sideways of the grooves is caused by fatigue. Grain pull-out is the mode of failure, occurring along the grains in rare cases. The abrasive wear is of with two different modes: two-body abrasion and three-body abrasion.

6.4.2 ADHESIVE WEAR

When two flat materials come in contact, the asperities of the two bodies in contact undergo bonding or adhesion with each other. Further relative motion shears off the bonded asperities to end up in adhesive wear. Shearing occurs either at the interface of the two asperities or at the weakest point of the two asperities, as suggested by the theory of sliding wear. The outcome of the wear gives rise to the irregular blocky debris particle wear. Another condition results when the successive layers of the asperity is sheared which made the wedge shaped debris.

6.4.3 FATIGUE WEAR

The continuous relative motion between two surfaces, either by sliding or rolling, induces the surface and subsurface fatigue due to the action of loading and unloading. The outcome of the wear give rise to the formation of pits and large fragments.

6.4.4 CORROSIVE WEAR

Corrosive wear is the wear resulting from the chemical or electrochemical interaction at the surface. In most cases, air is the corrosive medium that ends up in oxidation. The chemical interaction at the surface forms a thin film layer over the surface, and the action of the motion causes the layer to disintegrate into particles.

6.4.5 DELAMINATION

During the continuous repeated action of rolling or sliding, the subsurface cracks develop perpendicularly to the direction of motion. The subsurface cracks, further nucleates, and gives rise to the detachment of wear debris [12].

6.5 CHARACTERISTICS OF WORN SURFACE AND WORN DEBRIS

The wear mechanisms that influence material wear can be recognized through the microscopic examinations on the worn surface and worn debris. Such investigation displays the surface morphology of the worn surface, which helps in identifying the responsible wear mechanisms. The microscopic examinations on the worn surface and worn debris of the Mg-5.6Ti-3Al magnesium alloy is shown in the Figures 6.2 and 6.3, which displays the typical morphologies. Table 6.1 also shows the typical morphologies that may be observed in the worn surface and worn debris.

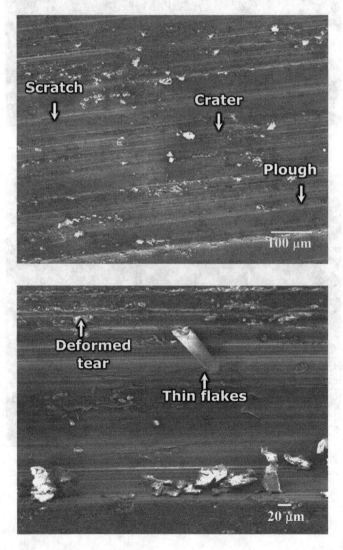

FIGURE 6.2 Typical worn surface of magnesium alloy. (a) abrasion (b) adhesion (c) melting (d) oxidation mechanism.   (Continued)

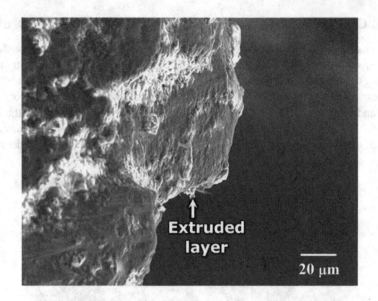

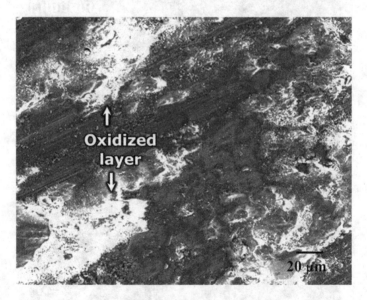

FIGURE 6.2 (Continued)

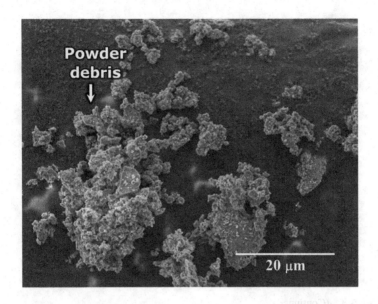

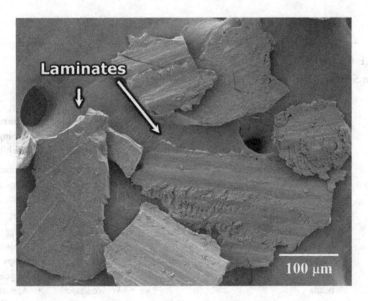

FIGURE 6.3 Typical wear debris of magnesium alloy. (a) oxidation (b) melting (c) abrasion and adhesive mechanism. (Continued)

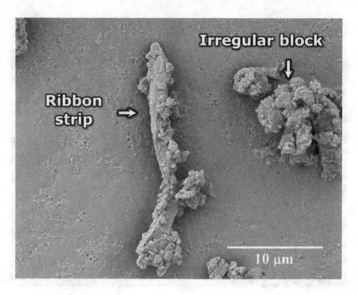

FIGURE 6.3   (Continued)

TABLE 6.1
Worn Surface and Wear Debris Morphology

	Wear Mechanism				
	Abrasive	Delamination	Oxidative	Adhesive	Thermal Softening and Melting
Worn surface	• Grooves • Scratches • Ploughs	• Craters • Channels on the worn surface	• White layers • Surface oxide layers	• Rows of furrows • Smearing and plastic deformation	• Forming flares and bulbs
Wear Debris	• Small fragments • Ribbon-like strips/bands	• Sheet-like flakes or • Laminates	• Powder debris particles	• Irregular and block-shaped (interfacial adhesion) • Wedge-shaped fragments (plastic shearing of successive layers) • Thin plates	• Large irregular lumps • Large sheets • Appearing smooth and featureless

6.6 TRIBO-CHARACTERISTICS OF METAL-BASED BIOIMPLANT MATERIALS

6.6.1 TITANIUM-BASED MATERIAL

Titanium is one of the best suited of implant materials owing to their lower density and biocompatibility. However, the higher coefficient of friction in titanium alloys gives rise to the increased wear of material, which ends up in the release of wear debris. Titanium is the most used dental implant material either pure or alloyed. A very thin layer of titanium dioxide formation occurs in the implanted titanium, and becomes disrupted due to mastication forces. This disruption induces a micro-gap, which leads to the relation motion and ends in the wear, particles, and ion release. The collective action of tribology and corrosion generally, referred to as tribo-corrosion, is responsible for such a process of material degradation. Thus the degraded particles induces the various adverse effects that lead to the failure of the implant. Figure 6.4 shows the schematic illustration of the factor and its effect on the implant. In a similar way, the degradation of implant material is unavoidable owing to the relative motion between them. The wear of material results in the loosening and failure of the implant. Thus the wear behavior of the implanted materials needs to be examined. Some of the research accomplishments on the wear behavior of titanium-based implant materials and its associated wear mechanisms are discussed. Table 6.2 summarizes the wear mechanisms of different titanium alloys under different conditions of wear testing. The wear parameters for the bioimplant material of grade 2 and grade 5 titanium alloy are optimized through the Taguchi technique bioimplant materials to find its suitability for the

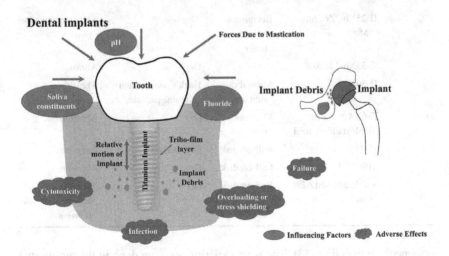

FIGURE 6.4 Factors influencing the tribology of implants and its effect.

TABLE 6.2

Wear Mechanisms for Titanium and Steel-Based Implant Materials

	Material	Type of Wear Tester	Conditions	Wear Mechanism
Titanium	Nitrided and oxynitrided Ti-6A-14V	Pin-on-plate	Dry and Ringer's solution	Adhesion, adhesive-oxidation
	Ti-6A-14V	Ball-on-plate	Simulated body fluid	Abrasion, adhesion and fatigue
	Nitrogen- and oxygen-implanted Ti-6A-14V	Pin/ball on disc	Hank's solution	Oxidation
	Oxygen implanted Ti-13Nb-13Zr	Reciprocating	Dry	Adhesive
	NiTi	Ball-on-disk	Ringer's simulated body fluid	Abrasion
	Ti-15Mo	Ball-on-plate	Simulated body fluid	Abrasion, adhesion and fatigue
	Ti-10Mo-xCu	Ball-on-disk	Dry	Abrasion and delamination
	Titanium Grade 2 and 5	Pin-on-disk	Dry	Abrasion, adhesion, delamination and oxidation
	Ti-35Zr-28Nb	Reciprocating wear tester	Simulated body fluid solution	Adhesion
	Ti-25Nb-3Zr-2Sn-3Mo	Reciprocating wear tester	Dry	Abrasion and adhesion
	Ti-35Nb-2Ta-3Zr	—	Dry	Abrasion
	Ti-30Zr	Microabrasion tester	Hank's solution and alumina particles	Abrasion
Steel	Ti-Co-Cr-coated 316L stainless steel	Microabrasion	Dry	Abrasion
	SS-316L	Ball-on-disk	Dry and wet	Adhesive
	AISI 316L	Ball-on-disk	Dry	Abrasion
	Boride diffused AISI 316L	Ball-on-disk	Dry	Adhesion, delamination and abrasion

orthopedic application [13]. The wear experiments were done in the pin-on-disk apparatus with a 10 mm diameter steel ball with L18 orthogonal array by considering the parameters of load, sliding velocity, and sliding distance. The sample made with the grade 5 titanium exhibited lower wear rate and friction coefficient compared to the grade 2 titanium. The worn surface analysis displayed the presence of grooves, a few pits, cracks, tears of lamina, and oxidized debris that evidence the abrasion, adhesion, delamination, and oxidation wear mechanisms.

The wear performance of the Ti6Al4V compound is experimented on in a ball-on-plate apparatus using the 5 mm diameter alumina ball under the simulated body fluid solution [14]. The experiment is performed at 50 N load, for a period of 180 minutes at a frequency of 1 Hz. The experimental result shows the 0.3 friction coefficient, which is found to be higher when compared with the friction coefficient of CoCrMo alloy and Ti15Mo alloy. The worn surface analysis displayed the occurrence of larger ploughs and spalling that evidenced the abrasion, adhesion, and fatigue wear mechanisms. The wear behavior of the Ti6Al4V samples treated with nitriding and oxynitriding were examined with the pin-on-plate apparatus reciprocating condition [15]. The wear experiments are performed at 0.016 and 0.103 MPa loads for 40 cycles/min frequency under dry conditions and Ringer's solution. The wear results showed the lesser coefficient of friction for the nitride titanium alloy compared to the oxynitrided sample with the values of 0.08 and 0.10, respectively. The worn surface analysis on the dry-operated samples displayed plastic deformed layers, micro protrusions, and adhesive craters of wear, which evidence the adhesion mechanism. The worn surface analysis done on the Ringer's solution samples displayed the adhesive-oxidation wear mechanism.

To advance the tribo-property of the Ti-6A-14V Ti alloy, the nitrogen and oxygen were implanted through the ion implantation technique by conventional and plasma immersion technique at varied temperatures, voltages, atoms dose, frequencies, and treatment times [16]. The tribo-behavior was examined with the pin-/ball-on-disc tribometer using the alumina ball of 3 mm diameter under the Hank's solution. While the surface analysis shows lower levels of aluminum and vanadium than the reference samples, there are no appreciable differences in the wear coefficients between the implanted and untreated samples. The treated titanium samples examined after the wear test displays the presence of titanium and oxygen, which shows the oxidation mechanism. Similarly, the Ti-13Nb-13Zr alloy was entrenched with the oxygen by the plasma absorption ion implantation technique [17]. The wear behavior of the base Ti-13Nb-13Zr alloy and oxygen-ion-implanted Ti-13Nb-13Zr alloy is examined in a reciprocating wear tester under a load of 3, 5, and 10 N with a 6 mm alumina ball for a frequency of 100 Hz/min for 20 minutes. The wear loss in volume is observed to be higher for the non-ion-implanted samples, and the oxygen ion implanted sample run at 3 N displayed lower wear loss. The friction coefficient of the oxygen-ion-implanted samples are observed to be lower when compared with the non-ion-implanted samples. The friction coefficient of the oxygen-ion-implanted sample is found to be lower up to certain time period, and beyond that, it increased due to the removal of the oxygen-implanted layer. The worn surface analysis exhibited the adhesive wear mechanism on the oxygen-implanted samples and abrasive wear mechanism on the non-oxygen-implanted samples.

The wear behavior of the Ti15Mo alloy is experimented in a ball-on-plate apparatus using the 5 mm diameter alumina ball under the simulated body fluid solution [14]. The experiment is performed at 50 N load, for a period of 180 minutes at a frequency of 1 Hz. The experimental result shows the friction coefficient of 0.18, which is found to be lower when compared with the friction coefficients of CoCrMo alloy and Ti-6Al-4V alloy. The worn surface analysis displayed the occurrence of larger ploughs and spalling that evidence the abrasion, adhesion, and fatigue wear mechanisms. The titanium-based alloy Ti-10Mo-xCu was produced through the powder metallurgy technique with the 0, 1, 3, 5 variations of copper powder [18]. Initially the titanium powders were coated with the polyethylene glycol, and then the required amount of molybdenum and copper powders were added, blended, and sintered to attain the titanium alloys. Further, the sintered alloys were subjected to wear testing in a ball-on-disk apparatus under the phosphate-buffered saline solution for a load of 1.5 N load. The sintered alloy samples revealed increased wear resistance with the increased copper content, and the alloy composition Ti-10Mo-5Cu unveiled the lowest wear rate. The worn surface analysis performed on the samples displayed the presence of parallel grooves, and the tear of lamina evidenced the abrasion and delamination wear mechanism. Besides the worn surface displayed, of the dark and grey regions, when subjected to the EDS analysis, the dark region showed higher oxygen content that evidenced the oxidation, and the grey region showed the elements of Ti, Mo, and Cu alone.

The NiTi alloy has been utilized as a bioimplant material, and the tribological performance of the alloy is examined with a ball-on-disk apparatus under the Ringer's pretend body fluid with the addition of silicon carbide abrasive particles [19]. The wear test is conducted with a zirconium oxide ceramic ball at a constant speed of 75 rpm and at varied loads, namely 0.2, 0.5, 1 and 2 N. The wear behavior of the NiTi alloy is greatly influenced by the load applied and the abrasive concentration. The wear rate is found to be decreased even at the increased load when the abrasive concentration exceeds 0.01 g/cm^3. At 0.03 g/cm^3, abrasive particle concentration, and 1.5 N load, the low specific wear rate is observed. The worn surface analysis examined on the sample run at 0.05 g/cm^3 abrasive particle concentration and 2 N load displayed the grooves, plough, ridges, and furrows that show the abrasion mechanism.

The titanium Ti35-Zr28-Nb alloy was developed through the powder metallurgy using Ti35-Zr28-Nb atomized powders [20]. The wear behavior of the powder sintered Ti35=Zr28=Nb alloy is experimented with the reciprocating wear tester in the simulated body fluid solution. The experiment was performed with the 0.03 m/s sliding speed and 3 N load using a 5 mm diameter silicon nitride ball. The wear results indicate that the wear resistance for the Ti35-Zr28-Nb alloy is higher compared to the pure titanium and somewhat closer to the wear resistance of Ti-6A-14V alloy. However, the friction coefficient is observed to be lower for Ti-6A-14V alloy, followed by Ti-35Zr-28Nb alloy and pure titanium. The worn surface analysis on Ti-35Zr-28Nb alloy displayed the existence of varied depths of furrows, plastic deformations, and the flaked debris that evidence the adhesion wear mechanism. The worn surface analysis on Ti displayed the existence of flaked groves and flaked debris abrasion and adhesion wear mechanisms. The worn surface analysis on Ti-6A-14V displayed the existence of grooves, and the tear of deformed layers layer evidenced the abrasive and adhesive wear mechanisms.

The wear behavior of the Ti-25Nb-3Zr-2Sn-3Mo titanium blend was enhanced nitriding through vacuum induction technology [21]. The wear experiments were performed with the nitride sample and base material in the reciprocating wear apparatus with a loads of 1, 5, and 10 N using the 7 mm diameter alumina ball. The wear results indicate that the wear resistance for the nitride Ti-25Nb-3Zr-2Sn-3Mo alloy is higher equated to the base material owing to the higher hardness in the nitride layer. In addition, the friction coefficient is observed to lower and stabilized for the nitride samples owing to the formation of TiN layers, and surface was uniform. On the worn surface analysis examined under 1 N load there is no obvious abrasion marks in the nitrided samples, whereas a few wear scars are observed in the friction pair. The worn surface analysis on the nitride samples exhibited the abrasion wear mechanism, and the base material shows the abrasion and adhesion wear mechanisms.

To increase the wear behavior and the antibacterial property of the titanium, the Ti-35Nb-2Ta-3Zr titanium alloy was developed through the spin coating technology [22]. The wear behavior of the developed titanium alloy was experimented under dry conditions with a 3 mm diameter steel ball for a 500 g load, 200 rpm speed, and 3.5 mm sliding displacement for 30 minutes. The friction coefficient of the developed sample is found to be unstable and exhibited the higher coefficient of friction. The worn surface analysis displayed the microplough, microcracks, and plastic deformation that evidence the abrasion mechanism. The wear behavior of the Ti-30Zr titanium alloy is examined with the microabrasion tester under Hank's solution and alumina particles [23]. The experiment is performed with the load of 1 to 5 N in steps of 1 N with 150 rpm speed for 240 seconds using the zirconia ball. The volume of wear is observed to be improved with the higher load, and the maximum volume of wear loss is observed at 5 N load. The friction coefficient is observed to be higher for the applied load of 1 N. The worn surface analysis displayed the existence of grooves, which evidence the abrasion mechanism.

6.6.2 STEEL-BASED MATERIAL

Due to the medical issues, the deformities and injuries are to be replaced with the support of biomedical implants. In the bioimplant materials, steel-based implant materials are those used long term, and still there is a space to enhance the properties of steel-based implant materials. Some of the research accomplishments on the wear behavior of steel-based implant materials and its associated wear mechanisms are discussed. The wear mechanisms of several steels under various wear testing settings are summarized in Table 6.2. Medical implants have long been made from 316L stainless steel because of its low carbon content and enhanced resistance to chemical corrosion. The 316L grade is considered the safest body metal in terms of biocompatibility when compared to other series alloys such as 301, 302, 303, and 304. Unlike 316L SS, which is uncoated or coated with TiN, the experiment's main goal is to assess the wear resistance characteristics of 316L-grade austenitic stainless steel (SS) that is coated with Ti-Co-Cr [24]. In the experiment, 21mm diameter cylindrical samples under 3N, 5N, and 7N loads are used for the microabrasion test. The Ti-Co-Cr-coated substrate outperformed other substrates in all stress scenarios, according to the trials, and had a low coefficient of friction. The reduced coefficient of friction was associated with the presence of the metals cobalt and chromium, which performed better than the coating materials' high coefficient of friction caused by the metal titanium. The surface micrographs of the untreated, TiN-coated, and Ti-Co-Cr-coated substrates exhibited wear scars following the microabrasion test performed under a 3 N load, as demonstrated by SEM analysis. The abrasion mechanism is supported by the micrograph of the Ti-Co-Cr-coated specimen, which shows fewer scratches and grooves. However, there was some wear and tear debris on the Ti-Co-Cr-coated substrate, which gave it a smoother exterior. As such, the covering provided a noticeable barrier between the specimen and the wear mechanism. The outcomes additionally illustrated the superior mechanical tolerance of Ti-Co-Cr-coated substrates at 3 N loads. The study aimed to compare the tribological behavior of uncoated bioimplant materials, Ti6Al4V and SS-316L, using a ball-on-disk wear testing machine in both dry and wet settings [25]. The findings showed that Ti6Al4V outperforms SS-316L in terms of wear failure rate. The wear resistance of the materials under investigation improved in the order of Ti-6A-14V and 316L. Adhesive was discovered to be the primary cause of wear for both Ti-6Al-4V and the 316L alloy. Due to material transfer brought on by adhesive wear (fracture and chipping), the counterface's contact surface became darker. The counterface used in the Ti-6A-14V alloy tests showed a more noticeable darkening on its contact surface when compared to the 316L. The authors looked into the tribological performance of AISI 316L that was boride dispersed [26]. The diffusional boriding treatments were performed for 2, 4, and 6 hours at 850, 950, and 1050 °C for each temperature. A ball-on-disk tribometer was utilised to examine the tribological reaction over a 10-km distance using an alumina ball with a 20 N load and 200 rpm sliding speed.

In comparison to the base material, the boride-diffused samples showed greater wear resistance, and it was discovered that these samples had a higher coefficient of friction. The abrasion wear mechanism in the untreated sample and the adhesion, delamination, and abrasion in the boride diffused steel samples were revealed by examinations of the worn surface. 316 stainless steel is improved in terms of mechanical and wear behavior by subjecting it to multiaxial forging at different effective cumulative strains, specifically 0, 1.4, 2.8, and 4.2 [27]. The 5 mm diameter sample pins are used in the pin-on-disk tester to test the tribological behavior of the forged samples at a load of 20 N and a sliding velocity of 1 m/s.

The forged samples' experimental results showed that, as strain increased, the wear rate and coefficient of friction decreased. For the samples forged at 0 effective cumulative strain, the worn surface examination revealed the presence of deep, closely spaced grooves as well as ribbon-like debris, which clearly showed the abrasion mechanism. Examining the worn surface in the 4.2 effective cumulative strain sample reveals compacted layers and debris in the form of wedges, which clearly show the adhesion mechanism. Through physical vapour deposition, the study investigates the tribological behavior of the CrAlTiN- and CrN/NbN-coated stainless steel 304 [28]. The tribological behavior was experimented on in the pin-on-disk tester under a load 15 N for 6 rpm speed with a 6 mm diameter pin. It is observed that wear rate of the CrAlTiN- and CrN/NbN-coated stainless steel 304 is lower compared to the substrate stainless steel 304. The coefficient of friction is also observed to be lower for the CrAlTiN- and CrN/NbN-coated stainless steel 304 compared to the substrate stainless steel 304.

6.6.3 Magnesium-Based Material

Magnesium is one of the most compatible implant material owing to its lower density and high strength. The major drawback is the low resistance to corrosion and wear. Hence the enhancement of the property of wear and corrosion is greatly needed. Some of the research accomplishments on the wear property of magnesium-based implant constituents and their associated wear mechanisms are discussed. Table 6.3 summarizes the wear mechanisms of different magnesium

TABLE 6.3
Wear Mechanisms for Magnesium Alloy and Cobalt-Alloy-Based Implant Materials

Material		Type of Wear Tester	Conditions	Wear Mechanism
Magnesium	AZ31B	Pin-on-disk	Dry condition	Abrasion, delamination, oxidation, and melting
	Mg-1.5Zn-0.6Zr	Universal friction and wear tester	Dry condition	Abrasion and delamination
	Mg-1.5Zn-0.6Zr-Sc	Universal friction and wear tester	Dry condition	Abrasion and delamination
	Mg-2Zn-0.2Mn	Pin-on-disk	Dry, deionized and SBF lubricant	Abrasion
	ZK60	Ball-on-disk tester	Dry and SBF lubricant	Abrasion and delamination
	ZK60-10HA	Ball-on-disk tester	Dry and SBF lubricant	Abrasion
	Mg-Zn-0.2Ca	Pin-on-disk	Dry and SBF lubricant	Abrasive
Cobalt	CoCrMo	Microabrasion tester	Calf serum solution	Abrasion
	Nitrided CoCrMo	Pin-on-disk	Dry condition	Abrasion and oxidation
	Borided CoCrMo	Ball-on-disk	Dry condition	Abrasion and surface fatigue
	CoCrMo	Ball-on-plate	Simulated body fluid solution (SBF)	Abrasion and fatigue

alloys under different conditions of wear testing. In the magnesium alloy, the AZ31B alloy is one of the most suitable material for biomedical applications, and the wear behavior of the hot rolled AZ31B alloy was examined by pin-on-disk experimentation [12]. The experimentations were performed with varied loads, sliding velocities, and at a constant sliding distance. The wear ratio is observed to increase with the increased load and sliding velocity. The wear behavior such as abrasion, delamination, oxidation, and melting are found to have significant influence on the wear mechanism of AZ31B alloy. The grooves parallel to the direction of sliding is observed at 20 N load, and the 0.25 m/s sliding velocity reveals the abrasion wear mechanism. The observation of fine particles of powders revealed the oxidation wear mechanism at 40 N load and 0.5 m/s sliding velocity. The energy dispersive analysis on the worn surface exhibited the strong peaks of oxygen, and it confirms the oxidation mechanism. At 40 N load and 1 m/s sliding velocity, the worn sample exhibits the surface cracks that reveal the delamination wear mechanism, and the energy dispersive analysis displayed the low-intensity oxygen peaks. The observation of the oxygen peaks and the surface cracks shows the transition in wear mechanism from oxidation to delamination with the increase in sliding velocity. At 40 N load and 2 m/s sliding velocity, the worn sample exhibits plastic deformed layers, which shows the transformation from mild wear to severe wear. Further, the increased load of 80 N and 2 m/s sliding velocity displays the melting mechanism within the thin layer of solidified material.

With increased weight percentages of scandium, namely 0, 0.2, 0.5, and 1%, the impact of the addition of scandium unusual earth metal on the tribological behavior of the Mg-1.5Zn-0.6Zr biodegradable magnesium alloy was investigated [29]. When more scandium is added, the friction coefficient is seen to decrease, and the wear resistance of the developed magnesium alloys shows an increase in wear resistance. The examination of the worn surface revealed the existence of ridges, cracks, plastic deformation, and grooves parallel to the direction of sliding, all of which were indicative of the abrasion and delamination processes. The increased addition of scandium displayed the smoother surface, which shows that the phenomenon of abrasion and delamination are suppressed.

The magnesium alloy of Mg-2Zn-0.2Mn alloy is produced with casting, and then it was hot-extruded to a bar of 6 mm diameter [30]. The wear behavior of the Mg-2Zn-0.2Mn alloy is experimented in the pin-on-disk tester with stainless steel as the counterpart. The experiments were carried out with the parameter loads of 2 and 5 N for the 200 rpm rotational speed over 30 minutes of sliding time under dry, deionized, and SBF lubricant. The wear rate of the magnesium alloy in the dry condition is found to be higher compared with the wear rate of sample experimented on with deionized water. The wear rate of the magnesium alloy in the dry condition is found to be lower compared with the wear rate of sample experimented on with deionized water SBF lubricant. The lowest friction coefficient is observed for the sample experimented on with deionized water for both 2 and 5 N loads. The worn surface of the sample experimented at 5 N load under the three conditions displayed scratches, grooves, and ploughs. But the grooves are found to be deeper for the samples experimented on in the dry condition and shallow grooves for the samples experimented on with deionized water and SBF lubricant.

The magnesium alloy ZK60 and ZK60 with 10 wt.% of hydroxyapatite is developed through powder metallurgy, and the wear behavior was experimented with the ball-on-disk tester under dry and SBF lubricant conditions [31]. The sample with the added hydroxyapatite exhibited the greater wear resistance related to the base magnesium alloy under both conditions. The worn surface analysis on the hydroxyapatite-added magnesium alloy displayed the abrasion and delamination mechanism under the dry condition and corrosion, abrasion, and slight delamination under the SBF condition. The base magnesium alloy displayed the abrasion mechanism under the dry condition and corrosion and abrasion under the SBF condition. The influence of 3 and 4 wt.% of zinc addition on the wear mechanism of Mg-Zn-0.2Ca magnesium alloy is experimented on in the pin-on-disk testing machine [32]. The experiment was carried out with the parameters load of 3 N for the 200 rpm rotational speed over 30 minutes of sliding time under the dry and SBF lubricant settings. The wear loss of the magnesium alloy in the dry condition is found to be lower compared with the SBF condition at both weight percentages of zinc. The friction coefficient is found to be lower for the samples experimented on in the SBF condition compared to the dry condition. The worn surface analysis on the Mg-3Zn-0.2Ca magnesium alloy sample shows the shallow grooves under the dry condition that evidence abrasive wear. The presence of cracks is observed for the Mg-3Zn-0.2Ca magnesium alloy sample under the SBF lubricated state.

6.6.4 Cobalt-Chromium-Based Material

Though cobalt-based implant materials exhibit the higher wear and corrosion resistance, the release of the cobalt and chromium ions leads to diverse effects. Greater understanding of the tribological behavior of cobalt-based implant materials will help to find the most suitable implant materials. Some of the research accomplishments on the wear mechanism of cobalt-based implant materials and its associated wear mechanisms are discussed. Table 6.3 summarizes the wear mechanisms of different cobalt chromium alloys under different conditions of wear testing. The wear behavior of the CoCrMo alloy is examined with and without the presence of silicon carbide abrasives in calf serum solution through a microabrasion tester [33]. The experimentations were performed at varied loads (0.5, 1, 2, 3, 5 N) and applied potentials (+200, 0, −200, −400, −600 mV/SCE). The experiments performed below −300 V with the presence of abrasive particles displayed microabrasion dominance, and above −300 V, the transition to microabrasion passivation is observed. The passivation–microabrasion is observed in the absence of abrasive particles. The worn surface of the CoCrMo alloy experimented on in the presence of an abrasive exhibits deep parallel grooves and agglomerated islands around the wear scar, which evidences the abrasion mechanism. The worn surface of the CoCrMo alloy experimented on without abrasive displays deep parallel grooves. The wear mechanism of the CoCrMo alloy is experimented on in a ball-on-plate apparatus using the 5 mm diameter alumina ball with simulated body fluid solution [14]. The experiment is performed at 50 N load for a period of 180 minutes at a frequency of 1 Hz. The experimental result shows a 0.25 friction coefficient, which looks to be inferior to the friction coefficient of Ti15Mo alloy and better than the friction coefficient of CoCrMo alloy. The worn surface analysis displayed the occurrence of shallow ploughs, small pits, and spalling that evident the abrasion and fatigue wear mechanisms.

To enhance the tribological property of Co28Cr6Mo cobalt alloy, nitrogen and oxygen was implanted through the ion implantation technique by conventional and plasma immersion technique at varied temperatures, voltages, atoms doses, frequencies, and treatment times [16]. The tribo-behavior was examined with the pin-/ball-on-disc tribometer using the alumina ball of 3 mm diameter with Hank's solution. There are no significant variations in the wear coefficients on the implanted samples compared to the untreated samples, and surface analysis exhibits the reduced level of aluminium and vanadium compared to the reference samples. The treated cobalt samples examined after wear testing display the presence of chromium and oxygen. The effect of nitriding on the wear mechanism of the CoCrMo alloy is analysed under the dry sliding condition through the pin-on-disk apparatus [16]. The nitriding was performed at a constant temperature and pressure of 400 °C, and 8.3×10^{-3} bar and at three voltage levels: -700, -900, and -1100 V. The wear behavior was experimented with a 6 mm diameter Al_2O_3 ball at a constant load of 5 N and at varied sliding distances of 0.5, 0.75, 1, and 2 km. The nitride samples exhibited the better wear resistance compared to the untreated alloy, and higher wear resistance is observed for the sample nitrided at -900 V with lower friction coefficient. The worn surface of the nitrides samples at -700 and -900V at 0.5 km sliding distance displayed shallow grooves and fine cracks, and the reason behind them could be the lower surface roughness. In addition, the worn surface is observed to be brighter, owing to the oxidation. The worn surface of the nitrides samples at -1100 V displayed the existence of deep and wide grooves due to the greater surface roughness. Thus the difference in the mechanism shows the two body abrasion mechanisms for the nitrides samples at -700 and -900 V and three body abrasion mechanisms for the nitride samples at -1100 V. Further, the worn surface nitrides samples at 2 km sliding distance exhibited the increased damage and oxidation in all three samples.

By using a ball-on-disk apparatus in dry sliding conditions, the impact of boriding on the CoCrMo alloy's wear mechanism is examined [34]. Three distinct temperatures were used to broide the samples: 1223 K for 6 hours, 1248 K for 8 hours, and 1273 K for 10 hours. Using an 11 mm diameter Al_2O_3 ball, wear behavior was tested over a 554 m sliding distance at 210 rpm sliding speed under a constant load of 40 N. The increase in infused layer thickness and the rise in boron infusion are influenced by temperature and time enhancements. When compared to the untreated alloy, the borided samples showed superior wear resistance; after 6 hours of treatment, the sample at 1223 K showed the highest wear resistance. In comparison to the untreated alloy, the boride-treated samples exhibit a higher coefficient of friction. The worn surface analysis showed that surface fatigue and abrasion were the main wear mechanisms, as shown by the presence of pits and grooves, respectively.

6.7 SUMMARY

The requirement for and significance of the tribological behavior of implant materials were revealed in this chapter. It is understood that the tribological behavior of the materials relies on the tribo-surface characteristics. Thus the significant observations of the tribo-surface characteristics of the implant materials like titanium-, magnesium-, steel-, and cobalt-chromium-based alloys were discussed in detail. Further it explored the morphology of the tribo-surface and wear debris in view of the wear mechanisms pictured with suitable scanning electron microscopic images. The wear of the implant material relies on the metallurgy, mechanical, and wear properties, which eventually hinder mechanisms. In addition, the wear parameters and the lubricated conditions are also responsible for variations in the tribo-surface characteristics and the transformation in the wear mechanisms.

REFERENCES

[1] L.C. Zhang, L.Y. Chen, A review on biomedical titanium alloys: Recent progress and prospect, Adv. Eng. Mater. 21 (2019) 1–29. https://doi.org/10.1002/adem.201801215.

[2] J. Villanueva, L. Trino, J. Thomas, D. Bijukumar, D. Royhman, M.M. Stack, M.T. Mathew, Corrosion, tribology, and tribocorrosion research in biomedical implants: Progressive trend in the published literature, J. Bio- Tribo-Corrosion. 3 (2017) 1–8. https://doi.org/10.1007/s40735-016-0060-1.

[3] A.P. Ramos, M.A.E. Cruz, C.B. Tovani, P. Ciancaglini, Biomedical applications of nanotechnology, Biophys. Rev. 9 (2017) 79–89. https://doi.org/10.1007/s12551-016-0246-2.

[4] Q. Chen, G.A. Thouas, Metallic implant biomaterials, Mater. Sci. Eng. R Reports. 87 (2015) 1–57. https://doi.org/10.1016/j.mser.2014.10.001.

[5] A.T. Sidambe, Biocompatibility of advanced manufactured titanium implants - A review, Materials (Basel). 7 (2014) 8168–8188. https://doi.org/10.3390/ma7128168.

[6] F. Khosravi, S.N. Khorasani, S. Khalili, R.E. Neisiany, E.R. Ghomi, F. Ejeian, O. Das, M.H. Nasr-Esfahani, Development of a highly proliferated bilayer coating on 316L stainless steel implants, Polymers (Basel). 12 (2020) 1–13. https://doi.org/10.3390/POLYM12051022.

[7] S.H. Teoh, Fatigue of biomaterials: A review, Int. J. Fatigue. 22 (2000) 825–837. https://doi.org/10.1016/S0142-1123(00)00052-9.

[8] M.Z. Ibrahim, A.A.D. Sarhan, F. Yusuf, M. Hamdi, Biomedical materials and techniques to improve the tribological, mechanical and biomedical properties of orthopedic implants – A review article, J. Alloys Compd. 714 (2017) 636–667. https://doi.org/10.1016/j.jallcom.2017.04.231.

[9] H.F. Li, J.Y. Huang, G.C. Lin, P.Y. Wang, Recent advances in tribological and wear properties of biomedical metallic materials, Rare Met. 40 (2021) 3091–3106. https://doi.org/10.1007/s12598-021-01796-z.

[10] S.F. E. L. Shi, Z.G. Guo, W.M. Liu, The recent progress of tribological biomaterials, Biosurf. Biotribol. 1 (2015) 81–97. https://doi.org/10.1016/j.bsbt.2015.06.002.

[11] S. Gang, F. Fengzhou, K. Chengwei, Tribological performance of bioimplants: A comprehensive review, Nanotechnol. Precis. Eng. 1 (2018) 107–122. https://doi.org/10.13494/j.npe.20180003.

[12] F. Mert, Wear behaviour of hot rolled AZ31B magnesium alloy as candidate for biodegradable implant material, Trans. Nonferrous Met. Soc. China. 27 (2017) 2598–2606. https://doi.org/10.1016/S1003-6326(17)60287-5.

[13] S.G. Solanke, V.R. Gaval, Optimization of wet sliding wear parameters of Titanium grade 2 and grade 5 bioimplant materials for orthopedic application using Taguchi method, J. Met. Mater. Miner. 30 (2020) 113–120. https://doi.org/10.14456/jmmm.2020.44.

[14] H. Wang, J. Zheng, X. Sun, Y. Luo, Tribo-corrosion mechanisms and electromechanical behaviours for metal implants materials of CoCrMo, Ti6Al4V and Ti15Mo alloys, Biosurf. Biotribol. 8 (2022) 44–51. https://doi.org/10.1049/bsb2.12031.

[15] I.M. Pohrelyuk, J. Padgurskas, O.V. Tkachuk, A.G. Lukyanenko, V.S. Trush, S.M. Lavrys, Influence of oxynitriding on antifriction properties of Ti–6Al–4V titanium alloy, J. Frict. Wear. 41 (2020) 333–337. https://doi.org/10.3103/S1068366620040108.

[16] C. Díaz, J. Lutz, S. Mändl, J.A. García, R. Martínez, R.J. Rodríguez, Improved bio-tribology of biomedical alloys by ion implantation techniques, Nucl. Instrum. Methods Phys. Res. Sect. B Beam Interact. Mater. Atoms. 267 (2009) 1630–1633. https://doi.org/10.1016/j.nimb.2009.01.118.

[17] L. Mohan, C. Anandan, Wear and corrosion behavior of oxygen implanted biomedical titanium alloy Ti-13Nb-13Zr, Appl. Surf. Sci. 282 (2013) 281–290. https://doi.org/10.1016/j.apsusc.2013.05.120.

[18] X. Lu, D. Zhang, W. Xu, A. Yu, J. Zhang, M. Tamaddon, J. Zhang, X. Qu, C. Liu, B. Su, The effect of Cu content on corrosion, wear and tribocorrosion resistance of Ti-Mo-Cu alloy for load-bearing bone implants, Corros. Sci. 177 (2020) 1–8. https://doi.org/10.1016/j.corsci.2020.109007.

[19] Y. Xue, Y. Hu, Z. Wang, Tribocorrosion behavior of NiTi alloy as orthopedic implants in Ringer's simulated body fluid, Biomed. Phys. Eng. Express. 5 (2019) 1–9. https://doi.org/10.1088/2057-1976/ab1db0.

[20] W. Xu, X. Lu, J. Tian, C. Huang, M. Chen, Y. Yan, L. Wang, X. Qu, C. Wen, Microstructure, wear resistance, and corrosion performance of Ti35Zr28Nb alloy fabricated by powder metallurgy for orthopedic applications, J. Mater. Sci. Technol. 41 (2020) 191–198. https://doi.org/10.1016/j.jmst.2019.08.041.

[21] X. Jiang, Y. Dai, Q. Xiang, J. Liu, F. Yang, D. Zhang, Microstructure and wear behavior of inductive nitriding layer in Ti–25Nb–3Zr–2Sn–3Mo alloys, Surf. Coat. Technol. 427 (2021) 127835. https://doi.org/10.1016/j.surfcoat.2021.127835.

[22] S. Liu, Q. Wang, W. Liu, Y. Tang, J. Liu, H. Zhang, X. Liu, J. Liu, J. Yang, L. Zhang, Y. Wang, J. Xu, W. Lu, L. Wang, Multi-scale hybrid modified coatings on titanium implants for non-cytotoxicity and antibacterial properties, Nanoscale. 13 (2021) 10587–10599. https://doi.org/10.1039/d1nr02459k.

[23] M. Liu, Z. Wang, C. Shi, L. Wang, X. Xue, Corrosion and wear behavior of Ti-30Zr alloy for dental implants, Mater. Res. Express. 6 (2019) 1–8.

[24] G. Godwin, S.J. Jaisingh, M.S. Priyan, S.C. Ezhil, Wear and corrosion behaviour of Ti-based coating on biomedical implants, Surf. Eng. 37 (2021) 32–41. https://doi.org/10.1080/02670844.2020.1730058.

[25] M.M. Sonekar, W.S. Rathod, An experimental investigation on tribologial behavior of bio-implant material (SS-316 l & Ti6Al4V) for orthopaedic applications, Mater. Today Proc.19 (2019) 444–447. https://doi.org/10.1016/j.matpr.2019.07.633.

[26] L.A. Arteaga-Hernandez, C.A. Cuao-Moreu, C.E. Gonzalez-Rivera, M. Alvarez-Vera, J.A. Ortega-Saenz, M.A.L. Hernandez-Rodriguez, Study of boriding surface treatment in the tribological behavior of an AISI 316L stainless steel, Wear. 477 (2021) 203825. https://doi.org/10.1016/j.wear.2021.203825.

[27] S.V. Muley, A.N. Vidvans, G.P. Chaudhari, S. Udainiya, An assessment of ultra fine grained 316L stainless steel for implant applications, Acta Biomater. 30 (2016) 408–419. https://doi.org/10.1016/j.actbio.2015.10.043.

[28] W. Huang, E. Zalnezhad, F. Musharavati, P. Jahanshahi, Investigation of the tribological and biomechanical properties of CrAlTiN and CrN/NbN coatings on SST 304, Ceram. Int. 43 (2017) 7992–8003. https://doi.org/10.1016/j.ceramint.2017.03.081.

[29] T. Li, X.T. Wang, S.Q. Tang, Y.S. Yang, J.H. Wu, J.X. Zhou, Improved wear resistance of biodegradable Mg–1.5Zn–0.6Zr alloy by Sc addition, Rare Met. 40 (2021) 2206–2212. https://doi.org/10.1007/s12598-020-01420-6.

[30] D.B. Liu, B. Wu, X. Wang, M.F. Chen, Corrosion and wear behavior of an Mg–2Zn–0.2Mn alloy in simulated body fluid, Rare Met. 34 (2015) 553–559. https://doi.org/10.1007/s12598-013-0052-y.

[31] J. Su, J. Teng, Z. Xu, Y. Li, Corrosion-wear behavior of a biocompatible magnesium matrix composite in simulated body fluid, Friction. 10 (2022) 31–43. https://doi.org/10.1007/s40544-020-0361-8.

[32] H. Li, D. Liu, Y. Zhao, F. Jin, M. Chen, The influence of Zn content on the corrosion and wear performance of Mg-Zn-Ca Alloy in simulated body fluid, J. Mater. Eng. Perform. 25 (2016) 3890–3895. https://doi.org/10.1007/s11665-016-2207-0.

[33] K. Sadiq, M.M. Stack, R.A. Black, Wear mapping of CoCrMo alloy in simulated bio-tribocorrosion conditions of a hip prosthesis bearing in calf serum solution, Mater. Sci. Eng. C. 49 (2015) 452–462. https://doi.org/10.1016/j.msec.2015.01.004.

[34] C.A. Cuao-Moreu, E. Hernández-Sanchéz, M. Alvarez-Vera, E.O. Garcia-Sanchez, A. Perez-Unzueta, M.A.L. Hernandez-Rodriguez, Tribological behavior of borided surface on CoCrMo cast alloy, Wear. 426–427 (2019) 204–211. https://doi.org/10.1016/j.wear.2019.02.006.

7 Metal-Based Additive-Manufactured Wear-Resistant Bioimplants

Bharat Kumar Chigilipalli[1], Shirisha Bhadrakali Ainapurapu[1], Borra N Dhanunjayarao[2], Arunakumari Mavuri[1], and Dhanunjay Kumar Ammisetti[3]

[1] Vignan's Institute of Information Technology Visakhapatnam, Andhra Pradesh, India

[2] Aditya Engineering College(A) Surampalem, Andhra Pradesh, India

[3] Lakireddy Bali Reddy College of Engineering Mylavaram, Andhra Pradesh, India

7.1 INTRODUCTION

Additive manufacturing (AM), commonly known as 3D printing, is growing rapidly in the medical field applications. Injuries during sports, accidents, age-related issues, and multiple or revision surgeries are increasing day by day. To meet these requirements, metal additive-manufactured bioimplants are highly suitable for attaining accuracy and design constraints. Selective laser melting (SLM), electron beam melting (EBM), direct metal laser sintering (DMLS), and binder jetting are mainly used for these purposes to attain high-dimensional accuracy of manufactured products [1–3]. This makes the AM process more suitable for surgical implants. The increasing demand of medical practitioners for surgical implants drives researchers to focus on optimising the functionality of bioimplant materials.

Bioimplant materials are kept inside the human body at least for more than 30 days [4]. They are helpful in providing support, reproducing the damaged tissues/bones, and improving tissue functionality by integrating with the human body. Some of the applications are neural/brain applications, cartilage/bone implants, dental and other structural implants, etc. [5–7]. Therefore, these materials should have chemical inertness, biocompatibility, bioactivity, wear resistance, and corrosion protection and are mainly selected for implantation. Blood, proteins, and body fluids such as Na+, Cl−, and K+ usually interact with metals, make the metal release ions, and make it hypersensitive and cession sensitive. To avoid such situations, surface modifications are usually implemented using various coating techniques. Chemical vapour deposition (CVD), physical vapour

DOI: 10.1201/9781003384847-7

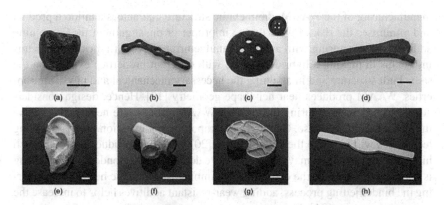

FIGURE 7.1 Additively deposited bioimplantable hybrid ceramic materials: (a–d) printed rigid ceramic crown, locking plate, acetabular cup, and bone plate, respectively; (e–h) external ear, trachea, meniscus, and ligaments, respectively [9].

deposition (PVD), electrochemical deposition methods and sol-gel methods are often used in medically implanted metallic materials. Bioinert materials such as titanium and titanium alloys, cobalt-chromium alloys, stainless steel, biocompatible ceramics, and bioactive materials are all the most widely used materials to serve the purpose [8]. These materials are bioinert materials that are highly wear resistant and are able to be manufactured through the 3D printing process, as shown in Figure 7.1. Bioactivity integration is always the main constraint for the selection of materials used in medical applications.

Along with all other necessary properties, bioimplants must be wear-resistant, and hence the selection, design, and manufacturing of these products are to be selected for that purpose. The material prepared by the 3D printing process can achieve high accuracy and will solve wear problems [10]. Currently, researchers are focusing on 3D printing and on secondary operations, such as applying texturing after 3D printing to improve dimensional accuracy and thereby improve wear resistance as proven by many researchers [11]. Biomedical devices like spinal/trauma fixation devices, lead wires, cardiovascular stents, dental and cardiovascular implants, etc. are majorly manufactured using 3D printing. Materials such as titanium, cobalt-chromium, biocompatible ceramics, and bioactive materials, etc. serve as bioimplant materials and are used in the AM process [8]. Postweld heat treatments will improve the wear resistance of additively deposited materials [12,13]. Researchers like Pradeep et al. have made texturing on 3D-printed samples and noticed an increase in the wear resistance of the deposited structure [14]. Also, the powder subjected to the ball milling process before being used for the SLM process helps to increase wear resistance [15]. Thus surface engineering and surface treatments improve the material properties [16,17].

Ainapurapu et al. have made a hybrid manufactured bimetallic structure using a wire arc additive manufacturing (WAAM) process on SS304L and a forging process on SS308L [18]. Considering individual patient conditions in the manufacturing of the WAAMed bimetallic structure guarantees a tailored product and minimises the risk of wear due to improper or misalignment fit. Combining additive manufacturing with another manufacturing process (hybrid manufacturing) helps in making a hybrid structure with different properties existing on the same built structure and in attaining the necessary mechanical and physical properties. WAAM produces near net-shape geometry [19]. Hence, design considerations during manufacturing through the WAAM process are necessary to make the structure more precise. Geometry and topology optimization using modelling techniques will improve the surface finish [20]. Materials produced through such high heat input process may frequently have defects; hence nondestructive testing is necessary to identify the defects before implementing in the human body. During the binder jetting process, adding wear-resistant additives helps to increase the material properties [21]. Researchers also concentrate on the in-process monitoring and postimplantation monitoring of the AM products to make the products more sustainable in the medical field [22].

The current review emphasises the materials used in biomedical products and various applications of the of 3D printing. This review critically discusses the wear resistance of 3D-printed products that are adopted in biomedical applications. Various secondary treatments and methods to improve the wear resistance of 3D-printed materials are also discussed.

7.2 METAL-BASED ADDITIVE MANUFACTURING TECHNIQUES

7.2.1 SELECTIVE LASER MELTING (SLM)

SLM is a popular AM technique for fabricating full-dense metallic materials with a high-energy laser source to make a layer-by-layer addition of metallic particles. The SLM process improves the material properties with the aid of high energy, high temperature, fast cooling rates, and asymmetric thermal gradients [23]. Therefore, researchers are now focusing on manufacturing bioimplants in the medical field using the SLM process. Also, the SLM process is the most effective method for manufacturing stainless steel, titanium alloys, nickel-based superalloys, etc. Even though these materials are proven to be best for use in the medical field, their wear properties have come into light and call for improvement.

Bartolomeu et al. [24] studied the tribological behavior of conventional casting and SLM SS316L in a phosphate-buffered saline solution and compared the results. The results proved that the SS316 using the SLM process is highly resistant to wear and concluded that these materials are highly recommended in bioimplants [25]. The addition of refractory metallic elements in Ti alloys will improve wear resistance [9]. Ti6Al4V dental prostheses and tissue engineering are possible through the SLM process, and hence the research is focusing on reducing the porosity and producing dense products [26,27]. However, eliminating the powder after completing the parts production is still a challenge.

7.2.2 Electron Beam Melting (EBM)

Another widely used metal AM method for manufacturing metal implants is electron beam melting. In EBM, the melting of powder is carried out using an electron beam as the energy source under vacuum conditions. Manufactured products such as hip and knee prostheses, surgical guides, skulls, screws and fracture fixation plates are widely manufactured using the EBM process [28,29]. AM has become the best option for fabricating medical devices with complex designs. Materials produced using EBM process are found to lower wear resistance compared to SLM-processed products. However, EBM-processed metallic bioimplants show remarkable toughness, rigidity, and impact resistance. During the EBM process, the pulverised material having good electrical conductivity will have no flow of electrons to restructure the material. Hence the selection of material is always crucial in the EBM process. The most used metal alloys are titanium alloys (Ti-6Al-4V, $\alpha + \beta$ alloys, and Ti-Al-Nb), cobalt–chrome alloys (Co-Ni-Cr, Co-Cr-Mo and Co-Cr-W-Ni), stainless steel (SS316L), and titanium–nickel alloys [28]. Mostly used Ti alloys are found to lower wear resistance; hence researchers found a solution for improving the wear rate and fatigue strength of EBAM-processed products using the Ti64 alloy in prosthesis materials [30]. Co-29Cr-6Mo alloy is harder and more wear resistant than titanium alloys. The addition of Nb improves the wear resistance of Ti alloy implants. Hence Ti-Nb-Zr alloys are good replaceable alloys for their wear resistance characteristics. Also, controlled cooling and high

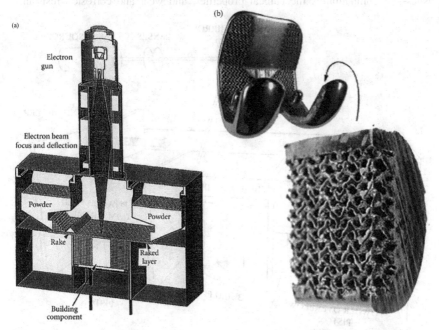

FIGURE 7.2   (a) Schematic view of the Arcam A2 electron beam melting (EBM) system and (b) wear-resistant Co-29Cr-6Mo femoral obtained via electron beam melting [29].

cooling rates help to improve EBAM-processed materials. EBM processed sample materials are shown in Figure 7.2.

7.2.3 DIRECT METAL LASER SINTERING (DMLS)

Direct metal laser sintering (DMLS) is the process of powder bed fusion using a computer-controlled high-power laser [31] beam for melting and fusing layers of metallic powder. First, a thin layer of powder with a specified thickness is provided to the working cylinder; in parallel, the powdered layer is scanned through the high-energy Yb-fibre laser system based on the defined pattern as this has a significant impact on accuracy [32]. Second, using two mirrors operated by galvanometers, the laser beam from the beam expander optics along the defined path is guided over the building area. The positions and regulation of the mirrors are checked with a home-in function feature (integrated autocalibration) which helps in reducing significantly the offset and gain drifts. Thus the F-Theta objective focuses the laser beam on the building area. Finally, the whole layer sintering process is iterated till the completion of the whole part. Further, solidification takes place with the melting of the powder at the laser beam track. Here, during the sintering, the steel platform provides structural support and heat dissipation. The process is operated in an argon atmosphere to eliminate oxidation. Figure 7.3 shows schematic view of DMLS Technology.

For biomedical applications, the materials used should possess defined characteristics—biocompatibility, mechanical properties, and wear and corrosion resistance

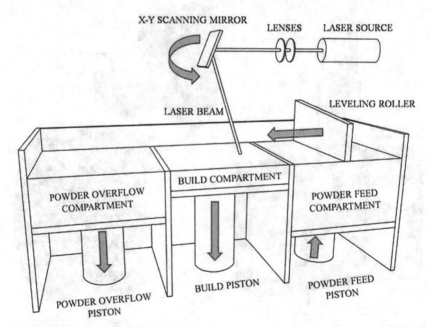

FIGURE 7.3   Scheme of DMLS technology [33].

[34,35]. An important prerequisite for materials to be used as biomaterials is osseointegration—establishing a structural and functional connection between the living bone and the surface of the implant, which is critical for implant stability [36,37]. The investigation of research is on improving osseointegration optimization and potential [38–42]. To enhance osseointegration and improve stability, the implant fabrication is done using titanium as biomaterial [43]. The methods of fabrication include sandblasting, acid-etching, anodization, discrete calcium-phosphate crystal deposition, and chemical modification [43]. Ti alloy composition helps in overcoming the titanium resistance occurring in surface treatment in various ways by changing the composition of the corrosive environment (intrabody environment). Ti alloys have improved mechanical properties, over titanium. Ti alloys are achieved when titanium is alloyed with other elements—aluminium, vanadium, palladium, zirconium, chromium, and copper; however, these components may not be tolerated by a human body environment. The methods used to produce implants are anodic oxidation, annealing, and abrasive blasting, which result in increasing surface resistance, corrosion, and wear resistance, respectively, and changing surface morphology as per individual requirements [44].

7.2.4 BINDER JETTING

Binder jetting is the process of printing high-value parts using an additive manufacturing process which is depicted in Figure 7.4. In this process, a printhead deposits selectively the liquid binding agent onto powdered particles, which are spread in thin layers. The powdered particles include foundry sand, ceramics, metal, or composites. For biomedical applications, studies reveal that titanium alloys, cobalt-based alloys, Co-Cr-based (Stellite) alloys, Ceramics such as tricalcium phosphates, hydroxyapatite, calcium sulphate, alumina, porcelain, ceramic composites, calcium phosphate ceramics play an important role as biomaterials to fabricate bone

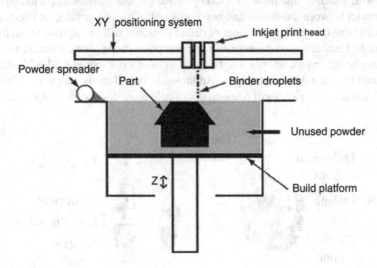

FIGURE 7.4 Binder jetting [47].

and teeth [45]. The materials produced with binder jetting are majorly used for orthopedic bioengineering, cortical bone, bone scaffolds, and implants. Binders play an equally important role in the binder jetting of printed bioimplants. Organic binders, inorganic binders, acid–base binders, Metal salts binders, solvent binders, phase-changing binders, and sintering inhibition binders are majorly used in binder jetting production. This binder jetting used for metallic materials will also allow post-heat treatment to improve the strength and wear resistance [46].

7.3 MATERIALS FOR WEAR-RESISTANT BIOIMPLANTS

7.3.1 TITANIUM ALLOYS

When making metal implants, titanium (Ti) alloys are among the most biocompatible materials to consider because they combine high strength, light weight, and corrosion resistance [48]. The shortcomings of these Ti alloy metal implants include low hardness and certain tribological properties in comparison to some other alloys (such as Co-Cr), as well as problems with stress shielding (which can be resolved by specifying implant porosity). Biomedical devices like spinal/trauma fixation devices, cardiovascular stents, and lead wires have long used commercial pure titanium. Ti-6Al-4V, a well-known medical-grade titanium alloy, has also been widely used in biomedical applications. which is still the most common titanium alloy used to make biomedical devices today. Comparing ultra-fine-grained (UFG) structures to their regularly grained counterparts reveals that UFG structures perform better mechanically and biologically. Investigations are still being carried out on how these processing routes can be used to create UFG structures to improve the mechanical and biological behavior of recently developed titanium alloys that contain only biocompatible alloying elements (such as Nb, Zr, and Ta). Commercially pure titanium and Ti-6Al-4V alloy with a surface treatment are used by dental implant manufacturers to enhance the contact between the device and bone cells [49]. Osteointegration, an interaction between bone cells and the surfaces of dental implants, will be improved with these materials. Lumbar fusion cages, osteosynthesis plates, bone plates, trabecular bone, hip prostheses, and mandibular implants are some of the Ti-based medical implants designed by using AM technologies. Additionally, one of the key aspects of bioimplants and still a major area of research in this field is the development of low-cost Ti

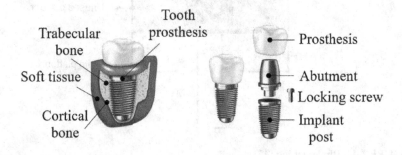

FIGURE 7.5 Dental implants model [50].

alloys with less weight. Dental implants and hip prostheses produced using additive manufacturing for biocompatibility are shown in Figure 7.5

The fabrication of Ti-based implants using traditional techniques (such as milling, forging, and machining) is fraught with difficulties. As a result, AM of Ti-based implants is a fantastic alternate manufacturing method for the quick creation of unique implants for replacing hard tissues. Laser powder bed fusion (LPBF), hot isostatic pressing (HIP), and fusion-based metal AM process are the various AM technologies used to manufacture Ti-based implants. Using these technologies, the microstructure of the Ti-based alloys can be altered, which leads to the attainment of higher strength and toughness. But there exists anisotropy that can be reduced by postannealing technologies [51].

Many implant-related factors in titanium-based implants could affect failure rates, particularly by affecting corrosion rate and wear resistance. The head size, material combination, and method of fixation of implants are those that have the greatest impact on the outcomes of total hip replacement [52]. Corrosion and tribological behavior of novel Ti-5Cu-xNb alloy were examined and suggested that β-type Ti-5Cu-xNb alloy is a promising candidate and is more suitable than the commercially used Ti and Ti-6Al-4V for dental applications. The development of Ni-Ti alloy-based biomedical implants, devices, and other components using AM techniques has increased significantly and has attracted the interest of numerous researchers [53]. Enhanced wear and corrosion performances were observed in commercially pure Ti fabricated using LPBF using low-cost ball milling near-spherical powder widening its applications in the fields of biomedical implants. Surface treatments like thermal oxidation increased the wear resistance of Ti-based biomedical implants [54]. Contemporary additive manufacturing (AM) methods, such as powder bed fusion (PBF) and directed energy deposition (DED), are used to address several problems that can arise with traditional manufacturing processes.

7.3.2 COBALT-CHROMIUM ALLOYS

Among the most successful materials for implant applications are Co-based alloys. These alloys were used as a hip replacement implant material in the early 1900s. Co-based alloys are used in bioimplant applications because they exhibit superior corrosion, wear, and mechanical properties. Studies conducted both in vivo and in vitro have shown that alloys based on cobalt have better biocompatibility. Cobalt-chromium (Co-Cr) alloys have a remarkable resistance to wear and are frequently used in dental and orthopedic implants. The production using AM guarantees intricate geometries and enhanced mechanical qualities. Although CoCr alloys have excellent mechanical properties, wear resistance, and biocompatibility, they do have some disadvantages. Due to contamination brought on by improper sterilisation and handling of CoCr alloys, which results in inflammation, allergic reaction, and aseptic loosening [55].

Orthopedic, dental, and cardiovascular implants frequently make use of cobalt-chromium (CoCr) alloys. Figure 7.6 shows CoCr implants for dental applications. CoCr alloys are among these materials that are increasingly used for orthopedic implants, primarily in total joint replacements (TJR), because

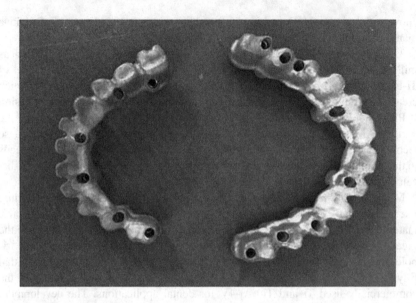

FIGURE 7.6 Double arch milling/postsintering Co-Cr frameworks [57].

of their excellent wear resistance in vivo and high stiffness. They can be used to create surgical implants for the hip, knee, shoulder, and surfaces of broken bones. Artificial knees and ankles are made of a Co-Cr-Mo alloy and ultra-high-molecular-weight polyethene (UHMWPE) [56].

EBM and SLM are the most widely used methods for obtaining AM metallic implants for Co-Cr-Mo alloy. Both technologies provide high levels of dimensional accuracy and corrosion resistance, and they are both members of the powder bed fusion group. Compared to SLM, EBM prints more quickly and is less expensive. SLM, in contrast to EBM, enables higher resolution, better surface finish, and more complex parts.

Various experiments were conducted to study the wear properties of Co-Cr biomedical implants. Through the plasma spray method, a niobium-tantalum (Nb-Ta) alloy coating on CoCr alloy with three different compositions was created. Coated surfaces were more protective than uncoated CoCr, and specifically alloy coatings provided better resistance than pure coatings. The alloy coatings had greater hemocompatibility and promoted cell proliferation in order to enhance the applicability of Co-Cr alloys in the biomedical field, various studies were conducted. High biocompatibility and antibacterial and antifouling properties can be achieved by implementing some coatings on these alloys. However, more study is required to fully comprehend the potential of Gr coatings in relation to implant design, manufacture, and use, as well as to guarantee their safety and effectiveness in a clinical setting [58].

7.3.3 STEEL

Steel alloy containing at least 10.5% chromium and 1.2% carbon is often used as bioimplant materials. Chromium offers stainless steel the benefit of being resistant

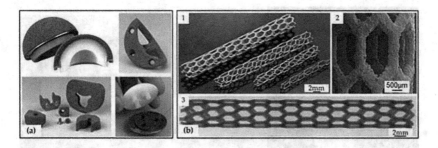

FIGURE 7.7   (a) Stainless steel orthopedic implants and (b) metal heart stents: (1) samples, (2) scanning electron microscope (SEM) picture, (3) X-ray graph [61].

to corrosion and wear resistance due to the formation of the chromium oxide layer, unlike regular steel. Additionally, stainless steel having other materials but in lower proportions, such as molybdenum or nickel, also improves wear resistance. The benefits of steel implants include their high acceptance, biocompatibility, high tensile strength and elastic modulus, low fabrication costs, availability, toughness, higher thermal conductivity, and consequently finer surface finish. The drawbacks include potential inflammatory reactions brought on by the release and long-term degradation of alloying elements. Cells may suffer consequences if Fe is released [59]

Steel biomedical implants are used most of the time for surgical instruments, short-term implants, and screws. Applications such as surgical instruments, orthopedic implants, and dental implants are also reported. These alloys can also be used as temporary biodegradable stents [60]. After undergoing some physical and chemical treatment, stainless steel can be used in fixed implants, such as those for artificial joints, to aid in bone repair. Especially SS316L can be used for orthopedic applications. SLM, PBF, EBM, and fused filament fabrication (FFF) are the various additive manufacturing technologies used for the fabrication of steel implants. Nickel ions that would otherwise leak out of implants due to local corrosion are kept in the stainless steel by sintering the material in a nitrogen atmosphere. To further confirm its biocompatibility, it is necessary to conduct cell culture studies, such as cytotoxicity assays or cell imaging. When hydroxyapatite is applied to stainless steel produced by SLM, the material's biocompatibility rises. An increase in chromium, molybdenum, and nickel elemental composition will greatly help to make the product wear resistant. The stainless steel used in cardiovascular and orthopedic implants is shown in Figure 7.7

7.3.4 BIOCOMPATIBLE CERAMICS

Biocompatible ceramics typically offer low abrasion along with good mechanical properties and are frequently used materials for prosthetics manufacturing. Ceramic materials have low electrical and thermal conductivities, a high resistance to corrosion, and biocompatibility [62]. Ceramic biomaterials are best suited for use in medical implants because of their extremely low toxicity and ability to form new bone tissues more effectively. Ceramics can mimic human tissue or can be

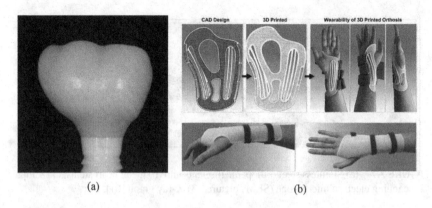

(a)   (b)

FIGURE 7.8   (a) Ceramic dental implants and (b) CAD design and wearability of 3D-printed lattice-based orthosis. Representative images of shape memory 3D-printed orthosis with reticular (upper images) and triangular (lower images) lattice structures [65,66].

reabsorbed by the body to promote the growth of healthy tissues. They are made of resorbable calcium phosphates, bioactive glass, glass ceramics, hydroxyapatite, calcium silicates, and zirconia radiation glasses [63].

Dental implants and some orthopedic implants are primarily made of ceramic are shown in Figure 7.8. Based on how the body responds, three types of ceramics are used in bone replacement and healing. The bioinert ceramic, which is almost inert in the body and creates a thin, fibrous layer at the connection, is the first option. The second type includes the bioactive ceramic, which can firmly adhere to bones. The bioresorbable ceramic is the third type, and it gradually degrades over time before being replaced by real bone [64]. Due to their low tensile strength, ceramics are only occasionally used in medical applications [64]. Scaffolds have also been built with ceramic materials. Binder jetting, fused filament fabrication are the additive manufacturing technologies mostly suited for ceramic implant manufacturing. Applying ZrO_2 as a coating in different weight percentages by using the powder metallurgy technique, can lead to an increase in the biocompatibility, corrosion, and wear resistance of various metal implants.

7.3.5   BIOACTIVE MATERIALS

An artificial substance that interacts with elements of living systems is referred to as a biomaterial in medicine. The biomaterial may be utilised alone or as a component of a complex system in therapeutic or diagnostic medical procedures. As biomaterials have advanced, the idea of "bioactive" materials has also done so. The interface between tissues and bioactive materials results in specific chemical bonding [67].

A unique class of materials called biomaterials is frequently used in bone tissue engineering. Due to their similar microstructure to osseous tissue and biologic-responsive qualities, including biocompatibility, osteoconductivity, osteoinductivity,

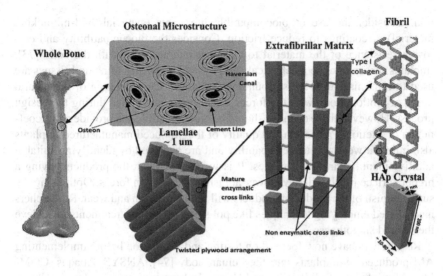

FIGURE 7.9 Microstructural representation of bone with size scales [72].

osseointegration, and superior mechanical properties, they have undergone extensive study and application in the biomedical field. Figure 7.9 indicates the microstructural representation of bone with size scales. Despite their many benefits, they still have a number of disadvantages, including wear, corrosion, the release of toxic ions, the inability to shield against stress, and, in some cases, the requirement to remove nonbiodegradable materials. Novel materials have been researched to overcome these restrictions, and hydroxyapatite (HA) has been widely used in these materials. Here synthesised hydroxyapatite (HAP) was prepared that exhibited excellent results in terms of biocompatible properties. These novel materials include 2D nanomaterials and their derivatives and have their application in bone tissue regeneration [68]. Recent studies show that the nanohydroxyapatite (n-HAp) structure is similar to human bone material and those along with their composites find its applications in scaffolds for bone regeneration [69]. Digital-light-processing-based resin was developed for 3D printing in curing different bone diseases [70]. VAT photopolymerization is used for manufacturing bioactive ceramic bone scaffolds [71].

7.4 DESIGN CONSIDERATIONS

Material selection and compatibility are the main criteria to improve the wear resistance of any manufactured product that is used in a specific application in the human body. Materials such as titanium alloys, cobalt-chromium alloys, or ceramic coatings are obvious choices for bioimplants. Surface coatings on bioimplant materials will enormously increase wear resistance along with corrosion resistance. Wear-resistant coatings like diamond-like carbon (DLC), specialised polymers, and ceramic coatings are applied to enhance surface hardness. Thus, self-lubricating materials, mechanisms, or coatings are employed to reduce friction. Consider the use of biocompatible lubricants (synovial-fluid-mimicking material) or coatings to reduce friction. Consider the biocompatibility and corrosion resistance of the material to ensure it interacts well with the body [73]. Implants that mimic the mechanical and physical properties of natural tissues are used to minimise stress on surrounding structures. Consideration of the natural range of motion along with the forces in the body are applied during the design process. However, these coatings should be biocompatible and provide a low coefficient of friction. Precession and quality of the produced/manufactured implants also improve wear resistance capability and are achieved by identifying suitable additive manufacturing techniques. It is well-known that the products having a higher surface finish will have lower abrasion and friction forces. Optimising the surface finish of the produced products will reduce friction and wear. Researchers have started employing techniques like polishing or surface treatments to achieve the desired smoothness.

Researchers have now focused on testing and simulation before implementing AM-produced bioimplants into the human body [74]. ANSYS, Abaqus, COMSOL Multiphysics, SolidWorks, and HyperMesh are majorly used for simulation purposes in bioimplants applications testing. By means of advanced testing and simulation techniques, the advancement of testing assesses wear resistance under realistic conditions, and these techniques have been improved. Predicting long-term life and performance by reducing material and human effort waste is possible using the simulation process. The simulation and design work to meet the patient's specific requirements surfaces day-to-day challenges to producing wear resistance design conditions. Bioimplant materials for prosthetic body parts and dental materials should designed in such a way that they distribute loads evenly by minimizing stress concentrations and wear points. Design features like radii, fillets, and proper design tolerances are considered to reduce the likelihood of abrasive wear. Mechanical properties are highly dependent on microstructural characteristics. Thus, controlling the grain size helps to improve the hardness and wear resistance of the metal [75], which is achieved through a heat treatment process. Proper heat treatment conditions applied on the 3D-printed bioimplanting products have better control over the grain size and grain structure. Regular monitoring and maintenance are necessary after the bioimplant implantation process in the human body. This helps to get regular updates of the designed product and thereby identify the unexpected issues raised with the new designs.

7.5 CHALLENGES AND FUTURE DIRECTIONS

From the preceding study, we can understand that various additive manufacturing methods are available for printing bioimplanting materials. However, all the materials and methods are not productive for giving good wear resistance products. To improve the quality of product, quality control measures in the AM process have to be adopted [1,69]. Powder quality control, layer thickness control, build orientation, heat treatment, in-situ monitoring, surface finish control, quality assured testing, and iterative design and its testing are various quality control measures to improve the build quality. However, these conditions must not violate regulatory compliance and may not vary with the product produced. Generally used bioimplants must be compatible with the human body; hence metallic materials produced through the AM process must possess biocompatibility. To achieve biocompatibility of implanted materials, advanced methods such as biocompatibility coatings, heat treatments, nanostructured materials, and testing facility has to be implemented. Thus secondary operations such as surface treatments, bioactive coatings, wear-resistant alloys, and surface engineering all help improve hardness and thereby improve wear resistance.

The AM process produces the required products with these techniques as per patient-specific design. However, the surface finish, which is crucial for deciding wear resistance, is always a challenging task for researchers to address. To achieve the required quality, geometry and topology optimization has to be carried before going to printing. Parameters optimisations have been carried out by many researchers to make improvements in the surface finish of the final objects [20]. Various machine learning models have been implemented for optimising and predicting the produced geometry. This helps to control the Ra values, which are directly proportional to wear resistance. In-process monitoring is now an advanced method to help researchers in producing accurate and desired geometry with a high surface finish that has direct control over the porosity of the end-products. To evaluate the products, nondestructive testing methods have to be implemented before using bioimplanting. Sometimes the produced products may have good surface quality, but mechanical products may be not up to the mark. Now the produced parts have to go for proper precise heat treatment to improve their properties. Even then, after the implanting, postimplantation monitoring is mandatory for such bioimplanting applications. Thus long-term surveillance of bioimplants is helpful to avoid hazardous issues that may come after the long period of implanting.

7.6 CONCLUSION

The demand for AM-based wear-resistant bioimplants is increasing day by day. Precision and versatility given by AM-produced parts give manufacturers and researchers the ability to create bioimplants with high accuracy and increased strength. Metal-based additive-manufactured wear-resisting bioimplants are steps towards advancing health care and improving the quality of orthopedic applications. Hence the improvement in the wear resistance of bioimplants is the main criterion for resisting dynamic forces, along with longevity and reducing the necessity for frequent replacements. Proper material selection, optimisation of design, and optimisation process parameters majorly affect porosity in terms of quality. However, the proper heat treatment process, biocoatings, and the addition of nanomaterials will increase the hardness, improving the wear resistance. The wear resistance of bioimplants is facing many challenges in real-time applications. Hence inline monitoring during manufacturing and postimplantation is now focusing on reducing material defects and improving wear resistance.

REFERENCES

1. Manjunath A, Anandakrishnan V, Ramachandra S, Parthiban K, Sathish S. Investigations on the effect of build orientation on the properties of wire electron beam additive manufactured Ti-6Al-4V alloy. Materials Today Communications. 2022; 33:104204.
2. Sathishkumar S, Paulraj J, Chakraborti P, Muthuraj M. Comprehensive review on biomaterials and their inherent behaviors for hip repair applications. ACS Applied Bio Materials. 2023; 6(11):4439–64.
3. Chigilipalli BK, Veeramani A. Investigation of microstructural properties and mechanical behavior of wire arc additively manufactured Incoloy 825. Journal of Materials Engineering and Performance. 2023; 33:2837–52.
4. Kolan KC, Leu MC, Hilmas GE, Brown RF, Velez M. Fabrication of 13–93 bioactive glass scaffolds for bone tissue engineering using indirect selective laser sintering. Biofabrication. 2011; 3(2):025004.
5. Prakasam M, Locs J, Salma-Ancane K, Loca D, Largeteau A, Berzina-Cimdina L. Biodegradable materials and metallic implants—a review. Journal of Functional Biomaterials. 2017; 8(4):44.
6. Wang X, Xu S, Zhou S, Xu W, Leary M, Choong P, et al. Topological design and additive manufacturing of porous metals for bone scaffolds and orthopaedic implants: a review. Biomaterials 2016; 83:127–41
7. Lee DJ, Lee JM, Kim EJ, Takata T, Abiko Y, Okano T, Green DW, Shimono M, Jung HS. Bio-implant as a novel restoration for tooth loss. Scientific Reports. 2017; 7(1):7414.
8. Goharian A, Abdullah MR. Bioinert metals (stainless steel, titanium, cobalt chromium). Trauma Plating Systems. 2017;115.
9. Liu G, He Y, Liu P, Chen Z, Chen X, Wan L, Li Y, Lu J. Development of bioimplants with 2D, 3D, and 4D additive manufacturing materials. Engineering. 2020; 6(11):1232–43.
10. Chigilipalli BK, Veeramani A. Investigations on dry sliding wear behavior of a wire arc additively manufactured nickel-based superalloy. Tribology Transactions. 2022; 65(5):912–23.
11. Pradeep GK, Duraiselvam M, Prasad KS, Mohammad A. Tribological behavior of additive manufactured γ-TiAl by electron beam melting. Transactions of the Indian Institute of Metals. 2020; 73:1661–7.
12. Sathishkumar S, Jawahar P, Chakraborti P. Influence of carbonaceous reinforcements on mechanical and tribological properties of PEEK composites–a review. Polymer-Plastics Technology and Materials. 2022; 61(12):1367–84.
13. Babu KT, Muthukumaran S, Kumar CB, Narayanan CS. Improvement in mechanical and metallurgical properties of friction stir welded 6061-t6 aluminum alloys through cryogenic treatment. Materials Science Forum. 2019; 969:490–5.
14. Pradeep GK, Duraiselvam M, Sivaprasad K. Tribological behavior of laser surface melted γ-TiAl fabricated by electron beam additive manufacturing. Journal of Materials Engineering and Performance. 2022; 31:1009–20.
15. Han Q, Setchi R, Evans SL. Synthesis and characterisation of advanced ball-milled Al-Al2O3 nanocomposites for selective laser melting. Powder Technology. 2016; 297:183–92.
16. Sathishkumar S, Jawahar P, Chakraborti P. Synthesis, properties, and applications of PEEK-based biomaterials. In Advanced Materials for Biomedical Applications 2022 Dec 13 (pp. 81–107). CRC Press.
17. Babu KT, Muthukumaran S, Kumar CB. A study on grain size, mechanical properties and first mode of metal transfer in underwater friction stir welded AA5052-O. Key Engineering Materials. 2018; 775:466–72.

18. Ainapurapu SB, Devulapalli VA, Theagarajan RP, Chigilipalli BK, Kottala RK, Cheepu M. Microstructure and mechanical properties of the bimetallic wire arc additively manufactured structure (BAMS) of SS304L and SS308L fabricated by hybrid manufacturing process. Transactions of the Indian Institute of Metals. 2023; 76(2):419–26.

19. Kumar CB, Anandakrishnan V. Experimental investigations on the effect of wire arc additive manufacturing process parameters on the layer geometry of Inconel 825. Materials Today: Proceedings. 2020; 21:622–7.

20. Chigilipalli BK, Veeramani A. An experimental investigation and neuro-fuzzy modeling to ascertain metal deposition parameters for the wire arc additive manufacturing of Incoloy 825. CIRP Journal of Manufacturing Science and Technology. 2022; 38:386–400.

21. Cui S, Lu S, Tieu K, Meenashisundaram GK, Wang L, Li X, Wei J, Li W. Detailed assessments of tribological properties of binder jetting printed stainless steel and tungsten carbide infiltrated with bronze. Wear. 2021; 477:203788.

22. Chigilipalli BK, Veeramani A. A machine learning approach for the prediction of tensile deformation behavior in wire arc additive manufacturing. International Journal on Interactive Design and Manufacturing. 2023:1–3.

23. Chigilipalli BK, Karri T, Chetti SN, Bhiogade G, Kottala RK, Cheepu M. A review on recent trends and applications of IoT in additive manufacturing. Applied System Innovation. 2023; 6(2):50.

24. Smith AF. The sliding wear of 316 stainless steel in air in the temperature range 20–500° C. Tribology International. 1985; 18(1):35–43.

25. Alvi S, Saeidi K, Akhtar F. High-temperature tribology and wear of selective laser melted (SLM) 316L stainless steel. Wear. 2020; 448:203228.

26. Bhadrakali AS, Sastry DV, Chigilipalli BK, Naik KS, Kakaravada TI, Acharya A, Kumar KL. Effect of heat input on microstructure and mechanical properties of bimetallic wire arc additive manufacturing of SS304L and ER308L prepared by hybrid manufacturing process. International Journal on Interactive Design and Manufacturing. 2023:1–2.

27. Sivasankar M, Arunkumar S, Bakkiyaraj V, Muruganandam A, Sathishkumar S. A review on total hip replacement. International Research Journal in Advanced Engineering Technology. 2016; 2(2):589–92.

28. Tamayo JA, Riascos M, Vargas CA, Baena LM. Additive manufacturing of Ti6Al4V alloy via electron beam melting for the development of implants for the biomedical industry. Heliyon. 2021; 7(5):e06892.

29. Murr LE, Gaytan SM, Martinez E, Medina F, Wicker RB. Next generation orthopaedic implants by additive manufacturing using electron beam melting. International Journal of Biomaterials. 2012; 2012:245727.

30. Javadhesari SM, Alipour S, Akbarpour MR. Biocompatibility, osseointegration, antibacterial and mechanical properties of nanocrystalline Ti-Cu alloy as a new orthopedic material. Colloids and Surfaces B: Biointerfaces. 2020; 189:110889.

31. Sarila VK, Moinuddin SQ, Cheepu M, Rajendran H, Kantumuchu VC. Characterization of microstructural anisotropy in 17–4 PH stainless steel fabricated by DMLS additive manufacturing and laser shot peening. Transactions of the Indian Institute of Metals. 2023; 76(2):403–10.

32. Chowdhury S, Yadaiah N, Prakash C, Ramakrishna S, Dixit S, Gupta LR, Buddhi D. Laser powder bed fusion: a state-of-the-art review of the technology, materials, properties & defects, and numerical modelling. Journal of Materials Research and Technology. 2022; 20:2109–72.

33. Palumbo B, Del Re F, Martorelli M, Lanzotti A, Corrado P. Tensile properties characterization of AlSi10Mg parts produced by direct metal laser sintering via nested effects modeling. Materials. 2017;10(2):144.

34. Maya-Johnson S, López D. Effect of the cooling rate in the corrosion behavior of a hot worked Ti-6Al-4V extra-low interstitial alloy. Materials & Design. 2014; 58:175–81.

35. Pavon J, Jimenez-Pique E, Anglada M, Lopez-Esteban S, Saiz E, Tomsia AP. Stress–corrosion cracking by indentation techniques of a glass coating on Ti6Al4V for biomedical applications. Journal of the European Ceramic Society. 2006; 26(7):1159–69.

36. Aljateeli M, Wang HL. Implant microdesigns and their impact on osseointegration. Implant Dentistry. 2013; 22(2):127–32.

37. Shalabi MM, Gortemaker A, Hof MV, Jansen JA, Creugers NH. Implant surface roughness and bone healing: a systematic review. Journal of Dental Research. 2006; 85(6):496–500.

38. Monjo M, Petzold C, Ramis JM, Lyngstadaas SP, Ellingsen JE. In vitro osteogenic properties of two dental implant surfaces. International Journal of Biomaterials. 2012; 2012.

39. Kottala RK, Balasubramanian KR, Jinshah BS, Divakar S, Chigilipalli BK. Experimental investigation and machine learning modelling of phase change material-based receiver tube for natural circulated solar parabolic trough system under various weather conditions. Journal of Thermal Analysis and Calorimetry. 2023:1–24.

40. Sesma N, Pannuti CM, Cardaropoli G. Retrospective clinical study of 988 dual acid-etched implants placed in grafted and native bone for single-tooth replacement. International Journal of Oral & Maxillofacial Implants. 2012; 27(5).

41. Kottala RK, Chigilipalli BK, Mukuloth S, Shanmugam R, Kantumuchu VC, Ainapurapu SB, Cheepu M. Thermal degradation studies and machine learning modelling of nano-enhanced sugar alcohol-based phase change materials for medium temperature applications. Energies. 2023; 16(5):2187.

42. Benalcázar-Jalkh EB, Nayak VV, Gory C, Marquez-Guzman A, Bergamo ET, Tovar N, Coelho PG, Bonfante EA, Witek L. Impact of implant thread design on insertion torque and osseointegration: a preclinical model. Medicina Oral, Patología Oral y Cirugía Bucal. 2023; 28(1):e48.

43. Mangano F, Chambrone L, Van Noort R, Miller C, Hatton P, Mangano C. Direct metal laser sintering titanium dental implants: a review of the current literature. International Journal of Biomaterials. 2014; 2014.

44. Orłowska A, Szewczenko J, Kajzer W, Goldsztajn K, Basiaga M. Study of the effect of anodic oxidation on the corrosion properties of the Ti6Al4V implant produced from SLM. Journal of Functional Biomaterials. 2023; 14(4):191.

45. Mirzaali MJ, Moosabeiki V, Rajaai SM, Zhou J, Zadpoor AA. Additive manufacturing of biomaterials—design principles and their implementation. Materials. 2022; 15(15):5457.

46. Mostafaei A, Elliott AM, Barnes JE, Li F, Tan W, Cramer CL, Nandwana P, Chmielus M. Binder jet 3D printing—process parameters, materials, properties, modeling, and challenges. Progress in Materials Science. 2021; 119:100707.

47. Mirzababaei S, Pasebani S. A review on binder jet additive manufacturing of 316L stainless steel. Journal of Manufacturing and Materials Processing. 2019;3(3):82.

48. Cheepu M, Susila P. Interface microstructure characteristics of friction-welded joint of titanium to stainless steel with interlayer. Transactions of the Indian Institute of Metals. 2020; 73:1497–501.

49. Nicholson JW. Titanium alloys for dental implants: a review. Prosthesis. 2020; 2(2):11.
50. Martinez-Mondragon M, Urriolagoitia-Sosa G, Romero-Ángeles B, Maya-Anaya D, Martínez-Reyes J, Gallegos-Funes FJ, Urriolagoitia-Calderón GM. Numerical analysis of zirconium and titanium implants under the effect of critical masticatory load. Materials. 2022;15(21):7843.
51. Kaoushik VM, Nichul U, Chavan V, Hiwarkar V. Development of microstructure and high hardness of Ti6Al4V alloy fabricated using laser beam powder bed fusion: a novel sub-transus heat treatment approach. Journal of Alloys and Compounds. 2023; 937:168387.
52. López-López JA, Humphriss RL, Beswick AD, Thom HH, Hunt LP, Burston A, Fawsitt CG, Hollingworth W, Higgins JP, Welton NJ, Blom AW. Choice of implant combinations in total hip replacement: systematic review and network meta-analysis. BMJ. 2017; 359.
53. Li Y, Yang C, Zhao H, Qu S, Li X, Li Y. New developments of Ti-based alloys for biomedical applications. Materials. 2014;7(3):1709–800.
54. Unune DR, Brown GR, Reilly GC. Thermal based surface modification techniques for enhancing the corrosion and wear resistance of metallic implants: a review. Vacuum. 2022: 111298.
55. Kassapidou M, Stenport VF, Johansson CB, Östberg AK, Johansson PH, Hjalmarsson L. Inflammatory response to cobalt-chromium alloys fabricated with different techniques. Journal of Oral & Maxillofacial Research. 2021; 12(4).
56. Bistolfi A, Giustra F, Bosco F, Sabatini L, Aprato A, Bracco P, Bellare A. Ultra-high molecular weight polyethylene (UHMWPE) for hip and knee arthroplasty: the present and the future. Journal of Orthopaedics. 2021; 25:98–106.
57. Heller H, Beitlitum I, Goldberger T, Emodi-Perlman A, Levartovsky S. Outcomes and complications of 33 soft-milled cobalt-chromium-ceramic full-arch screw-retained implant-supported prostheses: a retrospective study with up to 10-year follow-up. Journal of Functional Biomaterials. 2023; 14(3):157.
58. Saini M, Singh Y, Arora P, Arora V, Jain K. Implant biomaterials: a comprehensive review. World Journal of Clinical Cases. 2015; 3(1):52.
59. Khodaei T, Schmitzer E, Suresh AP, Acharya AP. Immune response differences in degradable and non-degradable alloy implants. Bioactive Materials. 2023; 24:153–70.
60. Moghadasi K, Isa MS, Ariffin MA, Raja S, Wu B, Yamani M, Muhamad MR, Yusof F, Jamaludin MF, bin Ab Karim MS, bin Yusoff N. A review on biomedical implant materials and the effect of friction stir based techniques on their mechanical and tribological properties. Journal of Materials Research and Technology. 2022; 17:1054–121.
61. Bai L, Gong C, Chen X, Sun Y, Zhang J, Cai L, Zhu S, Xie SQ. Additive manufacturing of customized metallic orthopedic implants: materials, structures, and surface modifications. Metals. 2019; 9(9):1004.
62. Festas AJ, Ramos A, Davim JP. Medical devices biomaterials–a review. Proceedings of the Institution of Mechanical Engineers, Part L: Journal of Materials: Design and Applications. 2020; 234(1):218–28.
63. Raghavendra SS, Jadhav GR, Gathani KM, Kotadia P. Bioceramics in endodontics–a review. Journal of Istanbul University Faculty of Dentistry. 2017; 51(3 Suppl 1):128–37.
64. Baino F, Novajra G, Vitale-Brovarone C. Bioceramics and scaffolds: a winning combination for tissue engineering. Frontiers in Bioengineering and Biotechnology. 2015; 3:202.

65. Nueesch R, Karlin S, Fischer J, Rohr N. In vitro investigation of material combinations for meso-and suprastructures in a biomimetic approach to restore one-piece zirconia implants. Materials. 2023; 16(4):1355.
66. Sala R, Regondi S, Pugliese R. Design data and finite element analysis of 3D printed poly (ε-Caprolactone)-based lattice scaffolds: influence of type of unit cell, porosity, and nozzle diameter on the mechanical behavior. Eng. 2021; 3(1):9–23.
67. Moghadam ET, Yazdanian M, Alam M, Tebyanian H, Tafazoli A, Tahmasebi E, Ranjbar R, Yazdanian A, Seifalian A. Current natural bioactive materials in bone and tooth regeneration in dentistry: a comprehensive overview. Journal of Materials Research and Technology. 2021; 13:2078–114.
68. Cao Z, Bian Y, Hu T, Yang Y, Cui Z, Wang T, Yang S, Weng X, Liang R, Tan C. Recent advances in two-dimensional nanomaterials for bone tissue engineering. Journal of Materiomics. 2023; 9:930–58.
69. Mo X, Zhang D, Liu K, Zhao X, Li X, Wang W. Nano-hydroxyapatite composite scaffolds loaded with bioactive factors and drugs for bone tissue engineering. International Journal of Molecular Sciences. 2023; 24(2):1291.
70. Zhang J, Hu Q, Wang S, Tao J, Gou M. Digital light processing based three-dimensional printing for medical applications. International Journal of Bioprinting. 2020;6(1):242.
71. Guo W, Li B, Li P, Zhao L, You H, Long Y. Review on vat photopolymerization additive manufacturing of bioactive ceramic bone scaffolds. Journal of Materials Chemistry B. 2023; 11:9572–96.
72. Siddiqui HA, Pickering KL, Mucalo MR. A review on the use of hydroxyapatite-carbonaceous structure composites in bone replacement materials for strengthening purposes. Materials. 2018; 11(10):1813.
73. Chigilipalli BK, Veeramani A. Investigation of the corrosion behavior of wire arc additively manufactured alloy 825. Transactions of the Indian Institute of Metals. 2023;76(2):279–86.
74. Kang CW, Fang FZ. State of the art of bioimplants manufacturing: part I. Advances in Manufacturing. 2018; 6:20–40.
75. Tejonadha Babu K, Muthukumaran S, Sathiya Narayanan C, Bharat Kumar CH. Analysis and characterization of forming behavior on dissimilar joints of AA5052-O to AA6061-T6 using underwater friction stir welding. Surface Review and Letters. 2020; 27(03):1950121.

8 Synthesis and Characterization of Ceramic-Based Wear-Resistant Bioimplants

R Govindan¹, GS Lekshmi², BS Mohan Kumar³, and S Thiruvengadam³

¹ Saveetha Institute of Medical and Technical Sciences
Chennai, Tamil Nadu, India

² Lodz University of Technology
Lodz, Poland

³ Rajalakshmi Engineering College
Chennai, Tamil Nadu India

8.1 INTRODUCTION

Biomaterials have made significant changes in the field of health care and bind tightly with hard and soft tissues, which stimulate tissue regeneration and repair. Various types of biomaterials, such as metals, ceramics, polymers, and their composites have been used for treating a wide range of health care issues. However, these materials have their own advantages and drawbacks. Polymers and ceramics suffer from inadequate mechanical strength and a rapid degradation rate compared to host tissues; thus they restrict their load-bearing applications. Metallic materials such as surgical-grade stainless steel (SS), titanium (Ti) alloys, magnesium alloys (Mg), and cobalt-chromium (Co-Cr) alloys are extensively studied metallic implants for biomedical applications. Due to their excellent mechanical properties of metallic materials, they can be used for load-bearing applications, especially orthopedic implants, dental materials, and prosthetic components. The mechanical properties of various metallic implants are shown in Figure 8.1. However, metallic materials suffer from lack of osteoconductivity, poor wear resistance, and corrosion resistance, which leads to the discharge of toxic corrosive ions and poor interaction with the host tissue. Conversely, these issues are typically associated with the surface nature, both the physical and chemical natures of the metallic implants, which play a unique role in the interaction between implant materials and the host environment.[1] As a result, it is urgent to search for/develop new materials and coating methods to fabricate biocompatible, bioactive, and mechanically strong bioimplant materials.

Bioceramic coating on a mechanically stronger and tougher metallic substrate is one of the strategies to overcome these issues. Ceramic coatings can significantly

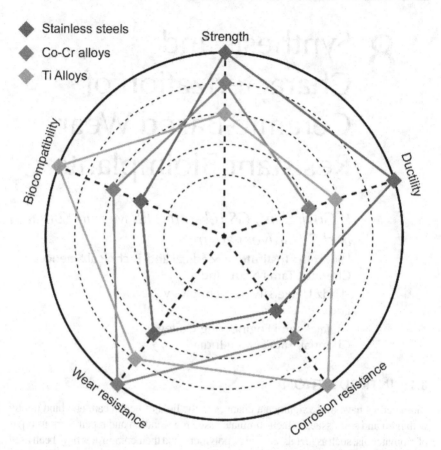

FIGURE 8.1 Comparison of various parameters of different metallic implants.[2]

enhance the biological properties on the surface of metallic materials, including antibiofilming, anticorrosion nature, thermal stability, excellent wear resistance, bioadhesion, bioactivity, and biocompatibility, these are the important properties of biomaterials.[3,4] Ceramic coating on a metallic surface is considered a rational strategy for biofunctionalizing the metallic surface with excellent cell–material interactions.[5] The ideal requirements for coating ceramic materials are biocompatibility, bioactivity, adequate fracture toughness and mechanical strength, and high corrosion resistance and wear resistance.[6] So far, no ideal material has been reported to as meeting these requirements. Specifically, both corrosion and wear in the biological environment have been considered crucial factors in the failure of metallic implant biomaterials.[7] It is noteworthy that the wear debris leads to inflammation, osteolysis, infection, pain, and inhibition.[8,9]

8.2 CHARACTERISTICS OF IDEAL IMPLANT BIOMATERIALS

The perfect graft biomaterials should possess biocompatibility (cell–material interaction) and antibacterial efficiency. Biocompatibility is a primary requirement

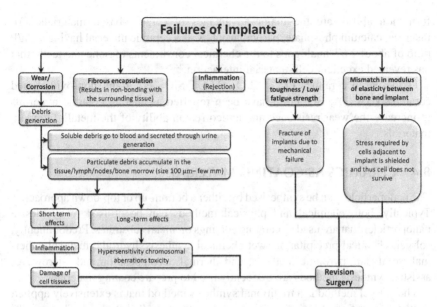

FIGURE 8.2   Various reasons for the failure of implant materials.[10]

for metallic implant materials, and implant materials should form a chemical bond with the host tissues/cells to form a carbonated-apatite layer under the physiological conditions.[11] Bacterial adherence on the metallic implants significantly affects the cell–material interaction.[12] *Pseudomonas aeruginosa (P. aeruginosa)* is an especially vigorous microbe that causes many infections.[13] Therefore, biocompatibility and an antibacterial nature are the requirement parameters for any artificial implants. However, many parameters affect implant failure, which requires secondary or revision surgeries (Figure 8.2).

8.3   CERAMICS AS COATING MATERIAL

Ceramics are inorganic materials that are usually produced at high temperatures. Ceramics including bioactive silicate/phosphate/borate glasses,[14–16] zirconium oxide [ZrO_2],[17] aluminium oxide [Al_2O_3],[18] and calcium phosphate family [hydroxyapatite (HA), β-tricalcium phosphate (β-TCP), etc.][19–21] materials are considered potential candidates for biomedical applications due to excellent biocompatibility. Generally, ceramic materials can be categorised into three types based on their interaction with host tissues, namely, bioinert, bioactive, and bioresorbable.[22,23] Bioinert ceramics do not form any chemical bonding with the host tissues; however, these ceramics form a physical bond while implanted with the host tissues. On the contrary, both bioactive and resorbable ceramics have facilitated the formation chemical bonds that support biointegration with the native site. In addition, resorbable ceramic materials are degraded over time and are swapped out by host tissues. Biocompatibility, bioactivity, low toxicity, excellent corrosion resistance, inhibition of disease transmission, and good new tissue formation ability are the major advantages of ceramic-based materials. For instance, calcium phosphate, particularly HA, is a ceramic material having a Ca/P ratio of about 1.67, analogous to the chemical constituents of bone and teeth, that has revealed excellent cell–material interaction.[24,25]

Oxide-based ceramics (TiO_2, ZrO_2, Al_2O_3, SiO_2, etc.,) and non-oxide-based ceramics (HA, FA, BG, etc.,) have been reported as coating ceramic materials to increase the wear resistance and anticorrosion ability of the metallic implant materials.

8.4 CERAMICS AS COATING MATERIAL

The nanoparticles can be synthesised by either a bottom-up or top-down approach.[26] Typically, both chemical and physical methods can be utilised to synthesise nanoparticles that are used as ceramic coatings on metal substrates. Predominantly, sol-gel, chemical precipitation, wet chemical synthesis, hydrothermal, solvothermal, solid-state pyrolytic methods, and thermal decomposition and microwave-assisted synthesis methods are frequently used to prepare coating materials.

The sol-gel method is a traditional synthesis method that is extensively applied for the preparation of various nanoparticles with controlled shapes.[27] These methods have numerous advantages, including nanoparticles of varying sizes, high purity and homogeneity, and ease of synthesis at low temperatures. The homogeneous sol is formed by the addition of two different precursors, and it transform into a gel, followed by the elimination of the solvent from the gel by drying at ambient temperature. For example, as demonstrated in Figure 8.3, the aqueous calcium reacts with phosphate precursors and forms sol at low temperatures. When the temperature is raised after a predetermined amount of time, the sol transforms into gel, resulting in the HA phase at high calcination temperatures. Wet chemical precipitation is a top-down approach. Soluble metal precursor transforms into insoluble product using a precipitating reagent, and the metal oxide is then obtained by annealing at appropriate temperatures. The metal oxides synthesised by wet chemical precipitation methods are in the small size range with a uniform distribution; the particles are highly pure in nature and poor crystallinity. Metal oxides such as ZnO, CeO_2, Fe_2O_3, and TiO_2 can be synthesised by the wet chemical precipitation method.[28]

Hydrothermal synthesis is an effective method utilised for the fabrication of metal oxide and nonoxide nanoparticles and is usually performed in an aqueous medium at an elevated temperature (usually 80–240 °C), pressure, and predetermined time (e.g., 1–20 hours).[30] In the hydrothermal synthesis, the aging process is performed at an elevated temperature and high pressure. The solvothermal synthesis is analogous to the hydrothermal method, instead of water; other solvents are used as the medium. Typically, the reactions are conducted at an elevated temperature (100–1000 °C) and an elevated pressure (1–10,000 bar).[31] Solvents such as diethanolamine, ethanol, methanol, 1,4-butanediol, toluene, and ethylene glycol are the typical examples for the synthesis of nanoparticles by the solvothermal method.[32] For instance, Mehdi et al. synthesised rod-like structured HA by a hydrothermal method.[33] The formation of rod-like HA comprises two steps: the nucleation step (formation of tiny crystal-like nuclei in a supersaturated medium) and the growth step (formation of rod-like HA under specific conditions [hydrothermal treatment]) (Figure 8.3).

Microwave-assisted synthesis is rapid heating achieved by microwave irradiation, which stimulates the reaction in short-time duration.[34] As schematically shown in Figure 8.3, microwave processing can be performed under any conditions for the preparation of HA. Various nanoparticles were synthesised using different microwave approaches, including microwave polyol synthesis, the direct microwave heating method, solid-state microwave irradiation, microwave-assisted hydrothermal methods, surfactant-free microwave-assisted mixing, etc.[35] In addition, various synthesis methods including microemulsion,[36] ball milling,[37] and sonochemical methods[38] can be applied to the synthesis of nanoparticles with different shapes and morphologies. Notably, the size and shape of the particles depend on their method of synthesis and the conditions used for the preparation of nanoparticles.

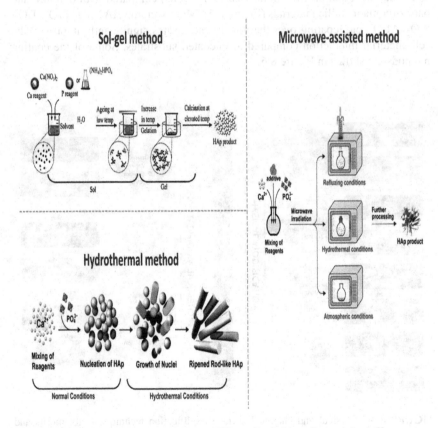

FIGURE 8.3 Schematic representation of HA synthesis by various methods.[29]

8.5 TYPES OF CERAMICS COATINGS

Various techniques, including sol-gel method, micro-arc oxidation (MAO), atomic layer deposition (ALD), the electrochemical method, magnetron sputtering, solution immersion, laser-cladding, chemical vapour deposition and dip coating method, have been used for ceramic coating on the metallic substrates. The ceramic coating on metallic substrate using the sol-gel method enhances the functionality of metallic substrate, especially biocompatibility of the implant materials. In addition, ceramic coating provides excellent corrosion resistance and antimicrobial activity compared with uncoated implants. Figure 8.4 displays the different physical and chemical surface modification techniques and their merits and demerits.

Among the various bioceramics, HA is considered to be better for coating bioceramics on metallic surfaces due to the mineral similarity to natural bone.[39] The HA-coated various metallic substrates improved biocompatibility over pristine metallic substrates.[40] For instance, Kim et al. reported HA-coated zirconia as a dental implant with improved durability.[41] HA-coated zirconia showed enhanced cell attachment and proliferation (MC3T3-E1 cells) compared with titanium and bare zirconia metallic materials (Figure 8.5). Moreover, the HA, SiO_2/ZrO_2, TiO_2, SiO_2, Al_2O_3, etc. coating over the metallic substrates significantly improved the cell–material interaction compared to uncoated substrates. Some of the coating methods are shown in Figure 8.6.

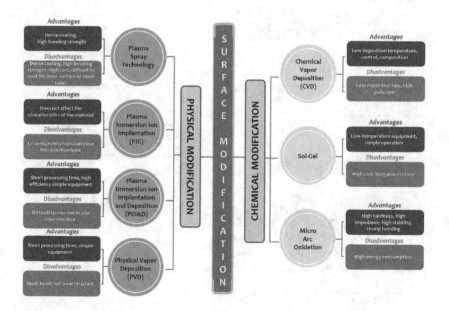

FIGURE 8.4 Physical and chemical surface modification techniques with merits and demerits.[10]

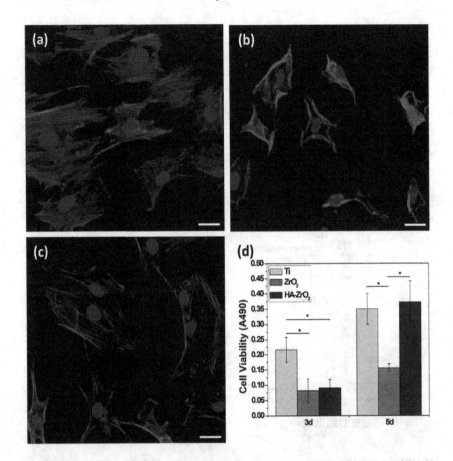

FIGURE 8.5   Confocal image of MC3T3-E1 cells attached on the surface of (a) Ti substrate, (b) zirconia substrate, (c) HA-coated zirconia substrates, and (d) MC3T3-E1 cells proliferation on the untreated and treated substrates. Scale bars: 30 µm.[41]

Micro-arc oxidation (MAO) is an effective method for coating ceramic materials on metallic substrates, which can provide adequate porosity, better bioadhesiveness, and bone forming ability, resulting in enhanced osseointegration.[42] The MAO process is an electrochemical method, which is conducted at very high voltages (100–600 V) for developing oxides and nonoxide layers on the Ti-based surface in the presence of electrolyte.[43] Huang et al. fabricated HA-coated Ti substrates by the MAO method with calcium acetate and β-GP as electrolyte.[44] The HA-coated commercial Ti substrate showed better cell attachment than the uncoated Ti substrates, which confirms that the HA coating significantly improved the cell–material interaction, which is favourable for metal implant-based orthopedic applications. The porous Cu-TiO$_2$ coatings were applied on the Ti substrate, which enhanced the corrosion resistance of titanium.[45]

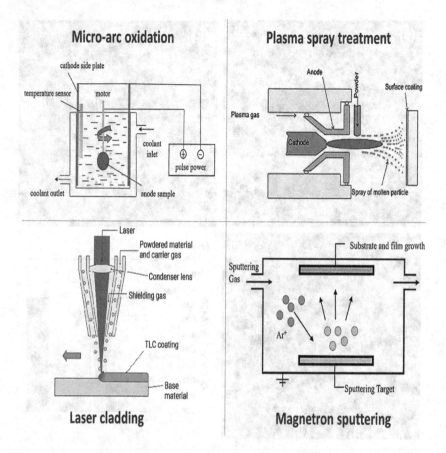

FIGURE 8.6 Schematic representation of various coating techniques.

Atomic layer deposition (ALD) is a surface functionalization method via traditional chemical vapour deposition of inorganic species on metallic substrates. ALD provides a uniform coating and self-controlled thickness over the metallic surface.[46] Kylmäoja et al. reported nanostructured HA-coated Ti with improved osseointegration properties.[47] Evidently, HA-coated Ti revealed excellent biocompatibility and bioavailability, resulting in better osseointegration. In the ALD, ceramics can be coated with layer-by-layer nanostructures that facilitate better cellular responses on metallic substrates.

Plasma spray deposition is an easy and well-established method to achieve ceramics-coated metallic substrates with a fine and uniform coating.[48] Heimann deposited Ca(Ti,Zr) hexaorthophosphate on a commercial Ti-6Al-4V substrate and studied its biomedical properties.[49] The coated Ti-6Al-4V substrate showed low solubility in simulated body fluid, an adequate porosity, a rational adhesion level on the Ti-6A-l4V implant surface, and a satisfactory osteogenic potential. Ganapathy et al. studied Al_2O_3 and 8 mole% of Yttrium-stabilised ZrO_2 hybrid-coated

Ti-6Al-4V alloy for orthopedic applications.[50] The tribological behaviors of the uncoated and Al_2O_3 and 8 mole% of yttrium-stabilised ZrO_2 hybrid substrates were estimated by a ball-on-plate wear tester in a biological environment (at 37 °C in SBF). The hardness and wear rate of the alumina-zirconia composite coatings were found to be 2.5- and 253-fold higher than those of the commercial Ti-6Al-4V alloy.

The electrochemical method is one of the most effective methods to coat oxide-based ceramics on the surface of metallic implants. The coating thickness and surface textures can be effectively controlled in the electrochemical method and also independent of the nature of the metallic substrate. Azzouz et al, coated 45S5 Bioglass® on the Ti-6Al-4V surface by electrophoretic deposition and studied its mechanical strength.[51] Song et al. reported HA-coated AZ91D Mg alloy synthesised by electrodeposition,[52] and HA coating significantly improved the rate of biodegradation of Mg alloy in the SBF solution. Hafedh et al. studied the wear and mechanical strength of the TiO_2-coated 316L stainless steel by electrophoretic deposition.[53] TiO_2-coated 316L stainless steel showed improved mechanical strength and wear resistance than uncoated 316L stainless steel substrate.

Roy et al. successfully deposited HA on commercial Ti substrates using RF magnetron sputtering and assessed their mechanical properties as well as biocompatibility nature.[54] The HA coating significantly enhanced the biocompatibility in both ex vivo and in vitro conditions. Moreover, when the coating thickness increased from 300 to 400 μm, adhesive bond strengths also increased from 4.8 to 24 MPa. Dinu et al. reported RF-magnetron sputtering HA-coated Mg substrates and evaluated their tribological behavior in a physiological environment.[55] They found higher wear resistance on HA-coated Mg substrates than uncoated substrates. Chen et al. described Ag-doped HA by magnetron sputtering and evaluated its antibacterial property.[56] The Ag-HA-coated substrate revealed excellent antibacterial activity against both *S. epidermidis* and *S. aureus* cells.

Laser cladding technology is a very effective technique for the fabrication of ceramic coatings over metallic surfaces due to its advantages such as rapid melting and solidification in terms of bond strength and good controllability in terms of thickness.[57] Liu et al. deposited Ca/P on a Ti-6Al-4V alloy and evaluated its bioactivity, biocompatibility, and wear resistance.[58] The Ca/P-coated substrate exhibited excellent bioactivity when immersed in the SBF and showed excellent biocompatibility with MG-63 cells when compared to pure substrate. The decreased volume wear was found to be Ca/P-ceramic-coated substrate with a 43.2% reduction compared to that of Ti6Al4V alloy, indicating that the Ca/P bioceramic coating showed excellent wear resistance. Behera et al. reported HA and functionally graded TiO_2-HA precursors on Ti–6Al–4V alloy with improved biocompatibility and bioactivity by laser cladding technology.[59] Implant materials prepared by laser cladding technology showed improved biocompatibility and bioactivity of Ti–6Al–4V. These studies clearly state that the laser cladding method effectively modifies the surface nature of metallic implants. Various techniques for the fabrication of metallic materials coated with different ceramics are given in Table 8.1.

TABLE 8.1

Various Techniques for the Fabrication of Metallic Materials Coated with Various Ceramics

Synthesis Route	Ceramics	Metal Substrate	Purpose	Ref.
Sol-gel	HA	Stainless steel	Corrosion resistance	60
	SiO_2/ZrO_2	Stainless steel	Biocompatibility	61
	TiO_2	Stainless steel	Antibacterial and sufficient Mechanical strength	62
Micro-arc oxidation	TiO_2/Al_2O_3	Ti-6Al-4V alloy	Wear resistance	63
Atomic layer deposition	TiO_2	Co-Cr	Antifungal	64
	Al_2O_3/TiO_2	Copper	Corrosion resistance	
Electrochemical method	HA	Mg alloy	Biodegradation performance	52
	Al_2O_3	Aluminium	Corrosion resistance	65
Plasma spray treatment	HA	Mg alloy	Corrosion resistance Bioactivity	66
	TiO_2	Titanium	Corrosion resistance	67
Magnetron sputtering	HA	Titanium	Corrosion resistance	68
	TiO_2	Stainless steel	Tribological properties	69
Laser cladding	Ca/P	Ti-6Al-4V alloy	Bioactivity, biocompatibility, wear resistance	58
	TiO_2/HA	Ti-6Al-4V alloy	Bioactivity, biocompatibility	59

8.6   METHODS FOR WEAR TEST

The methods that are used to study the wear and friction characteristics of metallic biomaterials are block-on-disk,[70,71] ball-on-disk[72,73] and pin-on-disk (Figure 8.7). These tests were performed at 37 ± 0.1 °C as a temperature and in SBF to mimic a biological environment.

The wear and friction of the ceramic coated biometallic substrates can be studied using methods mentioned above. In the pin-on-disc method, bioimplant materials can be tested with a pin shaped specimen that is pressed on the spinning grinding wheel with constant surface pressure. While, in the case of ball-on-disc, specimen is made in a ball shape instead of a pin with high pressure. The removal of coolant during the analysis is much less than that of pin-on-disk method. The block-on-disc, as its name suggests, block shaped specimen is used to study the friction and wear of metallic implant materials. Table 8.2 gives the summary of advantages and disadvantages of three wear test methods.

In addition, various characterization methods have been used to evaluate the wear and friction in terms of tribological behavior. Chemical analyses, surface analysis, and mechanical strength are important characterization techniques to

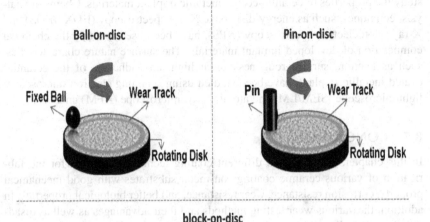

FIGURE 8.7   Schematic illustration of wear testing method.

TABLE 8.2
Merits and Demerits of Wear Test Methods

Methods	Merits	Demerits
Pin-on-disc	Surface pressures of the wheel remains constant even after completing the analysis. Simple method to analyse wear volume and wear rate of the materials	Pin alignment on rotating wheel is too difficult. Difficult to stand pin vertically. Long-term analysis.
Ball-on-disc	Possible to maintain high pressure during the analysis Contact surface is lesser than pin-on-disk method.	Lower contact ratio between ball and wheel Inaccuracy of wear volume of the ball determination
Block-on-disk	Simulation can be performed at high loading pressure, high temperature, and high speed.	

study the properties of ceramic-coated metallic implant materials. Chemical analysis techniques, such as energy-dispersive X-ray spectroscopy (EDXS/EDS) and X-ray photoelectron spectroscopy (XPS), have been used to study the chemical composition of developed implant materials. The surface nature characteristics, such as friction, surface roughness, scratching, and adhesion of the ceramic-coated metallic implant, have been studied using scanning electron microscope/ light microscope (SEM/LM) and atomic force microscope (AFM) analysis.

8.7 CONCLUSION

In this chapter, we discussed different coating techniques applied for the fabrication of various ceramic coatings on metal substrates with good mechanical property, corrosion resistance, wear resistance, and better biological properties. In addition, the various wear testing methods and their advantages as well as disadvantages were discussed. Evidently, the nature of ceramic materials and methods of coating techniques significantly influenced the cell–material interactions. The wear debris from metallic implants can be inhibited by the selection of appropriate ceramics and coating methods based on the end applications. Hence the coating of ceramics on metallic substrates with a suitable method can make excellent implant materials with good corrosion resistance and wear resistance.

8.7.1 AUTHORS' CONTRIBUTION

RG and GSL conceived the idea and wrote the manuscript. BSM and ST cooperated in revising the manuscript. All authors proofread the manuscript

REFERENCES

1. Amirtharaj Mosas KK, Chandrasekar AR, Dasan A, Pakseresht A, Galusek D. Recent advancements in materials and coatings for biomedical implants. *Gels*. 2022;8(5):323. doi:10.3390/gels8050323
2. Yan X, Cao W, Li H. Biomedical alloys and physical surface modifications: a mini-review. *Materials (Basel)*. 2021;15(1):66. doi:10.3390/ma15010066
3. Rodrigo-Navarro A, Sankaran S, Dalby MJ, del Campo A, Salmeron-Sanchez M. Engineered living biomaterials. *Nat Rev Mater*. 2021;6(12):1175–1190. doi:10.1038/s41578-021-00350-8
4. Xie C. Bio-inspired nanofunctionalisation of biomaterial surfaces: a review. *Biosurf Biotribol*. 2019;5(3):83–92. doi:10.1049/bsbt.2019.0009
5. Best SM, Porter AE, Thian ES, Huang J. Bioceramics: past, present and for the future. *J Eur Ceram Soc*. 2008;28(7):1319–1327. doi:10.1016/j.jeurceramsoc.2007.12.001
6. Priyadarshini B, Rama M, Chetan, Vijayalakshmi U. Bioactive coating as a surface modification technique for biocompatible metallic implants: a review. *J Asian Ceram Soc*. 2019;7(4):397–406. doi:10.1080/21870764.2019.1669861
7. Hussein M, Mohammed A, Al-Aqeeli N. Wear characteristics of metallic biomaterials: a review. *Materials (Basel)*. 2015;8(5):2749–2768. doi:10.3390/ma8052749
8. Li SJ, Yang R, Li S, et al. Wear characteristics of Ti–Nb–Ta–Zr and Ti–6Al–4V alloys for biomedical applications. *Wear*. 2004;257(9–10):869–876. doi:10.1016/j.wear.2004.04.001

9. Zhang L, Haddouti E-M, Welle K, et al. The effects of biomaterial implant wear debris on osteoblasts. *Front Cell Dev Biol.* 2020;8. doi:10.3389/fcell.2020.00352

10. Davis R, Singh A, Jackson MJ, et al. A comprehensive review on metallic implant biomaterials and their subtractive manufacturing. *Int J Adv Manuf Technol.* 2022;120(3–4):1473–1530. doi:10.1007/s00170-022-08770-8

11. Prasad K, Bazaka O, Chua M, et al. Metallic biomaterials: current challenges and opportunities. *Materials (Basel).* 2017;10(8):884. doi:10.3390/ma10080884

12. Malhotra R, Dhawan B, Garg B, Shankar V, Nag TC. A comparison of bacterial adhesion and biofilm formation on commonly used orthopaedic metal implant materials: an in vitro study. *Indian J Orthop.* 2019;53(1):148–153. doi:10.4103/ortho.IJOrtho_66_18

13. Panagea S, Winstanley C, Walshaw MJ, Ledson MJ, Hart CA. Environmental contamination with an epidemic strain of Pseudomonas aeruginosa in a Liverpool cystic fibrosis centre, and study of its survival on dry surfaces. *J Hosp Infect.* 2005;59(2):102–107. doi:10.1016/j.jhin.2004.09.018

14. Pourshahrestani S, Kadri NA, Zeimaran E, Towler MR. Well-ordered mesoporous silica and bioactive glasses: promise for improved hemostasis. *Biomater Sci.* 2019;7(1):31–50. doi:10.1039/C8BM01041B

15. Hyunh NB, Palma CSD, Rahikainen R, et al. Surface modification of bioresorbable phosphate glasses for controlled protein adsorption. *ACS Biomater Sci Eng.* 2021;7(9):4483–4493. doi:10.1021/acsbiomaterials.1c00735

16. Ege D, Zheng K, Boccaccini AR. Borate bioactive glasses (BBG): bone regeneration, wound healing applications, and future directions. *ACS Appl Bio Mater.* 2022;5(8):3608–3622. doi:10.1021/acsabm.2c00384

17. Tosiriwatanapong T, Singhatanadgit W. Zirconia-based biomaterials for hard tissue reconstruction. *Bone Tissue Regen Insights.* 2018;9:1179061X1876788. doi:10.1177/1179061X18767886

18. Rahmati M, Mozafari M. Biocompatibility of alumina-based biomaterials–a review. *J Cell Physiol.* 2019;234(4):3321–3335. doi:10.1002/jcp.27292

19. Wang P, Zhao L, Liu J, Weir MD, Zhou X, Xu HHK. Bone tissue engineering via nanostructured calcium phosphate biomaterials and stem cells. *Bone Res.* 2014;2(1):14017. doi:10.1038/boneres.2014.17

20. Zhang Y, Shu T, Wang S, et al. The osteoinductivity of calcium phosphate-based biomaterials: a tight interaction with bone healing. *Front Bioeng Biotechnol.* 2022;10. doi:10.3389/fbioe.2022.911180

21. Lu J, Yu H, Chen C. Biological properties of calcium phosphate biomaterials for bone repair: a review. *RSC Adv.* 2018;8(4):2015–2033. doi:10.1039/C7RA11278E

22. Vallet-Regí M. Ceramics for medical applications. *J Chem Soc Dalt Trans.* 2001;(2):97–108. doi:10.1039/b007852m

23. Salinas AJ, Vallet-Regí M. Bioactive ceramics: from bone grafts to tissue engineering. *RSC Adv.* 2013;3(28):11116. doi:10.1039/c3ra00166k

24. Shi H, Zhou Z, Li W, Fan Y, Li Z, Wei J. Hydroxyapatite based materials for bone tissue engineering: a brief and comprehensive introduction. *Crystals.* 2021;11(2):149. doi:10.3390/cryst11020149

25. DileepKumar VG, Sridhar MS, Aramwit P, et al. A review on the synthesis and properties of hydroxyapatite for biomedical applications. *J Biomater Sci Polym Ed.* 2022;33(2):229–261. doi:10.1080/09205063.2021.1980985

26. Guo T, Yao M-S, Lin Y-H, Nan C-W. A comprehensive review on synthesis methods for transition-metal oxide nanostructures. *CrystEngComm.* 2015;17(19):3551–3585. doi:10.1039/C5CE00034C

27. Parashar M, Shukla VK, Singh R. Metal oxides nanoparticles via sol–gel method: a review on synthesis, characterization and applications. *J Mater Sci Mater Electron*. 2020;31(5):3729–3749. doi:10.1007/s10854-020-02994-8

28. Nikam AV, Prasad BLV, Kulkarni AA. Wet chemical synthesis of metal oxide nanoparticles: a review. *CrystEngComm*. 2018;20(35):5091–5107. doi:10.1039/C8CE00487K

29. Sadat-Shojai M, Khorasani M-T, Dinpanah-Khoshdargi E, Jamshidi A. Synthesis methods for nanosized hydroxyapatite with diverse structures. *Acta Biomater*. 2013;9(8):7591–7621. doi:10.1016/j.actbio.2013.04.012

30. Mohan S, Vellakkat M, Aravind A, Reka U. Hydrothermal synthesis and characterization of zinc oxide nanoparticles of various shapes under different reaction conditions. *Nano Express*. 2020;1(3):030028. doi:10.1088/2632-959X/abc813

31. Walton RI. Subcritical solvothermal synthesis of condensed inorganic materials. *Chem Soc Rev*. 2002;31(4):230–238. doi:10.1039/b105762f

32. Li J, Wu Q, Wu J. Synthesis of nanoparticles via solvothermal and hydrothermal methods. In: *Handbook of Nanoparticles*. Springer International Publishing; 2016:295–328. doi:10.1007/978-3-319-15338-4_17

33. Sadat-Shojai M, Atai M, Nodehi A, Khanlar LN. Hydroxyapatite nanorods as novel fillers for improving the properties of dental adhesives: synthesis and application. *Dent Mater*. 2010;26(5):471–482. doi:10.1016/j.dental.2010.01.005

34. Zhu Y-J, Chen F. Microwave-assisted preparation of inorganic nanostructures in liquid phase. *Chem Rev*. 2014;114(12):6462–6555. doi:10.1021/cr400366s

35. Yin Z, Li S, Li X, et al. A review on the synthesis of metal oxide nanomaterials by microwave induced solution combustion. *RSC Adv*. 2023;13(5):3265–3277. doi:10.1039/D2RA07936D

36. Ganguli AK, Ganguly A, Vaidya S. Microemulsion-based synthesis of nanocrystalline materials. *Chem Soc Rev*. 2010;39(2):474–485. doi:10.1039/B814613F

37. Tsuzuki T. Mechanochemical synthesis of metal oxide nanoparticles. *Commun Chem*. 2021;4(1):143. doi:10.1038/s42004-021-00582-3

38. Xu H, Zeiger BW, Suslick KS. Sonochemical synthesis of nanomaterials. *Chem Soc Rev*. 2013;42(7):2555–2567. doi:10.1039/C2CS35282F

39. Fiume E, Magnaterra G, Rahdar A, Verné E, Baino F. Hydroxyapatite for biomedical applications: a short overview. *Ceramics*. 2021;4(4):542–563. doi:10.3390/ceramics4040039

40. Liu D-M, Yang Q, Troczynski T. Sol–gel hydroxyapatite coatings on stainless steel substrates. *Biomaterials*. 2002;23(3):691–698. doi:10.1016/S0142-9612(01)00157-0

41. Kim J, Kang I-G, Cheon K-H, et al. Stable sol–gel hydroxyapatite coating on zirconia dental implant for improved osseointegration. *J Mater Sci Mater Med*. 2021;32(7):81. doi:10.1007/s10856-021-06550-6

42. Wang Y, Yu H, Chen C, Zhao Z. Review of the biocompatibility of micro-arc oxidation coated titanium alloys. *Mater Des*. 2015;85:640–652. doi:10.1016/j.matdes.2015.07.086

43. Abbasi S, Golestani-Fard F, Rezaie HR, Mirhosseini SMM. MAO-derived hydroxyapatite/TiO_2 nanostructured multi-layer coatings on titanium substrate. *Appl Surf Sci*. 2012;261:37–42. doi:10.1016/j.apsusc.2012.07.044

44. Huang Y, Wang Y, Ning C, Nan K, Han Y. Hydroxyapatite coatings produced on commercially pure titanium by micro-arc oxidation. *Biomed Mater*. 2007;2(3):196–201. doi:10.1088/1748-6041/2/3/005

45. Wu H, Zhang X, Geng Z, et al. Preparation, antibacterial effects and corrosion resistant of porous $Cu–TiO_2$ coatings. *Appl Surf Sci*. 2014;308:43–49. doi:10.1016/j.apsusc.2014.04.081

46. Putkonen M, Sajavaara T, Rahkila P, et al. Atomic layer deposition and characterization of biocompatible hydroxyapatite thin films. *Thin Solid Films.* 2009;517(20):5819–5824. doi:10.1016/j.tsf.2009.03.013

47. Kylmäoja E, Holopainen J, Abushahba F, Ritala M, Tuukkanen J. Osteoblast attachment on titanium coated with hydroxyapatite by atomic layer deposition. *Biomolecules.* 2022;12(5):654. doi:10.3390/biom12050654

48. Tului M, Marino G, Valente T. Plasma spray deposition of ultra high temperature ceramics. *Surf Coatings Technol.* 2006;201(5):2103–2108. doi:10.1016/j. surfcoat.2006.04.053

49. Heimann RB. Plasma-sprayed bioactive ceramic coatings with high resorption resistance based on transition metal-substituted calcium hexaorthophosphates. *Materials (Basel).* 2019;12(13):2059. doi:10.3390/ma12132059

50. Ganapathy P, Manivasagam G, Rajamanickam A, Natarajan A. Wear studies on plasma-sprayed Al_2O_3 and 8mole% of Yttrium-stabilized ZrO_2 composite coating on biomedical Ti-6Al-4V alloy for orthopedic joint application. *Int J Nanomedicine.* 2015;2015:213–222. doi:10.2147/IJN.S79997

51. Azzouz I, Faure J, Khlifi K, Cheikh Larbi A, Benhayoune H. Electrophoretic deposition of 45S5 Bioglass® coatings on the Ti6Al4V prosthetic alloy with improved mechanical properties. *Coatings.* 2020;10(12):1192. doi:10.3390/coatings10121192

52. Song YW, Shan DY, Han EH. Electrodeposition of hydroxyapatite coating on AZ91D magnesium alloy for biomaterial application. *Mater Lett.* 2008;62(17–18):3276–3279. doi:10.1016/j.matlet.2008.02.048

53. Dhiflaoui H, Kaouther K, Larbi ABC. Wear behavior and mechanical properties of TiO_2 coating deposited electrophoretically on 316 L stainless steel. *J Tribol.* 2018;140(3). doi:10.1115/1.4038102

54. Roy M, Bandyopadhyay A, Bose S. Induction plasma sprayed nano hydroxyapatite coatings on titanium for orthopaedic and dental implants. *Surf Coatings Technol.* 2011;205(8–9):2785–2792. doi:10.1016/j.surfcoat.2010.10.042

55. Dinu M, Ivanova AA, Surmeneva MA, et al. Tribological behaviour of RF-magnetron sputter deposited hydroxyapatite coatings in physiological solution. *Ceram Int.* 2017;43(9):6858–6867. doi:10.1016/j.ceramint.2017.02.106

56. Chen W, Liu Y, Courtney H., et al. In vitro anti-bacterial and biological properties of magnetron co-sputtered silver-containing hydroxyapatite coating. *Biomaterials.* 2006;27(32):5512–5517. doi:10.1016/j.biomaterials.2006.07.003

57. Li HC, Wang DG, Hu C, Dou JH, Yu HJ, Chen CZ. Effect of Na_2O and ZnO on the microstructure and properties of laser cladding derived CaO-SiO_2 ceramic coatings on titanium alloys. *J Colloid Interface Sci.* 2021;592:498–508. doi:10.1016/j. jcis.2021.02.064

58. Liu B, Deng Z, Liu D. Preparation and properties of multilayer Ca/P bio-ceramic coating by laser cladding. *Coatings.* 2021;11(8):891. doi:10.3390/coatings11080891

59. Behera RR, Hasan A, Sankar MR, Pandey LM. Laser cladding with HA and functionally graded TiO_2-HA precursors on Ti–6Al–4V alloy for enhancing bioactivity and cyto-compatibility. *Surf Coatings Technol.* 2018;352:420–436. doi:10.1016/j. surfcoat.2018.08.044

60. Balamurugan A, Balossier G, Kannan S, Rajeswari S. Elaboration of sol–gel derived apatite films on surgical grade stainless steel for biomedical applications. *Mater Lett.* 2006;60(17–18):2288–2293. doi:10.1016/j.matlet.2005.12.126

61. Śmieszek A, Donesz-Sikorska A, Grzesiak J, Krzak J, Marycz K. Biological effects of sol–gel derived ZrO_2 and SiO_2/ZrO_2 coatings on stainless steel surface—in vitro model using mesenchymal stem cells. *J Biomater Appl.* 2014;29(5):699–714. doi:10.1177/0885328214545095

62. Villatte G, Massard C, Descamps S, Sibaud Y, Forestier C, Awitor KO. Photoactive TiO2 antibacterial coating on surgical external fixation pins for clinical application. *Int J Nanomedicine*. 2015;10:3367–3375. doi:10.2147/IJN.S81518

63. Yizhou S, Haijun T, Yuebin L, et al. Fabrication and wear resistance of TiO_2/Al_2O_3 coatings by micro-arc oxidation. *Rare Met Mater Eng*. 2017;46(1):23–27. doi:10.1016/S1875-5372(17)30071-1

64. Huang L, Jing S, Zhuo O, Meng X, Wang X. Surface hydrophilicity and antifungal properties of TiO_2 films coated on a Co-Cr substrate. *Biomed Res Int*. 2017;2017:1–7. doi:10.1155/2017/2054723

65. Vengatesh P, Kulandainathan MA. Hierarchically ordered self-lubricating superhydrophobic anodized aluminum surfaces with enhanced corrosion resistance. *ACS Appl Mater Interfaces*. 2015;7(3):1516–1526. doi:10.1021/am506568v

66. Gao YL, Liu Y, Song XY. Plasma-sprayed hydroxyapatite coating for improved corrosion resistance and bioactivity of magnesium alloy. *J Therm Spray Technol*. 2018;27(8):1381–1387. doi:10.1007/s11666-018-0760-9

67. Sun C, Hui R, Qu W, Yick S, Sun C, Qian W. Effects of processing parameters on microstructures of TiO_2 coatings formed on titanium by plasma electrolytic oxidation. *J Mater Sci*. 2010;45(22):6235–6241. doi:10.1007/s10853-010-4718-7

68. Surmeneva MA, Vladescu A, Surmenev RA, Pantilimon CM, Braic M, Cotrut CM. Study on a hydrophobic Ti-doped hydroxyapatite coating for corrosion protection of a titanium based alloy. *RSC Adv*. 2016;6(90):87665–87674. doi:10.1039/C6RA03397K

69. Krishna DSR, Sun Y. Thermally oxidised rutile-TiO_2 coating on stainless steel for tribological properties and corrosion resistance enhancement. *Appl Surf Sci*. 2005;252(4):1107–1116. doi:10.1016/j.apsusc.2005.02.046

70. Cvijović-Alagić I, Cvijović Z, Mitrović S, Rakin M, Veljović Đ, Babić M. Tribological behaviour of orthopaedic Ti-13Nb-13Zr and Ti-6Al-4V alloys. *Tribol Lett*. 2010;40(1):59–70. doi:10.1007/s11249-010-9639-8

71. Gialanella S, Ischia G, Straffelini G. Phase composition and wear behavior of NiTi alloys. *J Mater Sci*. 2008;43(5):1701–1710. doi:10.1007/s10853-007-2358-3

72. Suresh KS, Geetha M, Richard C, et al. Effect of equal channel angular extrusion on wear and corrosion behavior of the orthopedic Ti–13Nb–13Zr alloy in simulated body fluid. *Mater Sci Eng C*. 2012;32(4):763–771. doi:10.1016/j.msec.2012.01.022

73. Xu L, Xiao S, Tian J, Chen Y. Microstructure, mechanical properties and dry wear resistance of β-type Ti-15Mo-xNb alloys for biomedical applications. *Trans Nonferrous Met Soc China*. 2013;23(3):692–698. doi:10.1016/S1003-6326(13)62518-2

9 Synthesis and Characterization of Polymer-Based Wear-Resistant Bioimplants

Koray Şarkaya[1], Gülşah Akincioğlu[2], and Kemal Çetin[3]
[1] Pamukkale University
Denizli, Turkey
[2] Duzce University
Duzce, Turkey
[3] Necmettin Erbakan University
Konya, Turkey

9.1 INTRODUCTION

Humanity will continue to struggle with diseases and similar situations that threaten its health from the day it existed. In return for this struggle, medical science continues to develop daily. In this process, the developments in basic and material sciences provide multidisciplinary contributions to the development of modern medicine today. As a result of these contributions, new interdisciplinary sciences such as bioengineering and biomedical engineering have emerged. In this context, studies on the development of materials that will imitate the structural and functional properties of various tissues and organs and provide their natural function and simultaneously provide harmony with the organism are of great interest [1].

Biomaterials are synthetic or natural materials produced, used, and developed to fulfill or support the functions of organs or tissues in the human body to improve and maintain the quality of life of the living thing [2]. In line with various medical and biomedical needs, the demand and use of biomaterials are increasing worldwide (in Figure 9.1).

Biomaterials generally contain metallic, ceramic, or polymeric components. Among them, metals have the good durability and wear resistance needed to meet the mechanical demands of orthopedic implants, along with good corrosion resistance and high biocompatibility additives for bone implants [4]. However, both metals and ceramics have several disadvantages. In some situations, metals have a tendency to rust and to be toxic with metal ions, while ceramics are extremely fragile and have production challenges [5]. These factors lead to the prediction that the composite systems

DOI: 10.1201/9781003384847-9

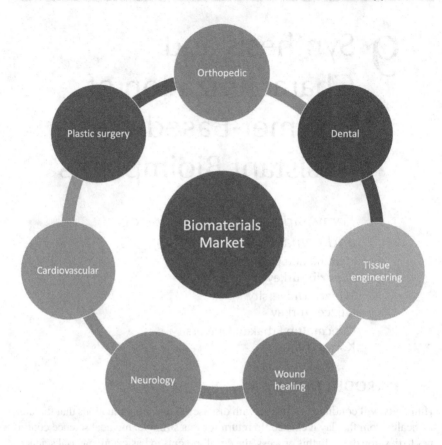

FIGURE 9.1   Distribution of biomaterials according to their usage areas by 2020 [3].

that can be created by combining metals or ceramics with polymers would be able to overcome the limitations of metals and ceramics for soft tissue applications [6,7].

Today, interest in materials made of polymers is growing every day in tandem with the advancement of technology. This situation also triggers the use of polymer-based biomaterials. The main property for a material to be accepted as a biomaterial is its biocompatibility. In addition, high strength and physicochemical properties, sterilizability, and corrosion resistance are expected behaviors [8]. On the other hand, polymers can be preferred in producing biomaterials due to their properties, such as being made in different sizes and shapes according to their intended use and resistance to corrosion with appropriate mechanical and physical properties [9]. Moreover, polymer-based biomaterials can be considered for many different purposes in biomedical fields, such as implants, wound dressing materials, controlled drug release systems, tissue engineering, and surgical threads [10]. However, the structure of polymers has a higher molecular weight as long-chain carbon structures are formed, and it is also more complex than compounds with smaller molecular structures. At this point, the properties of polymers must be fully understood and characterized to select the polymer part of a material to be

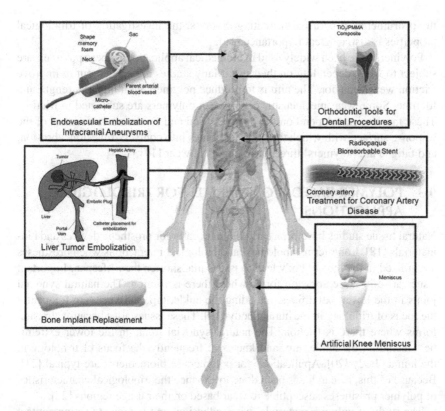

FIGURE 9.2 Some polymer types are used for biomedical applications with different functions [12].

designed as a biomaterial [11]. Figure 9.2 shows some polymers used in different forms for biomedical applications.

9.2 TRIBOLOGY

The science that studies the mechanisms of friction, wear, and lubrication of the relative behavior of interrelated surfaces is called tribology [13]. Biotribology, on the other hand, can be thought of as the state and application of tribological events in living things. Biotribology is a science that targets many applications in medicine and biomedical fields, such as the wearing of dental prostheses, the lubrication of contact lenses, the wear of artificial heart valves, the wear of screws and plates used in the healing of bone fractures, the lubrication of the pericardium and pleural surfaces, and the replacement of artificial joints [14]. Tribological behaviors are recognized as one of the most critical factors in many biological systems in how natural systems work, how diseases develop, and how medical interventions are administered. The living body is a perfectly organized complex system with all its tribological material properties [15]. On the other hand, to characterize the design and selection of materials suitable for the living body of the instruments to be used in treating diseases, the investigation of tribological properties is also of great importance [16].

Polymers have been widely used in biomedical applications. These polymers are subject to wear, depending on their use. Many studies are carried out to improve friction wear behavior. The aim is to produce polymers with higher strength and lifetime. Some wear mechanisms occur when polymers are subjected to friction. These mechanisms depend on the polymer used and on the characteristics of the response surface with which the polymer comes into contact. Adhesion, abrasion, and fatigue are polymers' three basic modes of wear [17].

9.3 POLYMER-BASED BIOMATERIALS FOR TRIBOLOGICAL APPLICATIONS

Natural tissue studies have been carried out recently for prosthetic devices and bio-materials [18]. Long-term tribological and biological interactions when prostheses are utilized in the human body lead to issues that shorten their lifespan. Important issues arise because abrasion forms where there is friction. The natural synovial joints in the lower extremities, including the ankle, hip, and knee, are frequently the focus of tribology in the human body [19]. These issues arise because abrasion forms where there is friction. The natural synovial joints in the lower extremities, including the ankle, hip, and knee, are frequently the focus of tribology in the human body [20]. Applications for polymers in biomedicine are typical [21]. Because of this, research has been done to enhance the tribological characteristics of polymer prostheses susceptible to wear based on their usage regions [22].

The study of polymer materials' wear, adhesion, and fatigue at friction contact is the foundation of polymer tribology. Basic polymers can be used in various tribological applications because of their structural qualities, most commonly as matrices and fillers in composite materials [23]. Human and animal systems are part of biomedical tribology, as is the growing development of replacement (prosthetic) devices to replace damaged tissues and organs [24]. Improving the tribological properties of biomedical materials gains importance in terms of increasing the life of prostheses and ergonomics [14]. For example, articular cartilage is a helpful rubber surface because of its favorable tribological characteristics, such as low wear rate and friction coefficient [25]. Osteoarticular illnesses are brought on by functional issues in the joints, which result in pain from the destruction of the cartilage tissue [26]. New techniques based on implants made of live tissue, in the case of grafts or prostheses, in the case of nonliving tissue, are required to correct and eradicate these deformations [27]. However, several unfavorable circumstances, such as tissue availability and reproducibility, the risk of disease transmission, size, and wear, are likely to arise when developing new techniques. As a result, many new studies are being conducted to replace joint cartilage or develop alternative methods to optimize joint replacement, while the importance and use of new-generation polymeric systems for this need are increasing daily.

Due to their advantageous characteristics like adsorption, oxygen permeability, biocompatibility, and flexibility, hydrogels are one of the most modern polymeric materials with a wide range of uses, especially in the environmental and biomedical fields [28]. Hydrogels have also been thoroughly studied for their potential to be mainly polymeric candidates for artificial cartilage since they are biocompatible and have tribological features comparable to the lubricating mechanisms observed in cartilage [29–31]. Hydrogels are widely used for cartilage tissues exhibiting poroelastic properties and treating arthritic joints. Due to the high wear in the joints, extensive studies have been carried out to solve this issue [32–35]. Therefore, hydrogels are suitable model systems for artificial articular cartilage.

Because of their potential for cartilage replacement and repair, poly(vinyl alcohol)- [36], poly(acrylamide)- [37], poly(vinyl pyrrolidone)- [38], and poly(2-hydroxyethyl methacrylate)- [29] based have gained much attention from researchers in recent years. Numerous facial repairs and cosmetic hydrogel-based treatments have received FDA approval regarding clinical translation [39,40]. The efficacy of hydrogel-based therapy has also been supported by clinical trials in several conditions, including advanced heart failure, type 2 diabetes, chronic renal disease, knee osteoarthritis, spinal fusion, and the spine [41]. For more widespread and practical biological applications, however, a lot of problems and difficulties need to be solved, and more clinical translation is required [42].

9.4 BIOIMPLANTS

The anatomical components of the human body can be treated, repaired, or replaced using biomaterials, which interact with human tissue and bodily secretions. Implants are a general term for biomaterials used in orthopedic or medical uses [43]. Every year, millions of patients can be treated and lead a healthier life by the implantation of devices such as orthopedics, heart, mouth, maxillofacial and plastic doctors, pacemakers, artificial hip joints, breast implants, dental implants, and implantable hearing aids [44]. So the use of medical devices and implants is becoming increasingly widespread, and thus their importance in improving the quality of life and saving lives is increasing daily.

The choice of materials used in the design of a medical implant is based on biocompatibility, biodegradability, adhesion, functionality, corrosion resistance, etc. [45]. Most studies to determine the choice of material used in implant construction and to better understand its interaction with living tissues offer alternatives for genotoxicity, carcinogenicity, cytotoxicity, irritation, sensitization, and sterilization [46]. These studies are based on the metallic, polymeric, ceramic biomaterials, and composite materials used in modern medical applications. Titanium alloys, cobalt-chromium alloys, and stainless steels are known as the most widely used orthopedic metal biomaterials [47]. Ceramic-based implants can be used in hip and knee arthroplasty surgeries, which are very common in orthopedics, in dental implants, as bone fillers to fill gaps in the bone, and as tissue scaffolds for tissue engineering [48].

9.4.1 POLYMERIC BIOIMPLANTS

Fabricating a three-dimensional scaffold's polymeric matrix is the critical function of biomimetic materials [49]. Recent developments in tissue engineering, controlled drug delivery, and regenerative medicine have created a need for recovering novel biomaterials, including thoroughly determining polymers' biodegradability and designing cutting-edge materials to manage degradability [50,51].

Polymers are extensively utilized in acetabular cups in bioimplantology. It is easy for stress concentration at the interface between two incongruent surfaces in incongruent joints, including the knee and ankle, to harm the nearby bones [52]. It is crucial for reducing various such stressors that the human body contains cartilage layers and synovial fluid [53]. However, residual stresses are challenging to eradicate and can significantly affect artificial joints of brittle metallic materials. Scientists began to concentrate on polymer materials as a result [54].

9.4.1.1 Polymers for Tissue Scaffolds

Tissue scaffolds are designed to temporarily substitute tissue defects, allowing for biomimetic structures similar to natural extracellular matrix structure and morphology [55]. The success of implants is related to the development of innovative materials and production methods. In addition, the designed tissue implant should show a tissue-like approach in terms of flexibility and should not change its post-implantation properties [56].

Polymers are one of the most widely used types of biomaterials in the design of tissue scaffolds for tissue repair [57]. The advantage of using polymeric materials in bone tissue is the ease of design and excellent controllability of the physicochemical properties of scaffolds, such as porosity, pore size, solubility, biocompatibility, enzymatic reactions, and allergic response [58,59]. In addition, the selection of the polymer to be used in production is based on factors such as the molecular weight of the polymer, solubility, swelling capacity, and biodegradability [60,61].

Using natural and synthetic polymers for bone tissue scaffolding is quite common. Natural polymers such as polysaccharides (chitosan, starch, alginate, hyaluronic acid, chitin) or proteins (collagen, gelatin, fibrin) can be used [62]. Natural polymers can be easily integrated into the body due to their high biocompatibility, biabsorbence, and favorable chemical structure for cell attachment. On the other hand, they also have disadvantages due to their weak mechanical strength and low stability in enzymatic and hydrolytic reactions [63].

Besides natural polymers, synthetic polymers are also used for bone tissue scaffolding. Poly(lactic acid), poly(glycolic acid), polycaprolactone, poly(vinyl alcohol), poly(ethylene glycol), and their copolymers are the most commonly used synthetic polymers in bone tissue engineering [64,65]. The advantages of synthetic polymers are that the desired scaffold architecture can be obtained with better mechanical properties and lower production costs than doped polymers [66]. However, there are also disadvantages, such as having lower biocompatibility compared to natural polymers and the emergence of toxic products that may cause inflammation after acidic degradation [67].

Bone consists of a combination of natural polymers and biological apatite. For this reason, composite systems in which polymers and bioceramics can be used together to produce bone tissue scaffolds are also a suitable option [68]. In this way, polymers have the high hardness and strength inherent in inorganic material [69]. On the other hand, since ceramics and glasses also have a fragile structure, the scaffolding attains a viscoelastic character using polymers [69]. As a result, polymer/ceramic composites have become promising materials for bone tissue engineering due to their improved mechanical and osteoconductivity [64].

9.4.1.2 Polymers for Cardiovascular Applications

Because of the superior biocompatibility and deformation capabilities of the polymers, they are preferable to metallic stents [70]. Polymers in cardiovascular applications occur in many areas, such as vascular grafts, stents, prosthetic heart valves, catheters, heart support devices, and hemodialysis [71].

For example, polyurethanes are widely used in cardiovascular practice due to their physicochemical and mechanical properties [72]. In addition, due to its bio-compatibility feature, it can be integrated with devices with blood contact [72]. On the other hand, although the polyurethane surface is highly resistant to microbes, it is similar to PTFE cardiovascular biomaterials in thrombosis formation [73]. Segmented polyurethanes are used in cardiovascular applications such as valve structures, pacemakers, and ventricular assist devices [74].

Polyesters are synonymous with polyethylene-terephthalate (PET). The trade name of PET is Dacron, and it is used in knitted or woven vascular grafts [73]. Textile-treated PET contains smaller pores than knitted PET, reducing blood leakage, and vascular graft applications show better results [75]. PET grafts are also coated with protein (albumin or collagen), reducing blood loss and showing better biocompatibility [74]. In addition, polyester is a widely preferred material in fusible stent production [76]. In this context, it is used with biodegradable polymers such as PGA, PDLA, and PLLA [77].

Polyolefins are used in tubing and preservation to provide low- and high-density blood reserves in the cardiovascular field [78]. It is also used to manufacture blood bags for blood storage [79]. Polyolefins can also be used as support material in constructing heart leaflets [80].

PTFEs, synthetic fluorocarbon polymers, are most commonly used in the cardiovascular field for vascular grafts and heart valves [81]. PTFE-containing materials are used in implantable prosthetic heart valve rings. PTFE sutures have been used in myxomatous mitral valve disease and mitral valve anterior and posterior leaflet prolapse [82]. However, it has also been successful in the vascular grafting of high-flow and large-diameter vessels such as the aorta [81].

9.5 BIOMATERIALS CHARACTERIZATIONS

Since surface chemistry is the most important feature that determines the interaction of biomaterials with tissues and cells, the surface chemistry of the biomaterial is one of the most critical factors in the efficient application of biomaterials implanted in the body [83]. Since the biological functions of biomaterials are greatly affected by the material's surface properties and chemical composition, it is vital to analyze the material's properties well [83]. Although the bulk properties of a material are highly suitable for a specific application, successful implant application is possible only if the surface properties are suitable [84].

The infrared (IR) spectroscopy technique is one of the primary analysis methods in the chemical examination of the surface properties of biomaterials. It is also applied in the detection of materials containing impurities in making the raw materials used in producing biomaterials [85]. The functional groups on the surface of biomaterials can be determined via IR analysis.

It is possible to determine the crystal structure of the component to be used as a biomaterial and its phases with the X-ray diffraction (XRD) analysis method [86]. It can be used frequently to determine the bioactivity of newly developed biomaterials [87]. The bioactivity of materials can be determined by forming hydroxy carbon-apatite structures on their surfaces, enabling them to bind with tissues after being kept in artificial body fluids with an ionic composition similar to physiological body fluids [88].

Nuclear magnetic resonance (NMR) spectroscopy is a method used to characterize bioorganic molecules by identifying the carbon-hydrogen content in molecules due to interactions with the nuclei of atoms. In addition, NMR spectroscopy is used to analyze monomer ratio, molecular weight, chain length, and branching for polymers [89]. In medicine, using magnetic resonance imaging (MRI) for soft tissue analysis to identify damaged or diseased tissue is an example of NMR applications [90].

The surface topography of the material (softness, hardness, roughness, and wettability), microstructure (porosity, pore size, pore shape), the interconnectivity of pores, and specific surface area) is essential if it is to be considered in determining its interaction with tissue [91]. According to this material feature, the interaction of the material to be implanted with the tissue may result in positive or negative results [92]. Electron microscopy methods can be applied to characterize the microstructural properties of a sample to be used as a biomaterial at 100 pm to 100 μm length scales. All of the defects of biomaterials, such as dislocations, cracks, and surface contamination layers, can be characterized by electron microscopy characterizing the details of the porous structures [93]. There are two general classes of electron microscopes: scanning electron microscope (SEM) and transmission electron microscope (TEM). Both of these methods can visualize the arrangement of atoms in different crystal structures [94].

The TEM method is known as a method that provides resolution at the atomic scale and is used to examine the material surface structure, elemental distribution, and morphology [95]. In addition, energy dispersion X-ray spectroscopy (EDS) and electron energy loss spectroscopy (EELS) systems, which analyze the X-rays and inelastic electrons emitted from the material, can also be used for the analytical characterization of the chemical structure of the material in the TEM device [96].

SEM is one of the most widely used methods in the characterization of biomaterials, in which biomaterial–tissue interactions can be understood by taking SEM images of the implanted biomaterials before and after implantation [97]. In addition, the SEM method is also used to examine the effect of mechanical force on the surface properties of materials used in orthopedics [98]. Similar to the applications of the TEM method, the chemical information of biomaterials can also be evaluated using characteristic X-rays or Auger electrons obtained from the sample under the electron beam [99]. Examining the surface morphological properties of the material with the support of SEM with different detectors has become suitable for determining properties such as surface reactivity, oxidation resistance, mechanical strength, and conductivity [100].

Field emission scanning electron microscope (FE-SEM), one of the improved versions of the SEM method, has a high separation power and can be used to determine the morphological structure of the material, particle sizes, and elemental analysis [101]. The energy scattering spectrometer (EDS) has detectors that collect the X-rays emitted from the material and enables the elemental content of the material to be analyzed. With EDS, the mapping method can determine which elements are concentrated in the target region on the SEM image [102]. Chemical analysis of the material can be done by analyzing the primary electrons and X-rays collected by the detectors [103]. In addition, crystallographic information about the material can be obtained by electron backscattering diffraction [104].

Atomic force microscopy (AFM) method can be applied to display these interactions at the nanometer level in three dimensions, where the biological response of tissues against implanted biomaterials occurs [105]. Unlike electron microscopes, an essential advantage of AFM is that the surface morphology of the biomaterial and surface roughness values can be obtained without surface treatment or coating that could damage or alter the material surface under investigation [106]. In this respect, displaying polymer materials in aqueous solution has benefits for biomaterials. For example, it allows the examination of the biomaterial surface in an environment similar to an environment where an implant can be found [107]. Thus it contributes to monitoring dynamic processes such as erosion, hydration, and adsorption that may occur at interfaces. The time required to obtain quality images can be changed depending on factors such as the scanning size and scanning speed applied in the analysis in the AFM method [108].

The surface area, particle size, and porosity of biomaterials can be characterized by quantitative measurement of adsorbed gases on solid surfaces. To calculate the surface area, the amount of nitrogen adsorbed to the material's surface by cooling or subsequent evaporation (desorption) is measured and calculated using the BET (Brauner-Emmett-Teller) equation [109]. Thus particle size can also be calculated in addition to calculating the surface area. For this purpose, the specific surface area is one of the most prominent characteristics in determining the morphological properties of porous materials [110]. The specific surface area provides a remarkable capacity for interaction with the tissue, attachment, and proliferation of cells [111]. The highly interconnected three-dimensional porosity enables multiple cells, vascularization, and diffusion of nutrients and oxygen to regenerate new functional tissues. Thus favorable compatibility of the scaffold with the tissue with which it interacts can be achieved quickly [112].

Many studies in tissue engineering aim to obtain polymeric scaffolds with very high and different porosity sizes while providing reasonable control of pore size and morphology [113]. For this reason, it is imperative to characterize the pore size and volume of the materials qualitatively because specific cells require pores of different sizes to ensure optimum attachment, growth, and motility [114]. One of the alternative methods used to characterize the surface of a material that can be implanted as a biomaterial is contact angle measurements [115]. Certain liquids can use a material's surface tension value to determine a substrate's wettability characteristic. Surface tension is calculated for a solid material by measuring the contact angle between the surface and the liquid drop on the surface. A low contact angle value indicates the hydrophobic nature of the material, while a high one indicates the surface's hydrophobic nature [116]. The primary purpose of modifying the biomaterial's surface to be implanted is to bring it to a state between the wettability of the surface and its water-repellent property [117]. Therefore, contact angle measurement provides a practical method to determine this range of values [118]. The adhesion of cell types can be determined under certain conditions, including bacteria, granulocytes, and erythrocytes via contact angle measurements [119–121].

Natural or synthetic biomaterials are expected to have various parameters that must be met before they are implanted into a living thing [122,123]. The size distribution and surface charge (zeta potential), purity, and molecular weight of the material to be implanted must be determined and meet the criteria [124]. In this context, Zetasizer is used to measure the particle size of systems dispersed from nanometers to micrometers in diameter using the dynamic light scattering (DLS) technique. Zetasizer systems are used to determine particle mobility and charge (Zeta potential) using the electrophoretic light scattering (ELS) technique and the molecular size of particles in solution using static light scattering (SLS) [125].

Measuring the response to temperature changes is essential in determining the physical properties of many biomaterials that increase their success in clinical applications [126]. In this context, thermal analysis methods are applied. Thermal analysis and calorimetric techniques are classified according to the measured physical, and the most frequently applied methods are thermogravimetric analysis (TGA), differential thermal analysis (DTA), and differential calorimetry analysis (DSC) techniques. The results obtained from these methods provide information about the chemical composition of the biomaterial and its thermodynamic, optical, and magnetic properties [127,128].

9.6 BIOCOMPATIBILITY AND TOXICITY OF BIOIMPLANTS

Biocompatibility is the most crucial factor in selecting biomaterials used in manufacturing implants for various medical applications [129]. Biocompatibility describes the interactions between the living system and the material included in this system [130]. If there is no reaction between the biomaterial and the tissue and at the same time, the material–tissue interface is stable, the biomaterial is defined as bioinert. Otherwise, if the interface is unstable, biocompatibility occurs between tissue and biomaterial, such as tissue damage, immunogenicity, inflammation, and toxicity [131]. As it can be understood from all these tissue response reactions, any object placed in the body, be it an implant or a transplanted organ or tissue, will likely trigger tissue response reactions that cause cytotoxicity since it will be perceived as a foreign body. For this reason, the biocompatibility of the biomaterial to be selected in the design process of an implant that will replace the function of any damaged tissue or organ placed in the body is vital for the organism [132].

The increasing use of biomaterials and medical devices makes the infectious conditions associated with these materials important [133,134]. It is defined as a problem in surgical branches due to the destruction of the tissue from contamination of the medical instruments placed in the body with microbes and infections that may cause the medical instrument to lose its function [135]. Infections resistant to antibiotics also result in the removal of infected implants. For these reasons, the patient's quality of life decreases, bringing a financial problem [136,137].

Infectious microorganisms associated with the biomaterial are mainly transmitted to the biomaterial from the skin. While the biomaterial is being placed, the bacteria found in the skin are also directed to the sterile tissue [138]. Another mechanism is airborne transmission. There are more or fewer microorganisms in the operating room's air, which may contaminate the implant surface before surgery [139]. The third way for microorganisms to reach the biomaterial is the hematogenous route [140]. For example, in dental implant treatment, the bacteria mixes with the blood and reaches the implant through the blood [141].

Biomaterial infections are characterized by biofilm formation. Microorganisms multiplying in a protected environment in a biofilm are protected from the body's immune response to infection and the antibiotic effect used in the treatment [142]. Biofilm-forming microorganisms often belong to more than one species or even a genus and coexist [143]. Bacteria, fungi, protozoa, viruses, and algae can be cited as examples of microorganisms that can form a biofilm [144]. There are many types of diseases, from joint and cardiac prosthetic infections, such as biofilm infections, to diabetic foot infections and gastrointestinal infections, such as cholera [145–147].

9.7 BIODEGRADABILITY OF POLYMER BIOIMPLANTS

Biodegradable scaffolds are essential for tissue regeneration because they provide cells with short-term support while they grow by using nutrients that have been supplied [148]. In situ tissue engineering uses a variety of scaffolds, including nanoscale materials, monolithic, fibrous, micro, and microporous gels, and 3D-printed scaffolds [149,150]. The prepared materials derived from natural, synthetic, or hybrid sources must be detached to confirm the continuance of signals and cells for rejuvenating certain organs or tissues [151,152]. For instance, many biomaterials have been used to treat damaged organs or impaired tissues while providing pain relief for broken bones [153,154].

Biomaterial biophysical features such as stiffness, structure, topography, and degradation can alter local tissue microenvironments via intracellular and intercellular signaling [155–157]. The pH or temperature can be changed, and the quantity of enzymes, cells, ions, or radical species can be regulated as part of these modifications to the tissue microenvironment [158]. Tissue-engineered biodegradable materials might theoretically serve their intended function while being implanted or integrating with the host afterward [159,160]. The biomaterial must integrate sympathetically with the recipient or transplanted cells to play a vital role in tissue regeneration via cell signaling, growth factor synthesis, and proliferation [161]. The extracellular matrix must also develop and differentiate [162]. For tissue regeneration in situ, biomaterial breakdown is desired [162]. For optimum tissue growth, the breakdown rate should coincide with the rate of tissue synthesis [163]. Since mechanical stiffness is lost due to biomaterial degradation, newly generated tissue should be capable of withstanding load transfer [164]. Additionally, inefficient healing can lead to tissue loss, implant loosening, and poor functionality of newly regenerated tissue if the biophysical properties of biomaterials and tissue are cytotoxic [165]. In general, it is possible to modify the in vivo milieu and control cellular fate by adjusting the biophysical properties of biomaterials [166].

9.8   LIMITATIONS AND CHALLENGES IN BIOMEDICAL APPLICATIONS

In recent studies, composites rather than individual materials used in biomedical implants and devices have received increased attention [167]. Which material performs well in various applications takes time to determine [4]. Also, these materials have yet to be subjected to researchers' in vivo comparison investigations and in vivo characterization experiments [168]. Many people are concurrently working to create new composites that will eventually satisfy the distinct mechanical and biocompatibility needs of every area of the body [82]. It is reasonable to conclude that using pure synthetic polymeric materials for medical implants and devices has peaked. In this area, it is currently favored to combine various materials to create composites that either have better mechanical strength and flexibility or have novel functionality, like the use of carbon fibers [12].

The use of cardiovascular biomaterials and its market share in the medical devices sector is increasing daily. Polymers are a practical choice in the use of cardiovascular materials [169]. In contrast, blood compatibility is one of the biggest problems, and, to overcome this, various surface modifications are being developed to develop biocompatible cardiovascular biomaterials [170–173].

The mechanical strength of biodegradable materials, the time required for their breakdown, and the waste products produced when they come into contact with people's bodies are all causes for concern [174]. The issue of biodegradability is also becoming more and more of a worry as nondegradable implants meet issues like stress shielding and wear debris and may require surgical removal [175]. Utilizing polymers that can dissolve in the body and reduce reliance on the implant while encouraging the growth and self-supportability of the muscle or bone around the implant can result in a more comfortable and helpful healing process [82]. Another substance that merits consideration is silk. Although silk fibroin polymers are biological, research has been done on producing synthetic silk for biomedical applications [176]. Silk fibroin films have been found to have good adhesion to mammalian cells, and biodegradable silk has long been utilized as a suture material [177]. As a result, they have been utilized as composites for bone production and improving cell attachment [178].

9.9 FUTURE CONCLUSIONS

Given the widespread attention that synthetic polymeric materials are receiving due to the increased emphasis on health care worldwide, the future of these materials in the medical sector is bright. Around the world, new composites are continually being created, including blends of natural and synthetic polymers that may be able to perform mechanical functions resembling those of the human body [179]. In addition, research is continuously being done to improve the functionality of devices and implants, particularly in biodegradability and MRI safety [180]. Given the enormous variety of compatible materials, the possibilities for material combinations as composites are practically limitless [181]. A more comprehensive range of applications is made possible by improvements in fabrication technology that make it possible to swiftly and affordably produce unique parts. What was once known to result in permanent dysfunction has been reduced to a limited impairment with increased comfort due to the proliferation of numerous medical devices and implants [82]. The biomedical industry has seen a critical turning point as a result. Finally, synthetic polymeric material advancements can improve living quality.

REFERENCES

[1] R.J. Narayan, The next generation of biomaterial development, Philos. Trans. R. Soc. A Math. Phys. Eng. Sci. 368 (2010) 1831–1837. doi:10.1098/RSTA.2010.0001.
[2] F. Barrère, T.A. Mahmood, K. de Groot, C.A. van Blitterswijk, Advanced biomaterials for skeletal tissue regeneration: Instructive and smart functions, Mater. Sci. Eng. R Reports. 59 (2008) 38–71. doi:10.1016/J.MSER.2007.12.001.
[3] Biomaterials Market Size to Hit US$ 390.92 Billion by 2027, (n.d.).
[4] S. Ramakrishna, J. Mayer, E. Wintermantel, K.W. Leong, Biomedical applications of polymer-composite materials: A review, Compos. Sci. Technol. 61 (2001) 1189–1224. doi:10.1016/S0266-3538(00)00241-4.
[5] M.F. Maitz, Applications of synthetic polymers in clinical medicine, Biosurface and Biotribology. 1 (2015) 161–176. doi:10.1016/J.BSBT.2015.08.002.
[6] P. Kadambi, P. Luniya, P. Dhatrak, Current advancements in polymer/polymer matrix composites for dental implants: A systematic review, Mater. Today Proc. 46 (2021) 740–745. doi:10.1016/J.MATPR.2020.12.396.
[7] M. Saad, S. Akhtar, S. Srivastava, Composite polymer in orthopedic implants: A review, Mater. Today Proc. 5 (2018) 20224–20231. doi:10.1016/J.MATPR.2018.06.393.
[8] A. Hudecki, G. Kiryczyński, M.J. Łos, Biomaterials, definition, overview, Stem Cells Biomater. Regen. Med. (2019) 85–98. doi:10.1016/B978-0-12-812258-7.00007-1.
[9] L.S. Nair, C.T. Laurencin, Biodegradable polymers as biomaterials, Prog. Polym. Sci. 32 (2007) 762–798. doi:10.1016/J.PROGPOLYMSCI.2007.05.017.
[10] D. Banoriya, R. Purohit, R.K. Dwivedi, Advanced application of polymer based biomaterials, Mater. Today Proc. 4 (2017) 3534–3541. doi:10.1016/J.MATPR.2017.02.244.

[11] N. Angelova, D. Hunkeler, Rationalizing the design of polymeric biomaterials, Trends Biotechnol. 17 (1999) 409–421. doi:10.1016/S0167-7799(99)01356-6.

[12] H.W. Toh, D.W.Y. Toong, J.C.K. Ng, V. Ow, S. Lu, L.P. Tan, P.E.H. Wong, S. Venkatraman, Y. Huang, H.Y. Ang, Polymer blends and polymer composites for cardiovascular implants, Eur. Polym. J. 146 (2021) 110249. doi:10.1016/J. EURPOLYMJ.2020.110249.

[13] B. Bhushan, P.L. Ko, Introduction to tribology, Appl. Mech. Rev. 56 (2003) B6–B7. doi:10.1115/1.1523360.

[14] Z.R. Zhou, Z.M. Jin, Biotribology: Recent progresses and future perspectives, Biosurf. Biotribol. 1 (2015) 3–24. doi:10.1016/J.BSBT.2015.03.001.

[15] H. Akça, O. İyibilgin, E. Gepek, M. Mühendisliği Bölümü, M. Fakültesi, S. Üniversitesi, T. Biyomedikal, M. ve Yarıiletken Malzemeler Uygulama ve Araştırma Merkezi, Biyomalzemeler ile İmplant Üretimi Sürecinin Biyotriboloji Yönünden Değerlendirilmesi, Duzce Univ. J. Sci. Technol. 8 (2020) 667–692. doi:10.29130/DUBITED.482400.

[16] A. Poliakov, V. Pakhaliuk, V.L. Popov, Current trends in improving of artificial joints design and technologies for their arthroplasty, Front. Mech. Eng. 6 (2020) 4. doi:10.3389/FMECH.2020.00004/BIBTEX.

[17] B.J. Briscoe, S.K. Sinha, Wear of polymers, Proc. Inst. Mech. Eng. J J. Eng. Tribol. 216 (2002) 401–413. doi:10.1243/135065002762355325.

[18] G.M. Raghavendra, K. Varaprasad, T. Jayaramudu, Biomaterials: Design, development and biomedical applications, Nanotechnol. Appl. Tissue Eng. 2015 (2015) 21–44. doi:10.1016/B978-0-323-32889-0.00002-9.

[19] X. Zhang, Y. Zhang, Z. Jin, A review of the bio-tribology of medical devices, Friction. 10 (2021) 4–30. doi:10.1007/S40544-021-0512-6.

[20] V.L. Popov, A.M. Poliakov, V.I. Pakhaliuk, Synovial joints. Tribology, regeneration, regenerative rehabilitation and arthroplasty, Lubricants. 9 (2021) 15. doi:10.3390/ LUBRICANTS9020015.

[21] P. Sahoo, S.K. Das, J. Paulo Davim, Tribology of materials for biomedical applications, Mech. Behav. Biomater. 2019 (2019) 1–45. doi:10.1016/B978-0-08-102174-3.00001-2.

[22] N. Vanparijs, L. Nuhn, B.G. De Geest, Transiently thermoresponsive polymers and their applications in biomedicine, Chem. Soc. Rev. 46 (2017) 1193–1239. doi:10.1039/C6CS00748A.

[23] N.K. Myshkin, S.S. Pesetskii, A.Y. Grigoriev, Tribology in industry polymer tribology: Current state and applications, Tribol Ind. 37 (2015) 284–290.

[24] S. Todros, M. Todesco, A. Bagno, Biomaterials and their biomedical applications: From replacement to regeneration, Processes. 9 (2021) 1949. doi:10.3390/ PR9111949.

[25] M.M. Blum, T.C. Ovaert, Investigation of friction and surface degradation of innovative boundary lubricant functionalized hydrogel material for use as artificial articular cartilage, Wear. 301 (2013) 201–209. doi:10.1016/J.WEAR.2012.11.042.

[26] M. Fusco, S.D. Skaper, S. Coaccioli, G. Varrassi, A. Paladini, Degenerative joint diseases and neuroinflammation, Pain Pract. 17 (2017) 522–532. doi:10.1111/ PAPR.12551.

[27] E.S. Fioretta, S.E. Motta, V. Lintas, S. Loerakker, K.K. Parker, F.P.T. Baaijens, V. Falk, S.P. Hoerstrup, M.Y. Emmert, Next-generation tissue-engineered heart valves with repair, remodelling and regeneration capacity, Nat. Rev. Cardiol. 18 (2020) 92–116. doi:10.1038/s41569-020-0422-8.

[28] L. Li, W. Smitthipong, H. Zeng, Mussel-inspired hydrogels for biomedical and environmental applications, Polym. Chem. 6 (2014) 353–358. doi:10.1039/C4PY01415D.

[29] K. Şarkaya, G. Akıncıoğlu, S. Akıncıoğlu, Investigation of tribological properties of HEMA-based cryogels as potential articular cartilage biomaterials, Polym. Technol. Mater. 61 (2022) 1174–1190. doi:10.1080/25740881.2022.2039190.

[30] M. Arjmandi, M. Ramezani, A. Nand, T. Neitzert, Experimental study on friction and wear properties of interpenetrating polymer network alginate-polyacrylamide hydrogels for use in minimally-invasive joint implants, Wear. 406–407 (2018) 194–204. doi:10.1016/j.wear.2018.04.013.

[31] J.K. Katta, M. Marcolongo, A. Lowman, K.A. Mansmann, Friction and wear behavior of poly(vinyl alcohol)/poly(vinyl pyrrolidone) hydrogels for articular cartilage replacement, J. Biomed. Mater. Res. Part A. 83A (2007) 471–479. doi:10.1002/JBM.A.31238.

[32] A.S. Oliveira, O. Seidi, N. Ribeiro, R. Colaço, A.P. Serro, Tribomechanical comparison between PVA hydrogels obtained using different processing conditions and human cartilage, Materials. 12 (2019) 3413. doi:10.3390/MA12203413.

[33] Y. Wu, X. Li, Y. Wang, Y. Shi, F. Wang, G. Lin, Research progress on mechanical properties and wear resistance of cartilage repair hydrogel, Mater. Des. 216 (2022) 110575. doi:10.1016/J.MATDES.2022.110575.

[34] A.S. Oliveira, S. Schweizer, P. Nolasco, I. Barahona, J. Saraiva, R. Colaço, A.P. Serro, Tough and low friction polyvinyl alcohol hydrogels loaded with anti-inflammatories for cartilage replacement, Lubricants. 8 (2020) 36. doi:10.3390/LUBRICANTS8030036.

[35] X. Zhao, W. Zhao, Y. Zhang, X. Zhang, Z. Ma, R. Wang, Q. Wei, S. Ma, F. Zhou, Recent progress of bioinspired cartilage hydrogel lubrication materials, Biosurf. Biotribol. 8 (2022) 225–243. doi:10.1049/BSB2.12047.

[36] V.M. Sardinha, L.L. Lima, W.D. Belangero, C.A. Zavaglia, V.P. Bavaresco, J.R. Gomes, Tribological characterization of polyvinyl alcohol hydrogel as substitute of articular cartilage, Wear. 301 (2013) 218–225. doi:10.1016/J.WEAR.2012.11.054.

[37] Y. Deng, J. Sun, X. Ni, B. Yu, Tribological properties of hierarchical structure artificial joints with poly acrylic acid (AA)—poly acrylamide (AAm) hydrogel and Ti6Al4V substrate, J. Polym. Res. 27 (2020) 1–9. doi:10.1007/S10965-020-02143-Z/FIGURES/10.

[38] Y. Shi, D. Xiong, J. Zhang, Effect of irradiation dose on mechanical and biotribological properties of PVA/PVP hydrogels as articular cartilage, Tribol. Int. 78 (2014) 60–67. doi:10.1016/J.TRIBOINT.2014.05.001.

[39] S. Cascone, G. Lamberti, Hydrogel-based commercial products for biomedical applications: A review, Int. J. Pharm. 573 (2020) 118803. doi:10.1016/J.IJPHARM.2019.118803.

[40] E. Caló, V. V. Khutoryanskiy, Biomedical applications of hydrogels: A review of patents and commercial products, Eur. Polym. J. 65 (2015) 252–267. doi:10.1016/j.eurpolymj.2014.11.024.

[41] A. Mandal, J.R. Clegg, A.C. Anselmo, S. Mitragotri, Hydrogels in the clinic, Bioeng. Transl. Med. 5 (2020) e10158. doi:10.1002/BTM2.10158.

[42] H. Cao, L. Duan, Y. Zhang, J. Cao, K. Zhang, Current hydrogel advances in physicochemical and biological response-driven biomedical application diversity, Signal Transduct. Target. Ther. 6 (2021) 1–31. doi:10.1038/s41392-021-00830-x.

[43] S. Affatato, A. Ruggiero, M. Merola, Advanced biomaterials in hip joint arthroplasty. A review on polymer and ceramics composites as alternative bearings, Compos. Part B Eng. 83 (2015) 276–283. doi:10.1016/J.COMPOSITESB.2015.07.019.

[44] A. Pandey, S. Sahoo, Progress on medical implant: A review and prospects, J. Bionic Eng. 20 (2022) 470–494. doi:10.1007/S42235-022-00284-Z.

[45] J. Song, B. Winkeljann, O. Lieleg, Biopolymer-based coatings: Promising strategies to improve the biocompatibility and functionality of materials used in biomedical engineering, Adv. Mater. Interfaces. 7 (2020) 2000850. doi:10.1002/ADMI.202000850.

[46] J.M. Anderson, F.J. Schoen, N.P. Ziats, In vivo assessment of tissue compatibility. In Biomaterials Science. An Introduction to Materials in Medicine, 2020, 869–877. doi:10.1016/B978-0-12-816137-1.00058-1.

[47] M.P. Staiger, A.M. Pietak, J. Huadmai, G. Dias, Magnesium and its alloys as orthopedic biomaterials: A review, Biomaterials. 27 (2006) 1728–1734. doi:10.1016/J.BIOMATERIALS.2005.10.003.

[48] W. Lattanzi, F. Miculescu, L. Vaiani, A. Boccaccio, A.E. Uva, G. Palumbo, A. Piccininni, P. Guglielmi, S. Cantore, L. Santacroce, I.A. Charitos, A. Ballini, Ceramic materials for biomedical applications: An overview on properties and fabrication processes, J. Funct. Biomater. 14 (2023) 146. doi:10.3390/JFB14030146.

[49] T. Lu, Y. Li, T. Chen, Techniques for fabrication and construction of three-dimensional scaffolds for tissue engineering, Int. J. Nanomedicine. 8 (2013) 337–350. doi:10.2147/IJN.S38635.

[50] B.M. Holzapfel, J.C. Reichert, J.T. Schantz, U. Gbureck, L. Rackwitz, U. Nöth, F. Jakob, M. Rudert, J. Groll, D.W. Hutmacher, How smart do biomaterials need to be? A translational science and clinical point of view, Adv. Drug Deliv. Rev. 65 (2013) 581–603. doi:10.1016/J.ADDR.2012.07.009.

[51] S.M. Choi, P. Chaudhry, S.M. Zo, S.S. Han, Advances in protein-based materials: From origin to novel biomaterials, Adv. Exp. Med. Biol. 1078 (2018) 161–210. doi:10.1007/978-981-13-0950-2_10/TABLES/1.

[52] C.W. Kang, F.Z. Fang, State of the art of bioimplants manufacturing: Part I, Adv. Manuf. 6 (2018) 20–40. doi:10.1007/S40436-017-0207-4.

[53] W. Lin, J. Klein, Recent progress in cartilage lubrication, Adv. Mater. 33 (2021) 2005513. doi:10.1002/ADMA.202005513.

[54] A. Tabatabaeian, A.R. Ghasemi, M.M. Shokrieh, B. Marzbanrad, M. Baraheni, M. Fotouhi, Residual stress in engineering materials: A review, Adv. Eng. Mater. 24 (2022) 2100786. doi:10.1002/ADEM.202100786.

[55] C.S.A. Bento, M.C. Gaspar, P. Coimbra, H.C. de Sousa, M.E.M. Braga, A review of conventional and emerging technologies for hydrogels sterilization, Int. J. Pharm. 634 (2023) 122671. doi:10.1016/J.IJPHARM.2023.122671.

[56] M. Mehrali, A. Thakur, C.P. Pennisi, S. Talebian, A. Arpanaei, M. Nikkhah, A. Dolatshahi-Pirouz, Nanoreinforced hydrogels for tissue engineering: Biomaterials that are compatible with load-bearing and electroactive tissues, Adv. Mater. 29 (2017) 1603612. doi:10.1002/ADMA.201603612.

[57] Y. Chen, Properties and development of hydrogels. In Hydrogels Based on Natural Polymers, 2019, 3–16. doi:10.1016/B978-0-12-816421-1.00001-X.

[58] W. Bonani, W. Singhatanadgige, A. Pornanong, A. Motta, Natural origin materials for osteochondral tissue engineering, Adv. Exp. Med. Biol. 1058 (2018) 3–30. doi:10.1007/978-3-319-76711-6_1.

[59] M.S. Shoichet, Polymer scaffolds for biomaterials applications, Macromolecules. 43 (2010) 581–591. doi:10.1021/MA901530R/ASSET/IMAGES/MEDIUM/MA-2009-01530R_0003.GIF.

[60] A.D. Padsalgikar, Emerging developments in polyurethane technology. Applications of Polyurethanes in Medical Devices, 2022, 209–245. doi:10.1016/B978-0-12-819673-1.00007-7.

[61] K.S. Ogueri, T. Jafari, J.L. Escobar Ivirico, C.T. Laurencin, Polymeric biomaterials for scaffold-based bone regenerative engineering, Regen. Eng. Transl. Med. 5 (2019) 128–154. doi:10.1007/S40883-018-0072-0/FIGURES/15.

[62] G.D. Mogoşanu, A.M. Grumezescu, Natural and synthetic polymers for wounds and burns dressing, Int. J. Pharm. 463 (2014) 127–136. doi:10.1016/J.IJPHARM.2013.12.015.

[63] S.A. Varghese, S.M. Rangappa, S. Siengchin, J. Parameswaranpillai, Natural polymers and the hydrogels prepared from them. In Hydrogels Based on Natural Polymers, 2020, 17–47. doi:10.1016/B978-0-12-816421-1.00002-1.

[64] B. Dhandayuthapani, Y. Yoshida, T. Maekawa, D.S. Kumar, Polymeric scaffolds in tissue engineering application: A review, Int. J. Polym. Sci. 2011 (2011). doi:10.1155/2011/290602.

[65] I. Oliveira, A.L. Carvalho, H. Radhouani, C. Gonçalves, J.M. Oliveira, R.L. Reis, Promising biomolecules, Adv. Exp. Med. Biol. 1059 (2018) 189–205. doi:10.1007/978-3-319-76735-2_8/COVER.

[66] A.M. Aghali, Poly(ethylene glycol) and co-polymer based-hydrogels for craniofacial bone tissue engineering, Orthop. Biomater. Adv. Appl. (2018) 225–246. doi:10.1007/978-3-319-73664-8_9/COVER.

[67] A. Iulian, L. Dan, T. Camelia, M. Claudia, G. Sebastian, Synthetic materials for osteochondral tissue engineering, Adv. Exp. Med. Biol. 1058 (2018) 31–52. doi:10.1007/978-3-319-76711-6_2/COVER.

[68] G.L. Koons, M. Diba, A.G. Mikos, Materials design for bone-tissue engineering, Nat. Rev. Mater. 5 (2020) 584–603. doi:10.1038/s41578-020-0204-2.

[69] J. Anita Lett, S. Sagadevan, I. Fatimah, M.E. Hoque, Y. Lokanathan, E. Léonard, S.F. Alshahateet, R. Schirhagl, W.C. Oh, Recent advances in natural polymer-based hydroxyapatite scaffolds: Properties and applications, Eur. Polym. J. 148 (2021) 110360. doi:10.1016/J.EURPOLYMJ.2021.110360.

[70] T. Hu, C. Yang, S. Lin, Q. Yu, G. Wang, Biodegradable stents for coronary artery disease treatment: Recent advances and future perspectives, Mater. Sci. Eng. C. 91 (2018) 163–178. doi:10.1016/J.MSEC.2018.04.100.

[71] N. Palani, Introduction to medical implants. In Toxicological Aspects of Medical Device Implants, 2020, 1–15. doi:10.1016/B978-0-12-820728-4.00001-0.

[72] A. Burke, N. Hasirci, Polyurethanes in biomedical applications, Adv. Exp. Med. Biol. 553 (2004) 83–101. doi:10.1007/978-0-306-48584-8_7/COVER.

[73] Y.H. Kuan, L.P. Dasi, A. Yoganathan, H.L. Leo, Recent advances in polymeric heart valves research, Int. J. Biomater. Res. Eng. 1 (2011) 1–17. doi:10.4018/IJBRE.2011010101.

[74] K.E. Styan, D.J. Martin, A. Simmons, L.A. Poole-Warren, In vivo biostability of polyurethane–organosilicate nanocomposites, Acta Biomater. 8 (2012) 2243–2253. doi:10.1016/J.ACTBIO.2012.03.004.

[75] M.T. Lam, J.C. Wu, Biomaterial applications in cardiovascular tissue repair and regeneration, Expert Rev. Cardiovasc. Ther. 10 (2014) 1039–1049. doi:10.1586/ERC.12.99.

[76] V. Shayani, K.D. Newman, D.A. Dichek, Optimization of recombinant t-PA secretion from seeded vascular grafts, J. Surg. Res. 57 (1994) 495–504. doi:10.1006/JSRE.1994.1175.

[77] W.J. Van der Giessen, A.M. Lincoff, R.S. Schwartz, H.M.M. Van Beusekom, P.W. Serruys, D.R. Holmes, S.G. Ellis, E.J. Topol, Marked inflammatory sequelae to implantation of biodegradable and nonbiodegradable polymers in porcine coronary arteries, Circulation. 94 (1996) 1690–1697. doi:10.1161/01.CIR.94.7.1690.

[78] A.G. Kidane, G. Burriesci, P. Cornejo, A. Dooley, S. Sarkar, P. Bonhoeffer, M. Edirisinghe, A.M. Seifalian, Current developments and future prospects for heart valve replacement therapy, J. Biomed. Mater. Res. Part B Appl. Biomater. 88B (2009) 290–303. doi:10.1002/JBM.B.31151.

[79] M.N. Helmus, J.A. Hubbell, Chapter 6 Materials selection, Cardiovasc. Pathol. 2 (1993) 53–71. doi:10.1016/1054-8807(93)90047-6.

[80] A.G. Kidane, G. Burriesci, M. Edirisinghe, H. Ghanbari, P. Bonhoeffer, A.M. Seifalian, A novel nanocomposite polymer for development of synthetic heart valve leaflets, Acta Biomater. 5 (2009) 2409–2417. doi:10.1016/J.ACTBIO.2009.02.025.

[81] S.K. Jaganathan, E. Supriyanto, S. Murugesan, A. Balaji, M.K. Asokan, Biomaterials in cardiovascular research: Applications and clinical implications, Biomed Res. Int. 2014 (2014). doi:10.1155/2014/459465.

[82] A.J.T. Teo, A. Mishra, I. Park, Y.J. Kim, W.T. Park, Y.J. Yoon, Polymeric biomaterials for medical implants and devices, ACS Biomater. Sci. Eng. 2 (2016) 454–472. doi:10.1021/ACSBIOMATERIALS.5B00429/ASSET/IMAGES/LARGE/AB-2015-00429V_0019.JPEG.

[83] Y.P. Jiao, F.Z. Cui, Surface modification of polyester biomaterials for tissue engineering, Biomed. Mater. 2 (2007) R24. doi:10.1088/1748-6041/2/4/R02.

[84] P. Roach, D. Eglin, K. Rohde, C.C. Perry, Modern biomaterials: A review—Bulk properties and implications of surface modifications, J. Mater. Sci. Mater. Med. 18 (2007) 1263–1277. doi:10.1007/S10856-006-0064-3/FIGURES/4.

[85] S. Joschek, B. Nies, R. Krotz, A. Göpferich, Chemical and physicochemical characterization of porous hydroxyapatite ceramics made of natural bone, Biomaterials. 21 (2000) 1645–1658. doi:10.1016/S0142-9612(00)00036-3.

[86] A.A. Bunaciu, E. gabriela Udriştioiu, H.Y. Aboul-Enein, X-ray diffraction: Instrumentation and applications, Crit. Rev. Analyt. Chem. 45 (2015) 289–299. doi:10.1080/10408347.2014.949616.

[87] M. Eckert, IUCr, Disputed discovery: The beginnings of X-ray diffraction in crystals in 1912 and its repercussions, Acta Crystallographica. 68 (2011) 30–39. doi:10.1107/S0108767311039985.

[88] L.L. Hench, H.A. Paschall, Direct chemical bond of bioactive glass-ceramic materials to bone and muscle, J. Biomed. Mater. Res. 7 (1973) 25–42. doi:10.1002/JBM.820070304.

[89] Q. Jiang, W. Huang, H. Yang, X. Xue, B. Jiang, D. Zhang, J. Fang, J. Chen, Y. Yang, G. Zhai, L. Kong, J. Guo, Radical emulsion polymerization with chain transfer monomer: An approach to branched vinyl polymers with high molecular weight and relatively narrow polydispersity, Polym. Chem. 5 (2014) 1863–1873. doi:10.1039/C3PY01437A.

[90] J.H.F. Bothwell, J.L. Griffin, An introduction to biological nuclear magnetic resonance spectroscopy, Biol. Rev. 86 (2011) 493–510. doi:10.1111/J.1469-185X.2010.00157.X.

[91] L. Zhu, D. Luo, Y. Liu, Effect of the nano/microscale structure of biomaterial scaffolds on bone regeneration, Int. J. Oral Sci. 2020 121. 12 (2020) 1–15. doi:10.1038/s41368-020-0073-y.

[92] B. Priyadarshini, M. Rama, Chetan, U. Vijayalakshmi, Bioactive coating as a surface modification technique for biocompatible metallic implants: A review, J. Asian Ceram. Soc. 7 (2019) 397–406. doi:10.1080/21870764.2019.1669861.

[93] R.F. Egerton, The scanning electron microscope. In Physical Principles of Electron Microscopy, 2005, 125–153. doi:10.1007/0-387-26016-1_5.

[94] B.J. Inkson, Scanning electron microscopy (SEM) and transmission electron microscopy (TEM) for materials characterization. In Materials Characterization Using Nondestructive Evaluation (NDE) Methods, 2016, 17–43. doi:10.1016/B978-0-08-100040-3.00002-X.

[95] S. Utsunomiya, R.C. Ewing, Application of high-angle annular dark field scanning transmission electron microscopy, scanning transmission electron microscopy-energy dispersive X-ray spectrometry, and energy-filtered transmission electron

microscopy to the characterization of nanopar, Environ. Sci. Technol. 37 (2003) 786–791. doi:10.1021/ES026053T/ASSET/IMAGES/LARGE/ES026053TF00007. JPEG.

[96] K.-L. Tai, C.-W. Huang, R.-F. Cai, G.-M. Huang, Y.-T. Tseng, J. Chen, W.-W. Wu, K.-L. Tai, G.-M. Huang, Y.-T.W. Tseng, -W Wu, C.-W. Huang, R.-F. Cai, J. Chen, -W W Wu, Atomic-scale fabrication of in-plane heterojunctions of few-layer MoS2 via in situ scanning transmission electron microscopy, Small. 16 (2020) 1905516. doi:10.1002/SMLL.201905516.

[97] P. Hill, H. Brantley, M. Van Dyke, Some properties of keratin biomaterials: Kerateines, Biomaterials. 31 (2010) 585–593. doi:10.1016/J.BIOMATERIALS.2009.09.076.

[98] X.M. Liu, S.L. Wu, Y.L. Chan, P.K. Chu, C.Y. Chung, C.L. Chu, K.W.K. Yeung, W.W. Lu, K.M.C. Cheung, K.D.K. Luk, Surface characteristics, biocompatibility, and mechanical properties of nickel-titanium plasma-implanted with nitrogen at different implantation voltages, J. Biomed. Mater. Res. Part A. 82A (2007) 469–478. doi:10.1002/JBM.A.31157.

[99] T.S. Sampath Kumar, Physical and chemical characterization of biomaterials, Charact. Biomater. (2013) 11–47. doi:10.1016/B978-0-12-415800-9.00002-4.

[100] D. Dwivedi, K. Lepková, T. Becker, Carbon steel corrosion: A review of key surface properties and characterization methods, RSC Adv. 7 (2017) 4580–4610. doi: 10.1039/C6RA25094G.

[101] K. Akhtar, S.A. Khan, S.B. Khan, A.M. Asiri, Scanning electron microscopy: Principle and applications in nanomaterials characterization. In Handbook of Materials Characterization, 2018, 113–145. doi:10.1007/978-3-319-92955-2_4/COVER.

[102] A. Laskin, J.P. Cowin, M.J. Iedema, Analysis of individual environmental particles using modern methods of electron microscopy and X-ray microanalysis, J. Electron Spectros. Relat. Phenomena. 150 (2006) 260–274. doi:10.1016/J.ELSPEC.2005.06.008.

[103] J. Ayache, L. Beaunier, J. Boumendil, G. Ehret, D. Laub, The different observation modes in electron microscopy (SEM, TEM, STEM). In Sample Preparation Handbook for Transmission Electron Microscopy, 2010, 33–55. doi:10.1007/978-0-387-98182-6_3.

[104] S. Nasrazadani, S. Hassani, Modern analytical techniques in failure analysis of aerospace, chemical, and oil and gas industries. In Handbook of Materials Failure Analysis: With Case Studies from the Oil and Gas Industry, 2016, 39–54. doi:10.1016/B978-0-08-100117-2.00010-8.

[105] K.D. Jandt, Atomic force microscopy of biomaterials surfaccs and interfaces, Surf. Sci. 491 (2001) 303–332. doi:10.1016/S0039-6028(01)01296-1.

[106] K. Kaczmarek, B. Konieczny, P. Siarkiewicz, A. Leniart, M. Lukomska-Szymanska, S. Skrzypek, B. Lapinska, Surface characterization of current dental ceramics using scanning electron microscopic and atomic force microscopic techniques, Coatings. 12 (2022) 1122. doi:10.3390/COATINGS12081122.

[107] K. Merrett, R.M. Cornelius, W.G. McClung, L.D. Unsworth, H. Sheardown, Surface analysis methods for characterizing polymeric biomaterials, J. Biomater. Sci. 13 (2012) 593–621. doi:10.1163/156856202320269111.

[108] D.G. Castner, B.D. Ratner, Biomedical surface science: Foundations to frontiers, Surf. Sci. 500 (2002) 28–60. doi:10.1016/S0039-6028(01)01587-4.

[109] K.E. Hart, L.J. Abbott, C.M. Colina, Analysis of force fields and BET theory for polymers of intrinsic microporosity, Mol. Simul. 39 (2013) 397–404. doi:10.1080/08927022.2012.733945/SUPPL_FILE/GMOS_A_733945_SM9008.PDF.

[110] K. Balagangadharan, S. Dhivya, N. Selvamurugan, Chitosan based nanofibers in bone tissue engineering, Int. J. Biol. Macromol. 104 (2017) 1372–1382. doi:10.1016/J.IJBIOMAC.2016.12.046.

[111] C. Wu, Y. Zhou, W. Fan, P. Han, J. Chang, J. Yuen, M. Zhang, Y. Xiao, Hypoxia-mimicking mesoporous bioactive glass scaffolds with controllable cobalt ion release for bone tissue engineering, Biomaterials. 33 (2012) 2076–2085. doi:10.1016/J. BIOMATERIALS.2011.11.042.

[112] S. Chung, M.W. King, Design concepts and strategies for tissue engineering scaffolds, Biotechnol. Appl. Biochem. 58 (2011) 423–438. doi:10.1002/BAB.60.

[113] L.M. Anovitz, D.R. Cole, Characterization and analysis of porosity and pore structures, Rev. Mineral. Geochem. 80 (2015) 61–164. doi:10.2138/RMG.2015.80.04.

[114] H.S. Bedi, P.K. Agnihotri, Interface and interphase in carbon nanotube-based polymer composites. In Handbook of Epoxy/Fiber Composites, 2022, 147–168. doi:10.1007/978-981-19-3603-6_9.

[115] W. Chen, Y. Liu, H.S. Courtney, M. Bettenga, C.M. Agrawal, J.D. Bumgardner, J.L. Ong, In vitro anti-bacterial and biological properties of magnetron co-sputtered silver-containing hydroxyapatite coating, Biomaterials. 27 (2006) 5512–5517. doi:10.1016/J.BIOMATERIALS.2006.07.003.

[116] T.T. Chau, W.J. Bruckard, P.T.L. Koh, A. V. Nguyen, A review of factors that affect contact angle and implications for flotation practice, Adv. Colloid Interface Sci. 150 (2009) 106–115. doi:10.1016/J.CIS.2009.07.003.

[117] T.S. Meiron, A. Marmur, I.S. Saguy, Contact angle measurement on rough surfaces, J. Colloid Interface Sci. 274 (2004) 637–644. doi:10.1016/J.JCIS.2004.02.036.

[118] R. Akbari, C. Antonini, Contact angle measurements: From existing methods to an open-source tool, Adv. Colloid Interface Sci. 294 (2021) 102470. doi:10.1016/J. CIS.2021.102470.

[119] Y. Zhao, C. Tian, Y. Liu, Z. Liu, J. Li, Z. Wang, X. Han, All-in-one bioactive properties of photothermal nanofibers for accelerating diabetic wound healing, Biomaterials. 295 (2023) 122029. doi:10.1016/J.BIOMATERIALS.2023. 122029.

[120] H. Ma, Y. Sun, Y. Tang, Y. Shen, Z. Kan, Q. Li, S. Fang, Y. Lu, X. Zhou, Z. Li, H. Ma, Y. Sun, Y. Tang, Z. Kan, S. Fang, X. Zhou, Z. Li, Y. Shen, Y. Lu, Robust electrospun nanofibers from chemosynthetic poly(4-hydroxybutyrate) as artificial dural substitute, Macromol. Biosci. 21 (2021) 2100134. doi:10.1002/ MABI.202100134.

[121] S. Dhingra, V. Gaur, V. Saini, K. Rana, J. Bhattacharya, T. Loho, S. Ray, A. Bajaj, S. Saha, Cytocompatible, soft and thick brush-modified scaffolds with prolonged antibacterial effect to mitigate wound infections, Biomater. Sci. 10 (2022) 3856–3877. doi:10.1039/D2BM00245K.

[122] T. Aydemir, J.I. Pastore, E. Jimenez-Pique, J.J. Roa, A.R. Boccaccini, J. Ballarre, Morphological and mechanical characterization of chitosan/gelatin/silica-gentamicin/bioactive glass coatings on orthopaedic metallic implant materials, Thin Solid Films. 732 (2021) 138780. doi:10.1016/J.TSF.2021.138780.

[123] S.Y. Rahnamaee, S.M. Dehnavi, R. Bagheri, M. Barjasteh, M. Golizadeh, H. Zamani, A. Karimi, Boosting bone cell growth using nanofibrous carboxymethylated cellulose and chitosan on titanium dioxide nanotube array with dual surface charges as a novel multifunctional bioimplant surface, Int. J. Biol. Macromol. 228 (2023) 570–581. doi:10.1016/J.IJBIOMAC.2022.12.159.

[124] N.H. Shahemi, S. Liza, Y. Sawae, T. Morita, H. Shinmori, Y. Yaakob, Effects of surface wettability and thermal conductivity on the wear performance of ultrahigh molecular weight polyethylene/graphite and ultrahigh molecular weight polyethylene/graphene oxide composites, Polym. Adv. Technol. 33 (2022) 1916–1932. doi:10.1002/PAT.5651.

[125] X. Meng, H. Xiong, F. Ji, X. Gao, L. Han, Z. Wu, L. Jia, J. Ren, Facile surface treatment strategy to generate dense lysozyme layer on ultra-high molecular weight polyethylene enabling inhibition of bacterial biofilm formation, Colloids Surf. B Biointerfaces. 225 (2023) 113243. doi:10.1016/J.COLSURFB.2023.113243.

[126] A. Vedadghavami, F. Minooei, M.H. Mohammadi, S. Khetani, A. Rezaei Kolahchi, S. Mashayekhan, A. Sanati-Nezhad, Manufacturing of hydrogel biomaterials with controlled mechanical properties for tissue engineering applications, Acta Biomater. 62 (2017) 42–63. doi:10.1016/J.ACTBIO.2017.07.028.

[127] H. Liu, H.H.Y. Tong, Z. Zhou, Feasibility of thermal methods on screening, characterization and physicochemical evaluation of pharmaceutical cocrystals, J. Therm. Anal. Calorim. 147 (2022) 12947–12963. doi:10.1007/S10973-022-11762-1.

[128] S. Sherif Stino, Thermal analysis of dental materials, Biomater. J. 1 (2022) 15–23. doi:10.5281/znodo.582940.

[129] S. Bauer, P. Schmuki, K. von der Mark, J. Park, Engineering biocompatible implant surfaces: Part I: Materials and surfaces, Prog. Mater. Sci. 58 (2013) 261–326. doi:10.1016/J.PMATSCI.2012.09.001.

[130] L. Ghasemi-Mobarakeh, D. Kolahreez, S. Ramakrishna, D. Williams, Key terminology in biomaterials and biocompatibility, Curr. Opin. Biomed. Eng. 10 (2019) 45–50. doi:10.1016/J.COBME.2019.02.004.

[131] D.F. Williams, On the mechanisms of biocompatibility, Biomaterials. 29 (2008) 2941–2953. doi:10.1016/J.BIOMATERIALS.2008.04.023.

[132] D. Williams, Concepts in biocompatibility: New biomaterials, new paradigms and new testing regimes, Biocompat. Perform. Med. Devices. (2012) 3–17. doi:10.1533/9780857096456.1.1.

[133] E. Rezvani Ghomi, N. Nourbakhsh, M. Akbari Kenari, M. Zare, S. Ramakrishna, Collagen-based biomaterials for biomedical applications, J. Biomed. Mater. Res. Part B Appl. Biomater. 109 (2021) 1986–1999. doi:10.1002/JBM.B.34881.

[134] J.A. Del Olmo, L. Ruiz-Rubio, L. Pérez-Alvarez, V. Sáez-Martínez, J.L. Vilas-Vilela, Antibacterial coatings for improving the performance of biomaterials, Coatings. 10 (2020) 139. doi:10.3390/COATINGS10020139.

[135] A. Hrycko, P. Mateu-Gelabert, C. Ciervo, R. Linn-Walton, B. Eckhardt, Severe bacterial infections in people who inject drugs: The role of injection-related tissue damage, Harm Reduct. J. 19 (2022) 1–13. doi:10.1186/S12954-022-00624-6/FIGURES/1.

[136] D. Ronin, J. Boyer, N. Alban, R.M. Natoli, A. Johnson, B.V. Kjellerup, Current and novel diagnostics for orthopedic implant biofilm infections: A review, APMIS. 130 (2022) 59–81. doi:10.1111/APM.13197.

[137] D.P. Perrault, A. Sharma, J.F. Kim, G.C. Gurtner, D.C. Wan, Surgical applications of materials engineered with antimicrobial properties, Bioengineering. 9 (2022) 138. doi:10.3390/BIOENGINEERING9040138.

[138] G. Kaur, G. Narayanan, D. Garg, A. Sachdev, I. Matai, Biomaterials-based regenerative strategies for skin tissue wound healing, ACS Appl. Bio Mater. 5 (2022) 2069–2106. doi:10.1021/ACSABM.2C00035/ASSET/IMAGES/LARGE/MT2C00035_0008.JPEG.

[139] C.E. Edmiston, G.R. Seabrook, R.A. Cambria, K.R. Brown, B.D. Lewis, J.R. Sommers, C.J. Krepel, P.J. Wilson, S. Sinski, J.B. Towne, Molecular epidemiology of microbial contamination in the operating room environment: Is there a risk for infection?, Surgery. 138 (2005) 573–582. doi:10.1016/J.SURG.2005.06.045.

[140] D. Campoccia, L. Montanaro, C.R. Arciola, A review of the clinical implications of anti-infective biomaterials and infection-resistant surfaces, Biomaterials. 34 (2013) 8018–8029. doi:10.1016/J.BIOMATERIALS.2013.07.048.

[141] H.J. Busscher, H.C. Van Der Mei, G. Subbiahdoss, P.C. Jutte, J.J.A.M. Van Den Dungen, S.A.J. Zaat, M.J. Schultz, D.W. Grainger, Biomaterial-associated infection: Locating the finish line in the race for the surface, Sci. Transl. Med. 4 (2012). doi:10.1126/SCITRANSLMED.3004528.

[142] S. Veerachamy, T. Yarlagadda, G. Manivasagam, P.K. Yarlagadda, Bacterial adherence and biofilm formation on medical implants: A review, Proc. Inst. Mech. Eng. Part H J. Eng. Med. 228 (2014) 1083–1099. doi:10.1177/0954411914556137.

[143] S. Liu, C. Gunawan, N. Barraud, S.A. Rice, E.J. Harry, R. Amal, Understanding, monitoring, and controlling biofilm growth in drinking water distribution systems, Environ. Sci. Technol. 50 (2016) 8954–8976. doi:10.1021/ACS.EST.6B00835/ASSET/IMAGES/LARGE/ES-2016-00835V_0004.JPEG.

[144] M. Novak Babič, C. Gostinčar, N. Gunde-Cimerman, Microorganisms populating the water-related indoor biome, Appl. Microbiol. Biotechnol. 104 (2020) 6443–6462. doi:10.1007/S00253-020-10719-4/FIGURES/2.

[145] D. Lebeaux, A. Chauhan, O. Rendueles, C. Beloin, From in vitro to in vivo models of bacterial biofilm-related infections, Pathogens. 2 (2013) 288–356. doi:10.3390/PATHOGENS2020288.

[146] M. Magana, C. Sereti, A. Ioannidis, C.A. Mitchell, A.R. Ball, E. Magiorkinis, S. Chatzipanagiotou, M.R. Hamblin, M. Hadjifrangiskou, G.P. Tegos, Options and limitations in clinical investigation of bacterial biofilms, Clin. Microbiol. Rev. 31 (2018). doi:10.1128/CMR.00084-16/ASSET/7465720B-A925-4E65-8A57-D34D277E08A3/ASSETS/GRAPHIC/ZCM0031826280005.JPEG.

[147] M.A. Rather, K. Gupta, P. Bardhan, M. Borah, A. Sarkar, K.S.H. Eldiehy, S. Bhuyan, M. Mandal, Microbial biofilm: A matter of grave concern for human health and food industry, J. Basic Microbiol. 61 (2021) 380–395. doi:10.1002/JOBM.202000678.

[148] E.C. Novosel, C. Kleinhans, P.J. Kluger, Vascularization is the key challenge in tissue engineering, Adv. Drug Deliv. Rev. 63 (2011) 300–311. doi:10.1016/J.ADDR.2011.03.004.

[149] R. Zeinali, L.J. Del Valle, J. Torras, J. Puiggalí, Recent progress on biodegradable tissue engineering scaffolds prepared by thermally-induced phase separation (TIPS), Int. J. Mol. Sci. 22 (2021) 3504. doi:10.3390/IJMS22073504.

[150] D. Lei, Y. Yang, Z. Liu, B. Yang, W. Gong, S. Chen, S. Wang, L. Sun, B. Song, H. Xuan, X. Mo, B. Sun, S. Li, Q. Yang, S. Huang, S. Chen, Y. Ma, W. Liu, C. He, B. Zhu, E.M. Jeffries, F.L. Qing, X. Ye, Q. Zhao, Z. You, 3D printing of biomimetic vasculature for tissue regeneration, Mater. Horizons. 6 (2019) 1197–1206. doi:10.1039/C9MH00174C.

[151] B.N. Brown, S.F. Badylak, Extracellular matrix as an inductive scaffold for functional tissue reconstruction, Transl. Res. 163 (2014) 268–285. doi:10.1016/J.TRSL.2013.11.003.

[152] C.J. Koh, A. Atala, Tissue engineering, stem cells, and cloning: Opportunities for regenerative medicine, J. Am. Soc. Nephrol. 15 (2004) 1113–1125. doi:10.1097/01.ASN.0000119683.59068.F0.

[153] S. Kumar, M. Nehra, D. Kedia, N. Dilbaghi, K. Tankeshwar, K.H. Kim, Nanotechnology-based biomaterials for orthopaedic applications: Recent advances and future prospects, Mater. Sci. Eng. C. 106 (2020) 110154. doi:10.1016/J.MSEC.2019.110154.

[154] F.M. Chen, X. Liu, Advancing biomaterials of human origin for tissue engineering, Prog. Polym. Sci. 53 (2016) 86–168. doi:10.1016/J.PROGPOLYMSCI.2015.02.004.

[155] X. Wan, Z. Liu, L. Li, X. Wan, Z. Liu, L. Li, Manipulation of stem cells fates: The master and multifaceted roles of biophysical cues of biomaterials, Adv. Funct. Mater. 31 (2021) 2010626. doi:10.1002/ADFM.202010626.

[156] M.A. Fernandez-Yague, S.A. Abbah, L. McNamara, D.I. Zeugolis, A. Pandit, M.J. Biggs, Biomimetic approaches in bone tissue engineering: Integrating biological and physicomechanical strategies, Adv. Drug Deliv. Rev. 84 (2015) 1–29. doi:10.1016/J.ADDR.2014.09.005.

[157] A.K. Gaharwar, I. Singh, A. Khademhosseini, Engineered biomaterials for in situ tissue regeneration, Nat. Rev. Mater. 2020 59. 5 (2020) 686–705. doi:10.1038/s41578-020-0209-x.

[158] H.S. Yoo, T.G. Kim, T.G. Park, Surface-functionalized electrospun nanofibers for tissue engineering and drug delivery, Adv. Drug Deliv. Rev. 61 (2009) 1033–1042. doi:10.1016/J.ADDR.2009.07.007.

[159] A. Nesic, S. Meseldzija, G. Cabrera-Barjas, A. Onjia, Novel biocomposite films based on high methoxyl pectin reinforced with zeolite Y for food packaging applications, Foods. 11 (2022) 360. doi:10.3390/FOODS11030360.

[160] J.T. Oliveira, R.L. Reis, Polysaccharide-based materials for cartilage tissue engineering applications, J. Tissue Eng. Regen. Med. 5 (2011) 421–436. doi:10.1002/TERM.335.

[161] H. Xia, H. Li, W. Gao, X. Fu, R.H. Fang, L. Zhang, K. Zhang, Tissue repair and regeneration with endogenous stem cells, Nat. Rev. Mater. 2018 37. 3 (2018) 174–193. doi:10.1038/s41578-018-0027-6.

[162] Z.S. Xiao, S. Ahmad, Y. Liu, G.D. Prestwich, Synthesis and evaluation of injectable, in situ crosslinkable synthetic extracellular matrices for tissue engineering, J. Biomed. Mater. Res. Part A. 79A (2006) 902–912. doi:10.1002/JBM.A.30831.

[163] J.R. Porter, T.T. Ruckh, K.C. Popat, Bone tissue engineering: A review in bone biomimetics and drug delivery strategies, Biotechnol. Prog. 25 (2009) 1539–1560. doi:10.1002/BTPR.246.

[164] S. Prasadh, R.C.W. Wong, Unraveling the mechanical strength of biomaterials used as a bone scaffold in oral and maxillofacial defects, Oral Sci. Int. 15 (2018) 48–55. doi:10.1016/S1348-8643(18)30005-3.

[165] A. Oryan, A. Moshiri, A. Meimandi-Parizi, Implantation of a novel tissue-engineered graft in a large tendon defect initiated inflammation, accelerated fibroplasia and improved remodeling of the new Achilles tendon: A comprehensive detailed study with new insights, Cell Tissue Res. 355 (2014) 59–80. doi:10.1007/S00441-013-1726-3/TABLES/5.

[166] X. Cun, L. Hosta-Rigau, Topography: A biophysical approach to direct the fate of mesenchymal stem cells in tissue engineering applications, Nanomaterials. 10 (2020) 2070. doi:10.3390/NANO10102070.

[167] A.L. Vega-Avila, O. Perales-Perez, R. Valentín Rullan, Biopolymers nanofibers for biomedical applications and environmental applications. In Electrospun Biomaterials and Related Technologies, 2017, 109–147. doi:10.1007/978-3-319-70049-6_4.

[168] P.G. Coelho, J.M. Granjeiro, G.E. Romanos, M. Suzuki, N.R.F. Silva, G. Cardaropoli, P. Van Thompson, J.E. Lemons, Basic research methods and current trends of dental implant surfaces, J. Biomed. Mater. Res. Part B Appl. Biomater. 88B (2009) 579–596. doi:10.1002/JBM.B.31264.

[169] M. Bernard, E. Jubeli, M.D. Pungente, N. Yagoubi, Biocompatibility of polymer-based biomaterials and medical devices – regulations, in vitro screening and risk-management, Biomater. Sci. 6 (2018) 2025–2053. doi:10.1039/C8BM00518D.

[170] P.K. Chu, J.Y. Chen, L.P. Wang, N. Huang, Plasma-surface modification of biomaterials, Mater. Sci. Eng. R Reports. 36 (2002) 143–206. doi:10.1016/S0927-796X(02)00004-9.

[171] K. Zhang, T. Liu, J.A. Li, J.Y. Chen, J. Wang, N. Huang, Surface modification of implanted cardiovascular metal stents: From antithrombosis and antirestenosis to endothelialization, J. Biomed. Mater. Res. Part A. 102 (2014) 588–609. doi:10.1002/JBM.A.34714.

[172] S.K. Jaganathan, A. Balaji, M.V. Vellayappan, A.P. Subramanian, A.A. John, M.K. Asokan, E. Supriyanto, Review: Radiation-induced surface modification of polymers for biomaterial application, J. Mater. Sci. 50 (2015) 2007–2018. doi:10.1007/S10853-014-8718-X/FIGURES/4.

[173] M.F. Maitz, M.C.L. Martins, N. Grabow, C. Matschegewski, N. Huang, E.L. Chaikof, M.A. Barbosa, C. Werner, C. Sperling, The blood compatibility challenge. Part 4: Surface modification for hemocompatible materials: Passive and active approaches to guide blood-material interactions, Acta Biomater. 94 (2019) 33–43. doi:10.1016/J.ACTBIO.2019.06.019.

[174] C. Mukherjee, D. Varghese, J.S. Krishna, T. Boominathan, R. Rakeshkumar, S. Dineshkumar, C.V.S. Brahmananda Rao, A. Sivaramakrishna, Recent advances in biodegradable polymers – Properties, applications and future prospects, Eur. Polym. J. 192 (2023) 112068. doi:10.1016/J.EURPOLYMJ.2023.112068.

[175] J.L. Wang, J.K. Xu, C. Hopkins, D.H.K. Chow, L. Qin, Biodegradable Magnesium-based implants in orthopedics—A general review and perspectives, Adv. Sci. 7 (2020) 1902443. doi:10.1002/ADVS.201902443.

[176] S. Kapoor, S.C. Kundu, Silk protein-based hydrogels: Promising advanced materials for biomedical applications, Acta Biomater. 31 (2016) 17–32. doi:10.1016/J.ACTBIO.2015.11.034.

[177] Y. Zhao, Z.S. Zhu, J. Guan, S.J. Wu, Processing, mechanical properties and bio-applications of silk fibroin-based high-strength hydrogels, Acta Biomater. 125 (2021) 57–71. doi:10.1016/J.ACTBIO.2021.02.018.

[178] X. Yao, S. Zou, S. Fan, Q. Niu, Y. Zhang, Bioinspired silk fibroin materials: From silk building blocks extraction and reconstruction to advanced biomedical applications, Mater. Today Bio. 16 (2022) 100381. doi:10.1016/J.MTBIO.2022.100381.

[179] N. Goonoo, A. Bhaw-Luximon, G.L. Bowlin, D. Jhurry, An assessment of biopolymer- and synthetic polymer-based scaffolds for bone and vascular tissue engineering, Polym. Int. 62 (2013) 523–533. doi:10.1002/PI.4474.

[180] B.D. Ulery, L.S. Nair, C.T. Laurencin, Biomedical applications of biodegradable polymers, J. Polym. Sci. Part B Polym. Phys. 49 (2011) 832–864. doi:10.1002/POLB.22259.

[181] M.J.T. Raaijmakers, N.E. Benes, Current trends in interfacial polymerization chemistry, Prog. Polym. Sci. 63 (2016) 86–142. doi:10.1016/J.PROGPOLYMSCI.2016.06.004.

10 Synthesis and Characterization of UHMWPE Wear-Resistant Bioimplants

R Padmavathi¹ and V Kanchana²
¹ Vel Tech Multi Tech Dr. Rangarajan Dr. Sakunthala
Engineering College
Chennai, Tamil Nadu, India
² Sree Sastha Institute of Engineering and Technology
Chennai, Tamil Nadu, India

10.1 INTRODUCTION

One of the most effective surgical procedures since the 1960s is total joint replacement (TJR). The very most important material combinations today for prosthetic hip or knee joints are metal on polymer material, ceramic on polymer material, and metal on metal, notably lightweight ones [1].

Bioimplants have been extensively used throughout history to help increase many organisms' longevity and quality of life. Because of an aging population and advances in medical technology, surgical procedures like bone grafting and dental implants are becoming more commonplace worldwide. The study of the characteristics and uses of materials that are employed in biological systems is the focus of biomaterials research, which also focuses on tissue and organ replacement that fulfill the functions of human body parts [2].

Devices are made using biomaterials, which interact with biological systems to cohabit for longer service with little failure. Williams in 1981 described biomaterials as "nonviable materials used in medical devices, intended to interact with the biological systems." These are used in repair, replacement, or damaged parts of the musculoskeletal system (bones, joints, and teeth). Due to its comparatively high strength, low friction, high wear, and chemical resistance in corrosive conditions, ultrahigh-molecular-weight polyethylene (UHMWPE) is utilized for the production of implants like artificial joints and facial surgery, among other things. The primary factor in this material's widespread use as a bioimplant material is that it shares chemical properties and physical and mechanical properties with biological tissues [3].

Due to a lack of scientific knowledge in those times, diverse materials, such as stone, ivory, and gold, were used for failed bone replacements when looking at bioimplants on a macro level (including bone replacements). Bioimplants did not start integrating with the fast advancing scientific procedures of that time until the 1700s. Due to these significant advancements, the research and scientific knowledge that was being made would soon lead to the modern procedures that are used today [4]. Different polyethylene (PE) grades can function quite differently from one another depending on their density and branching.

Instead of being dependent on molecular mass, UHMWPE is also a semi-crystalline polymer that has an interfacial all-trans phase made up of fully crystalline and entirely amorphous phases. It possesses great biocompatibility, toughness, durability, and wear resistance. UHMWPE's relevance for obtaining remarkable performance in complete joint arthroplasties is therefore undeniable. It is frequently utilized as a bearing material with ceramic or metallic counter surfaces [5].

In conclusion, it is currently unknown why surface texturing might improve performance and why certain pattern patterns might harm the related tribiological performance. Furthermore, the impact of the five pattern parameters—shape, dimension, depth, area density, and distribution—in the field of orthopedic implants has not yet been sufficiently studied in depth. In this chapter, the preparation and characterization of UHMPE polymer based bioimplants materials are discussed.

10.2   IMPORTANCE OF WEAR RESISTANCE IN POLYMER BIOIMPLANTS

Artificial joints are made of biomaterials with great wear resistance, which suggests that bearing pairs would produce few wear particles, solving the main issue with bioimplants and extending the lifespan of artificial joints. Additionally, less volume loss can lessen the chance of wearing through the PE cup, which will strengthen the stability of prosthetics [6,7]. Since its inception as an implant material for orthopedic more than 40 years ago. The use of UHMWPE as a bearing material in total knee and hip replacement prostheses has gained significant attention. Despite being widely used, implanted knee and hip prosthesis with UHM-WPE components continue to have a short clinical lifespan due to the tribological and mechanical properties of the polymer [8].

UHMWPE has gained worldwide recognition as a bearing material used in total knee and hip replacement prostheses since it was first developed more than 40 years ago as an orthopedic implant material. Because of the tribological and mechanical characteristics of UHMWPE, implanted knee and hip prostheses—despite their widespread use—continue to have a limited clinical lifespan [9–11].

Over the course of the history and development of bioimplants, numerous materials have been created. The following are the primary needs for these materials:

1. Biocompatibility
2. Equivalence of mechanical performance to that of the bones
3. Price

The most crucial prerequisite for a material used in bioimplants is that it must be biocompatible with the human body, meaning that it must integrate without having a negative effect on the host body. Different materials that can be used in bioimplants have been developed based on these needs. Ceramic, polymer, and metallic systems can be used as classifiers of bioimplant materials [12].

The human body has used polymer-based biomaterials since they were first created, usually in the form of synthetic polymers. Due to their strength, inertness, and biocompatibility, polymer biomaterials have been used in clinical practice to relieve the load of damaged or infected bone and to enhance patient quality of life. Polymer biomaterials are used in a variety of tissues, including the dermis, musculoskeletal system, nervous system, and cardiovascular system. Before selecting any material, it must possess a specific set of characteristics, including surface topography, free energy, and functional group [13–15].

Since the 1970s, PEs have mostly been employed as a bearing material in prosthetic hip and knee joints. In these applications, where biocompatibility and resistance to the aqueous saline body environment, as well as wear resistance and relative toughness, are essential. UHMWPE with linear or cross-linked morphologies are frequently utilized. Additionally, UHMWPE has a low coefficient of friction, superior wear resistance, and self-lubrication. Young patients find the 10- to 15-year lifespan of UHMWPE-based bioimplants to be undesirable. Additionally, the cost of the revision hip replacement is significantly higher than the cost of the initial treatment. As a result, there is a strong need to increase the durability of artificial joints made of UHMWPE. Since the early 1970s, cross-linked polyethylene (XLPE) has gradually grown in popularity. Numerous studies have shown that cross-linking can assist in lowering the wear rate of polyethylene in vivo. Aseptic loosening brought on by polyethylene wear particles cannot be completely prevented, despite the fact that cross-linked polyethylene has a lower wear rate than ordinary polyethylene.

Much work has gone into extending the service lives of TJR and improving the microstructure of UHMWPE to produce superior wear performance. In general, there are two ways to improve wear properties: (1) changing the chemical structure through techniques like ion doping, cross-linking by irradiation, or chemical routes and (2)changing the physical microstructure through thermal heat treatment or compression under high pressure. Since thermomechanical techniques don't alter the chemical structure, which could have an impact on the characteristics, they may be favored for changing the qualities [16–18].

The hip joint is a ball-and-socket joint, and the congruence of the implants, pelvic muscles, and capsule is what gives it stability. The components of the artificial hip have been designed to allow for a wide range of motion without the neck of the prosthesis rubbing against the rim of the acetabular cup, which would cause dislocation. Implants' design features must allow them to withstand loads up to eight times their own weight [19–21].

UHMWPE's molecular weight, which currently ranges in average between 2 and 6 million, contributes to its wear resistance. The prosthesis motion and load bearing generate wear debris on the articulating surface and at the interfaces where there is micromotion. It is currently recognized that UHMWPE wear is the main cause of aseptic loosening and late revision of hip implants. Around 100 million microscopic UHMWPE wear particles are released into the tissues surrounding the hip joint every day of patient movement, according to studies. This worn debris can set off a chain reaction of adverse tissue reactions that ultimately lead to aseptic loosening of the components and osteolysis (death of bone). The hypothesis put forth by the researchers suggests that an enhancement in the femoral head's surface quality could be the cause of the observed rise in clinical wear performance [22–24].

Since there are now no such models specifically for wear attributes, empirical relationships cannot be exploited in a design framework. The challenge arises from the need to evaluate too many variables, including mechanical characteristics, toughness, fracture, material systems and their microstructure, components, shape, load, and wear testing procedures [25,26].

When there are no third-body particles present, the following mechanism underlies the formation of wear debris in UHMWPE:

1. The joint articulation creates a multidirectional stress field at the wear surface.
2. The principal stress component happens in the direction of flexion and extension.
3. The secondary stress component happens in the direction of abduction/ adduction for the hip and in the direction of tibial rotation for the knee.
4. Preferential orientation of molecules happens in the direction of the principal stress component.
5. Transverse softening causes surface rupture between the orientated molecules.
6. Orientation causes strain softening in the transverse direction, which is concurrent with the secondary stress component.
7. Surface rupture causes the development of fibrillar or filmy wear particles by transferring load to the subsurface shear plane [27].

10.3 METHODS FOR SYNTHESIZING UHMWPE IMPLANTS AND THEIR CHARACTERIZATION

A type of polymer referred to as a linear homopolymer is UHMWPE. PE is a polymer created from the monomer ethylene (C_2H_4), a gas with a molecular weight of 28. Polyethylene has the general chemical formula (C_2H_4)n, where n is the degree of polymerization. For an ultra-high molecular weight polyethylene, the molecular chain can consist of as much as 2,00,000 ethylene repeat units. In other words, there are up to 4,00,000 carbon atoms in the molecular chain of UHMWPE. UHMWPE is a material having high strength, little creep, little coefficient of friction, little abrasion, and little wear resistance. Due to its exceptional qualities, UHMWPE is widely employed in both military and nonmilitary applications, including belts, joints, racquets, ropes, and composite materials. Additionally, it has a lower density than water, excellent chemical resistance, minimal moisture absorption, high specific strength and modulus, and superior impact and abrasion resistance [28,29].

Before the 1940s, molasses, a by-product of the sugar industry, was the main source of ethylene for the polymerization process. Molasses's ethanol was dehydrated to produce ethylene. Since the development of the steam-cracking process, the great majority of ethylene production has been dependent on petroleum sources, including naphtha, ethane, and, to a lesser extent, propane and butane. Numerous lower alkanes and olefins are among the reaction's gaseous by-products, and the mixture can be divided via selective absorption and low-temperature fractional distillation. Olefins can also be produced by cracking gas oil but with a lower yield. Since breakdown reactions that take place at high temperatures are also exothermic and might result in an explosion if the reaction gets out of control, the heat of polymerization during the polymerization process must be carefully managed [30].

UHMWPE is a complicated material, and treating it during synthesis is much more difficult. Designing suitable metal catalysts and cocatalysts, identifying appropriate reaction conditions that tend to accelerate chain propagation while slowing down chain transfer, moderating the metal catalyst's Lewis acidity to lessen hydride elimination, and modifying the steric and electronic properties of the metal center are all parts of this process. Despite these challenges, a number of UHMWPE-producing catalytic systems have been devised, new processing methods have been created, and specialized applications have recently appeared [31].

Modern PE was created in 1993 as a result of an attempt by Eric Fawcett and Reginald Gibson to condense ethylene with benzaldehyde at Imperial Chemical Industries. Since then, numerous varieties of PE have been created for use in commerce, and research is ongoing on the synthesis of PE using various catalysts.

There are five very different ways to make high polymers of ethylene: the high-pressure processes, Ziegler–Natta processes, Phillips processes, Standard Oil (Indiana) procedures, and metallocene processes are only a few examples of industrial processes. The conventional heterogeneous Ziegler–Natta method can be used to create UHMWPE from ethylene gas (C_2H_4) in a solvent with titanium tetrachloride ($TiCl_4$) acting as a catalyst (Figure 10.1). Chain propagations and chain terminations, of which propagations and terminations are particularly significant, are among the typical polymerization processes of UHMWPE. Catalyst activation is not required for all systems. Karl Ziegler and Giulio Natta made the initial discovery of transition metal-based catalysts for the controlled

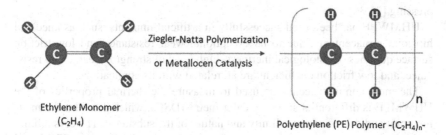

Ethylene Monomer
(C_2H_4)

Ziegler-Natta Polymerization
or Metallocen Catalysis

Polyethylene (PE) Polymer -(C_2H_4)n-

FIGURE 10.1   Synthesis of Polyethylene from Ethylene.

synthesis of PE. Ziegler–Natta catalysts for the manufacture of UHMWPE have been studied for a very long time, and they are among the primary catalysts utilized for olefin polymerizations in industries today. Magnesium chloride is frequently utilized to support this kind of catalyst, while titanium is frequently employed as the metal center of the catalysts. Other cocatalysts, like triethyl aluminum, are typically needed to activate ZN catalysts so that coordination sites between metal centers and ethylene double bonds can be formed. Following this, monomer additions are repeated to increase the molecular weight of the final products. One benefit of ZN catalysts over other kinds of catalysts is the synthesis of linear UHMWPE as a result of the low tendency of bimolecular hydrogen transfer at low pressure of ethylene [32].

Medical-grade UHMWPE has three grade-categorized materials depending on the molecular weight (Mw) and also manufacturer process. The polymer has a long-chain aliphatic hydrocarbon type ($-CH_2-CH_2-CH_2-CH_2-$) and is thus thermoplastic in nature. Low values for the glass transition temperature (Tg) would be expected as a result of the carbon-carbon bonds' flexibility. However, the Tg has limited physical relevance because it is linked to the motion of relatively long segments in amorphous materials, and there are few of these segments in crystalline polymers.

A C-C covalent bond forms the structure of UHMWPE, which is structured in both ordered and disordered regions, or crystalline and amorphous, respectively. The crystal's structure is orthorhombic, and its crystalline phase consists of chains folded into strongly oriented lamellae. Within the amorphous phase, the nearly 10–50 nm thick and 10–50 nm long lamellae are oriented arbitrarily, with molecules connecting each lamellae to the next.

The outstanding qualities of UHMWPE include low density, high strength, high modulus, good resistance to chemicals and abrasion, high energy absorption, impact strength, low friction coefficient, and more [33,34].

There are a variety of qualities to take into account while creating a new UHMWPE material for implant applications. It is possible to measure the UHMWPE powder's properties to make sure that different production lots are all the same. Manufacturers will test the solid polyethylene slab to assess the quality of the consolidation and to ascertain whether any unfavorable effects have occurred after consolidation, where the PE powder is compressed into a solid slab of material using ram extrusion, compression molding, or other techniques, such as isostatic pressing [35,36].

UHMWPE has been used successfully in artificial implants, such as knee and hip joint replacements, due to its exceptional wear resistance and low-friction surface qualities. Its biological inertness, high level of strength, wear, creep resistance, and low friction coefficient are all related with its applications.

The most common technique used to measure the thermal properties of the UHWMPE is differential scanning calorimetry (DSC), which provides the melting point and degree of crystallinity and nature of the substance. The crystallinity of the first heat melting endotherm and a heat of fusion of 289 J/g were 77% based on an integration range of 50–160 °C. The crystallinity of the second heat dropped to 58% [37].

Mw, molecular weight distribution (MWD), branching, melting temperature, and polymer state (entangled versus disentangled) are significant molecular characteristics of UHMWPE. DSC has been utilized a lot to gather insightful data about UHMWPE. At a heating rate of 10 °C/min, the nascent UHMWPE sample exhibits a strong melting peak at a temperature of roughly 140 °C. The nature of developing UHMWPE and its entangled/disentangled state can be better understood through the use of a combination of DSC and melt rheology characterization methods. The Mw and MWD of UHMWPE (in the range of 2–10 million g/mol) were more precisely determined using melt rheology. This method was discovered to be effective for spotting branching [38].

10.4 PROCESS PARAMETERS INFLUENCES ON WEAR BEHAVIORS OF UHMWPE IMPLANTS

Several joint replacement devices can use UHMWPE as a bearing material because of its mechanical and tribological properties. UHMWPE is used for buttons to resurface the patella in total knee arthroplasty, counterfaces inserted into the glenoid in shoulder arthroplasty, sleeves to allow semiconstrained rotation in elbow and wrist arthroplasty designs, and sleeves. In order to process UHMWPE, the powder is normally first made into a consolidated form and then machined into the desired final shape. UHMWPE cannot be processed using typical melt processing techniques like injection molding, blow molding, etc. due to the physical cross-linking of chains with extremely high molecular weights known as entanglement, which raises the melt's viscosity. Unlike PEs with lower molecular weights, UHMWPE does not melt or flow as easily. So, to process embryonic UHMWPE, techniques including gel spinning, compression molding, ram extrusion, sintering, and direct compression molding are applied [39].

10.4.1 MILLING AND MACHINING OF UHMWPE

The implant maker may purchase UHMWPE stock material as resin or as converted stock material. In the first scenario, the manufacturer is responsible for converting the resin, whereas in the second scenario, UHMWPE merely needs to be machined into final components. The manufacturer has a variety of resin grades to choose from, each having a distinct molecular weight and somewhat varied physical and mechanical qualities after conversion, in addition to the many shape options.

The final component's shape may, to some extent, dictate the shape of the UHMWPE stock. Knee implants that are comparatively flat can be milled using slab stock that has been mass-produced utilizing compression molding. Compression-molded stock may be desirable since it is more isotropic in its resistance to crack propagation and in its polymer morphology because knee implants are subjected to complicated multiaxial loads in real life. Since acetabular shell bearing inserts frequently come from big center-feed lathes, axis symmetric components like those may benefit from the use of extruded rod UHMWPE stock. However, if needed, compression-molded slabs can be cut into rods and used in axisymmetric products. On the other hand, extruded rod stock can be cut into pucks and machined to produce relatively flat geometries like knee implants.

The grade of UHMWPE resin, more particularly the molecular weight of the precursor resin, raises further concerns about stock selection. Device manufacturers have long been supplied bulk compression-molded slabs of the lower-molecular-weight Hoechst resins (GUR 1020/1120) via converters. The higher-molecular-weight Hoechst resins (GUR 1050/1150), in contrast, have often been available to producers only as extruded rods, but, more recently, converters have begun to offer GUR 1050 in compression-molded sheet form as well. Due to the compression-molded stock's higher resin grade, historical references comparing implant ram extrusion with compression molding frequently ignore the complicating factor of resin grade. This is one component of the resin selection problem.

10.4.2 Direct Compression Molding

Direct compression molding (DCM), also known as net shape compression molding, effectively converts the resin into a finished or semifinished item for the manufacturer of the polyethylene insert by using special molds (Figure 10.2).

The extraordinarily smooth surface finish obtained with no machining marks at the articulating surface is one benefit of DCM. Additionally, since the projected surface area of each individual part mold is very modest in comparison to the area of big molds used to compression-mold sheets, greater processing pressures may be obtained, if needed.

Direct compression molding has been used to make acetabular and tibial inserts for over 20 years. The technique may have been employed in the past because the production of knee implants required complicated curves that the cutting and milling tools available at the time were unable to precisely create due to a lack of numerical control. The yield strength can be enhanced by 40% when compression molding is carried out at exceptionally high pressures

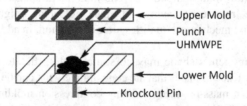

FIGURE 10.2 Schematic representation of compression molding of UHMWPE.

of more over 300 MPa without significantly affecting the impact strength or toughness [40].

The tibia component in a total knee replacement and the cemented all-polyethylene acetabular component are two instances of UHMWPE that was directly compressed into shape.

10.4.3 Ram Extrusion of UHMWPE

Midway in the 1980s, converters started ram extruding with Hoechst GUR 415 resin, which had a higher average molecular weight and a lower extraneous particle count compared to 1900 and which was simpler to extrude than GUR 412. Orthopedics employed extruded rods made of GUR 412, 415, and (less frequently) 1900 CM (a grade of 1900 resin containing calcium stearate). As a result, it is challenging to make generalizations regarding the types of resin used in implants without tracking down the lot numbers utilized by a certain manufacturer. Only a few converters now provide the orthopedic market with medical grade GUR 1020 and 1050 ram-extruded UHMWPE. While Ortho-plastics' medical grade extrusion is located in England, MediTECH, Westlake Plastics, and Orthotech all have facilities for medical grade extrusion in the United States.

An extruder receives a continuous feed of UHMWPE powder (Figure 10.3). A hopper that lets powder into a heated reception chamber, a horizontal reciprocating ram, a heated die, and an output make up the extruder's basic components. The ram and the back pressure of the molten UHMWPE keep the UHMWPE under pressure inside the extruder. The frictional force of the molten resin as it is pressed horizontally through the outlet against the heated die wall surface produces the back pressure. The UHMWPE rod is gradually cooled outside the outlet in a series of electric heating mantles. Extrusion can produce rods up to 12 inches in diameter; however, because bigger rod diameters require longer cooling times, the rate of production is influenced by the rod size. Most frequently, rods with a diameter of 20–80 mm are employed in orthopedic applications. The average output rate is about mm/minute.

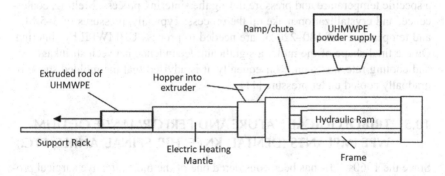

FIGURE 10.3 Schematic of a ram extruder.

10.4.4 Hot Isostatic Pressing of ArCom UHMWPE

One orthopedic manufacturer (Biomet, Inc., Warsaw, Indiana, USA) uses the other conversion technique, known as hot isostatic pressing, to turn resin into stock material. The first phase in this multistep conversion process, known by the company as ArCom, is the creation of a cylindrical compact using cold isostatic pressing, which removes the majority of the air. In order to stop the degradation of the UHMWPE, the compressed green rods are then sintered in a hot isostatic pressure (HIP) furnace in an argon-filled bag. Due to the hydrostatic sintering procedure, the resulting ArCom rod stock is nearly isotropic and might be regarded as a compression-molded version of the resin. After that, the isomolded rod stock is utilized to create completed implants using turning or milling processes [6].

10.4.5 Gel Extrusion and Spinning

UHMWPE and oil are combined in a number of processes, with the oil serving as a diluent rather than a solvent. The UHMWPE particles absorb the oil, expand, and solidify into gels. The resulting gel can then be extruded using adapted plastic screw extruders and fiber lines, unlike UHMWPE alone.

After the oil has been extracted from the sheets, a porous material suitable for filter membranes or separators for battery electrode plates has been produced. Most modern vehicle lead acid batteries are made with UHMWPE electrode plate separators, which were made in this way. Fibers can also be produced by orienting gel filaments before extracting the oil. It is possible to successfully pull the flexible and random chains of linear polymers into highly directed and extended conformations.

In the lab, total draw ratios of up to 350 have been attained. The highest specific tensile properties of any polymeric fiber are produced by this so-called gel spun UHMWPE. A maximum tensile modulus of 220 GPa and a maximum tensile strength of 6.0 GPa have been recorded in systematic tests of gel spun UHMWPE fibers [9].

10.4.6 Sintering

UHMWPE that is powdery or granular is compressed into the appropriate shape at a specific temperature and pressure during the sintering process. Melting, coalescence, and crystallization make up the process. Typically, pressures of 3–5 MPa and temperatures of 180–220 °C are needed to process UHMWPE by sintering. On the final shape of the mold, a significant dependence between shrinkage rate and cooling rate was seen. Consequently, it is advised that the molded shape be gradually cooled under pressure [11].

10.5 TRIBOLOGICAL NATURE AND PERFORMANCE OF UHM-WPE IMPLANTS (DENTAL, KNEE, HIP, SPINAL, ANKLE, ETC.)

Since the 1960s, TJR has been considered one of the most effective surgical procedures. Metal-on-polymer, ceramic-on-polymer, and metal-on-metal are now the three most used material combinations for artificial hip and knee joints.

UHMWPE is a popular and effective material for TJRs. Because wear is still a significant clinical issue, UHMWPE's wear resistance is the limiting factor in its application. Experimental studies have shown that, when done under the right circumstances, the introduction of ionizing radiation (gamma rays) can increase wear resistance of UHMWPE [12].

Any hip- or knee-related condition makes walking extremely difficult and severely disables the patient. The femoral head and the acetabulum in the pelvis form the spherical hip joint.

Regarding the clinical effectiveness of total joint replacements over the long term, UHMWPE wear has attracted significant attention. Two separate wear mechanisms that are active in total hip and complete knee replacements have been identified through clinical retrieval analysis. While the majority of the wear debris generated by the acetabular component is less than a micron in size and frequently particulate or fibrous in nature, the tibial component generates substantially bigger, thin flake-like wear debris [41].

UHMWPE has been used successfully in artificial implants, such as knee and hip joint replacements, due to its exceptional wear resistance and low-friction surface qualities. Its biological inertness, high levels of strength, wear, creep resistance, and low friction coefficient are all factors in its utilization. However, the wear debris produced by joint motions may result in osteolysis and implant loosening, which would add to the primary reason for joint revision. Since UHMWPE outperforms other polymers in terms of wear resistance, high fracture toughness, and biocompatibility as an articulating counterface for arthroplasties, it is the industry standard [20].

10.6 SURFACE MODIFICATIONS METHODS TO ENHANCE WEAR RESISTIVITY

UHMWPE is not appropriate for use in medical applications due to its low melting point (130–136 °C). However, limitations may be circumvented by using composite materials for reinforcement, such as carbon nanotubes. The generation of free radicals during gamma irradiation is another disadvantage of UHMWPE. When exposed for a long time, these radicals are prone to react with oxygen and rupture polymer chains. They may also cause the crystalline part of the substance to degrade. The main reasons for the high wear rate of medical implants are their biomechanics, impingement, and loosening when utilized in joints and hip arthroplasty. The major treatment for these problems is the use of highly cross-linked ultra-high-molecular-weight polyethylene because it lowers material wear debris and osteolysis as a result.

The surface modification of pristine UHMWPE or the reinforcing of base UHMWPE material with ceramic/composites can both be used to get over UHMWPE's limitations in biomedical applications. Next, we'll go through two techniques to modify UHMWPE for use in biomedical applications.

1. Surface modifications to pure UHMWPE by means of an electron beam, immersion in carbon ions, or cold atmospheric plasma with air present.
2. Composite materials such as hydroxyapatite (HAP), multiwalled carbon nanotubes (MWCNT), gallic acid (GA), dodecyl gallate (DG), nanographene

oxide, diamond-like carbon (DLC) films, vinyl triethoxysilane, which serves as a coupling agent, and gallic acid (GA) and dodecyl gallate (DG) are used to reinforce UHMWPE matrix reinforcement. Improved bulk and surface qualities, including low wear rate, high tensile strength, biocompatibility, oxidation resistance, and low coefficient of friction, are the result of these reinforcements added to the UHMWPE matrix.

The functionalization of pure-medical-grade UHMWPE has been achieved by surface treatment of polymeric material with an electron beam in the presence of air, which results in enhancement of the surface properties of polymer [42–44].

10.7 FUTURE DIRECTIONS AND ADVANCEMENTS IN UHMWPE BIOIMPLANTS

Researchers have created a tensile and biocompatible biomaterial with potential use as a medical implant as a result of the rise in various medical causalities and the steadily rising global elderly population. Researchers' in-depth investigations have uncovered various materials, such as UHMWPE, that are used as a main component in the production of biomaterials. This material has been seen to have some limitations, such as a limited lifespan for medical implants and low wear resistance, but an alternative approach to controlling implant aging has been developed, focusing on reinforcing UHMWPE with various fibers or chemicals capable of functionalizing the material and enhancing its properties. Mechanical characteristics, wear resistance, biocompatibility, cytocompatibility, wettability, and surface characteristics of biomaterials are among the functionalized attributes.

Bioimplant manufacturing frequently combines the processes of material selection, bioimplant design and manufacture, and surface modification by micro-/nanotexturing or nanomaterial coating. Utilizing functionalized UHMWPE, the future of the medical implant industry is focused on offering simple, affordable treatments for orthopedic problems that are experienced internationally.

Utilizing functionalized UHMWPE, the future of the medical implant industry is focused on offering simple, affordable treatments for orthopedic problems that are experienced internationally [45,46].

10.8 CONCLUSION

Due to the rise in various medical causalities and the gradually increasing number of older people worldwide, researchers have developed a tensile and biocompatible biomaterial that may be used as a medical implant. Extensive study has shown a variety of materials, including UHMWPE, that are key components in the biomaterials production process. The field of high-performance specialty polymer research, development, and commercialization has grown significantly in the last several years. Because of its acceptable strength properties for a polymer such as its high wear resistance, low coefficient of friction, chemical resistance in harsh media, and fracture toughness. UHMWPE can be used widely in a range of engineering fields and under a variety of operating conditions. The wear resistance of metal-polymer tribo-joints can be increased by a factor of five when UHMWPE-based materials are used. In recent years, several micro- and nanocomposites based on UHMWPE have been produced. However, the exact mechanisms underlying the great wear resistance of compositions built on matrices with high molecular weight are still not well understood. The impact of supramolecular structural factors on the wear resistance of microcomposites is a topic of discussion in particular.

REFERENCES

1. Gang Shen, Jufan Zhang, Ruslan Melentiev, Fengzhou Fang 2021. Study on tribological performance of groove-textured bioimplants. *Journal of the Mechanical Behavior of Biomedical Materials* 119: 104514.
2. A. Sumayli 2021. Recent trends on bioimplant materials: A review. *Materials Today: Proceedings* 46: 2726–2731.
3. S. V. Panin, L. A. Kornienko, N. Sonjaitham, M. V. Tchaikina, V. P. Sergeev, L. R. Ivanova, S. V. Shilko 2012. Wear-resistant ultrahigh-molecular-weight polyethylene-based nano- and microcomposites for implants. *Journal of Nanotechnology* 2012: 729756.
4. Muzamil Hussain, Rizwan Ali Naqvi, Naseem Abbas, Shahzad Masood Khan, Saad Nawaz, Arif Hussain, Nida Zahra, Muhammad Waqas Khalid 2020. Ultra-high-molecular-weight-polyethylene (UHMWPE) as a promising polymer material for biomedical applications: A concise review. *Polymers* 12: 323.
5. Pierangiola Bracco, Anuj Bellare, Alessandro Bistolfi, Saverio Affatato 2017. Ultra-high molecular weight polyethylene: Influence of the chemical, physical and mechanical properties on the wear behavior. A review. *Materials* 10: 791.
6. Steven M. Kurtz 2009. The origins of UHMWPE in total hip arthroplasty. In *UHMWPE Biomaterials Handbook*, 33–44. William Andrew, Applied Science Publishers.
7. Stephen Spiegelberg, Adam Kozak, Gavin Braithwaite 2016. Characterization of physical, chemical, and mechanical properties of UHMWPE. *UHMWPE Biomaterials Handbook* (3rd Edition). *Ultra High Molecular Weight Polyethylene in Total Joint Replacement and Medical Devices*, 531–552. William Andrew, Applied Science Publishers.
8. Oscar Olea-Mejia, Witold Brostow, Eli Buchman 2010. Wear resistance and wear mechanisms in polymer + metal composites. *Journal of Nanoscience and Nanotechnology* 10: 8254–8259.
9. Theo A. Tervoort, Jeroen Visjager, Paul Smith 2002. On abrasive wear of polyethylene. *Macromolecules* 35: 8467–8471.
10. Sudhakar Padmanabhan, Krishna R. Sarma, Kishor Rupak, Shashikant Sharma 2010. Synthesis of ultrahigh molecular weight polyethylene: A differentiate material for specialty applications. *Materials Science and Engineering B* 168: 132–135.
11. Veronica Manescu, Iulian Antoniac, Aurora Antoniac, Gheorghe Paltanea, Marian Miculescu, Ana-Iulia Bita, Stefan Laptoiu, Marius Niculescu, Alexandru Stere, Costel Paun, Mihai Bogdan Cristea 2022. Failure analysis of ultra-high molecular weight polyethylene tibial insert in total knee arthroplasty. *Materials* 15: 1–20.

12. Gang Shen, Fengzhou Fang, Chengwei Kang 2018. Tribological performance of bioimplants: A comprehensive review. *Nanotechnology and Precision Engineering* 1: 107–122.
13. Mary Beth Turell, Anuj Bellare2004. A study of the nanostructure and tensile properties of ultra-high molecular weight polyethylene. *Biomaterials* 25: 3389–3398.
14. M. C. Sobieraj, C. M. Rimnac 2009, Ultra high molecular weight polyethylene: Mechanics, morphology, and clinical behavior. *Journal of the Mechanical Behavior of Biomedical Materials* 2(5): 433–443.
15. Alessandro Ralls, Pankaj Kumar, Mano Misra, Pradeep L. Menezes 2020. Material design and surface engineering for bio-implants. *JOM* 72: 684–696.
16. Deepika Shekhawat, Amit Singh, Ashray Bhardwaj, Amar Patnaik 2021. A short review on polymer. *Metal and Ceramic Based Implant Materials* 1017: 012038.
17. Jun Fu, Bassem W. Ghali, Andrew J. Lozynsky, Ebru Oral, Orhun K. Muratoglu 2011. Wear resistant UHMWPE with high toughness by high temperature melting and subsequent radiation cross-linking. *Polymer* 52: 1155–1162.
18. Gladius Lewis 2001. Properties of crosslinked ultra-high-molecular-weight polyethylene. *Biomaterials* 22: 371–401.
19. Gang Shen, Jufan Zhang, Chengwei Kang, Fengzhou Fang 2021. Study on surface texture patterns for improving tribological performance of bioimplants. *Surface & Coatings Technology* 422: 127567.
20. Domingos Lusitâneo Pier Macuvele, Janaína Nones, Jonas V. Matsinhe, Marla M. Lima, Cíntia Soares, Márcio A. Fiori, Humberto G. Riella 2017.Advances in ultrahigh molecular weight polyethylene/hydroxyapatite composites for biomedical applications: A brief review. *Materials Science and Engineering* C76: 1248–1262.
21. Piotr Olesik, Marcin Godzierz, Mateusz Kozio 2019. Preliminary characterization of novel LDPE-based wear-resistant composite suitable for FDM 3D printing. *Materials* 12: 2520.
22. Adiye Emel Sokullu Urkaç 2006. Characterization of ultrahigh molecular weight polyethylene (UHMWPE) modified by metal-gas hybrid ion implantation technique. Thesis.
23. S. M. Kurtz, O. K. Muratoglu, M. Evans, A. A. Edidin 1999. Advances in the processing sterilization and crosslinking of ultra-high molecular weight polyethylene for total joint arthroplasty. *Biomaterials* 20: 1659–1688.
24. Giuseppe Forte, Sara Ronca 2017. Synthesis of disentangled ultra-high molecular weight polyethylene: Influence of reaction medium on material properties. *International Journal of Polymer Science* 2017: 7431419.
25. D. S. Li, H. Garmestani, S. Ahzi, M. Khaleel, D. Ruch 2009. Microstructure design to improve wear resistance in bioimplant UHMWPE materials. *Journal of Engineering Materials and Technology* 131: 041211.
26. Huan Zhang, Shicheng Zhao, Zhong Xin, Chunlin Ye, Zhi Li, Jincheng Xia2019. Wear resistance mechanism of ultrahigh-molecular-weight polyethylene determined from its structure—property relationships. *Industrial & Engineering Chemistry Research* 58(42): 19519–19530.
27. G. E. Selyutin, Yu. Yu. Gavrilov, E. N. Voskresenskaya, V. A. Zakharov, V. E. Nikitin, V. A. Poluboyarov 2010. Composite materials based on ultrahigh molecular polyethylene: Properties, application prospects. *Chemistry for Sustainable Development* 18: 301–314.
28. John M. Kelly 2002. Ultra-high molecular weight polyethylene. *Journal of Macromolecular Science Part C-Polymer Reviews* C42 (3): 355–371.
29. Ketan Patel, Samir H. Chikkali, Swaminathan Sivaram2020.Ultrahigh molecular weight polyethylene: Catalysis, structure, properties, processing and applications. *Progress in Polymer Science* 109: 101290.

30. Frantisek Cerny, Mohamed Ali Khalil Ibrahim, Jan Suchanek, Svatava Konvickova, Vladimir Jech, Zdenek Horak 2012. Improvement of UHMWPE properties for bio-implants by gamma irradiation. *Materials Science Forum* 700: 207–210.
31. Zhaoxiang Liu, Haochen Zhang 2022. Ultra-high molecular weight polyethylene: Preparation and applications. *Journal of Physics: Conference Series* 2229: 012006.
32. Yanping Wang, Ruiling Cheng, Linli Liang, Yimin Wang 2005. Study on the prep-aration and characterization of ultra-high molecular weight polyethylene–carbon nanotubes composite fiber. *Composites Science and Technology* 65: 793–797.
33. A. Wang, D. C. Sun, S.-S. Yau, B. Edwards, M. Sokol, A. Essner, V. K. Polineni, C. Stark, J. H. Dumbleton 1997. Orientation softening the deformation and wear of ultra-high molecular weight polyethylene. *Wear* 203–204: 230–241.
34. A. El-Domiaty, M. El-Fadaly, A.Es. Nassef 2002. Wear characteristics of ultrahigh molecular weight polyethylene (UHMWPE). *Journal of Materials Engineering and Performance* 11(5): 577.
35. A. Valenza, A. M. Visco, L. Torrisib, N. Campo 2004. Characterization of ultra-high-molecular-weight polyethylene (UHMWPE) modified by ion implantation. *Polymer* 45: 1707–1715.
36. D. M. Rein, Y. Cohen, J. Lipp, E. Zussman 2009. Preparation of ultra-high molec-ular weight polyethylene fibers, electrospun with carbon nanotubes, *Materials Science*, 1–8.
37. O. V. Gogoleva, P. N. Petrova, S. N. Popov, A. A. Okhlopkova 2015. Wear resistant composite materials based on ultrahigh molecular weight polyethylene and basalt fibers. *Journal of Friction and Wear* 36 (4): 301–305.
38. Ketan Patel, Samir H. Chikkali, Swaminathan Sivaram 2020. Ultrahigh molecular weight polyethylene: Catalysis, structure, properties, processing and applications. *Progress in Polymer Science* 109: 101290.
39. A. Bertoluzza, C. Fagnano, M. Rossi, A. Tinti, G. L. Cacciari 2000. Micro-Raman spectroscopy for the crystallinity characterization of UHMWPE hip cups run on joint simulators. *Journal of Molecular Structure* 521: 89–95.
40. H. S. Dobbs 1982: Characterization of molecular weight polyethylene. *Biomaterials* 3: 49–51.
41. A. Wang, D. C. Sun, C. Stark, J. H. Dumbleton 1995. Wear mechanisms of UHMWPE in total joint replacements. *Wear* 181–183: 241–249.
42. Nikhil Avinash Patil, James Njuguna, Balasubramanian Kandasubramanian 2020. UHMWPE for biomedical applications: Performance and functionalization. *European Polymer Journal* 125: 109529.
43. S. V. Panina, L. A. Kornienko, T. Nguen Suan, L. R. Ivanova, M. A. Poltaranin, S. V. Shilko 2014. Wear resistance of composites based on ultrahigh molecular weight polyethylene filled with graphite and molybdenum disulfide microparticles. *Journal of Friction and Wear* 35(4): 290–296.
44. Wei Li, Haiyan Hu 2018. Study on preparation of ultrahigh molecular weight poly-ethylene fibers. *Advances in Computer Science Research* 78: 15–18.
45. S. Sathishkumar, J. Paulraj, P. Chakraborti, M. Muthuraj 2023. Comprehensive review on biomaterials and their inherent behaviors for hip repair applications. *ACS Applied Bio Materials* 11, 4439–4464.
46. Aravind Bhat Kalambettu, Padmavathi Rajangam, Sangeetha Dharmalingam 2012. The effect of chlorotrimethylsilane on bonding of nano hydroxyapatite with a chitosan–polyacrylamide matrix. *Carbohydrate Research* 352: 143–150.

11 Wear Debris Implications on Bioimplants

Artificial Hip Joints

S Sathishkumar[1], P Jawahar[1], Prasun Chakraborti[1],
M Muthusivaramapandian[1], S Indiran[2],
P Sathishkumar[2], and Suchart Siengchin[2]
[1] National Institute of Technology
Agartala, Tripura, India
[2] King Mongkut's University of Technology
North Bangkok, Thailand

11.1 INTRODUCTION

People in the developing world might enjoy high living standards, yet the general health is declining for several reasons, especially hip failures. The hip is the second largest weight-bearing bone in the human body, and its joint is a ball-and-socket structure made up of four distinct parts: the femoral stem, the femoral head, the cartilage liner, and the acetabulum (Sivasankar et al., 2016). Figure 11.1

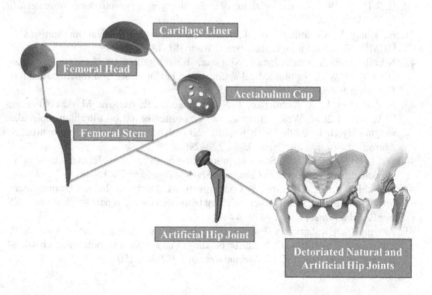

FIGURE 11.1 Deteriorated hip joint and artificial hip joint with wear debris.

DOI: 10.1201/9781003384847-11

represents natural and artificial hip joints with debris. While osteoarthritis, rheumatoid arthritis, and osteonecrosis are common causes of hip failure, other factors, such as childhood illness and injury, can also contribute (Kelmer et al., 2021). The metals (Bolognesi & Ledford, 2015) (cobalt alloy, [Co] stainless steel [316L], titanium alloy [Ti], ceramics [Goswami et al., 2021] (alumina [Al_2O_3], zirconia [ZrO_2], zirconia-toughened alumina [ZTA]), and polymers (Banoriya et al., 2017) (nylon (PTFE), ultra-high-molecular-weight-polyethylene (UHMWPE), and polyether ether Ketone (PEEK) are great feasible implant materials used for various hip repair applications (Sathishkumar et al., 2023).

Tribology is intertwined with the human body, which may be observed in teeth, bones, heart valves, skin, and eyes. As a result, every human should understand tribology's fundamental mechanisms and how to deal with difficulties that arise (Zhou & Jin, 2015). The wear-related feature of bioimplants occurs when the implant has two mating surfaces (for example, cortical bone with infused implants.

A complete in vitro examination of implant friction, wear, and bodily lubricant behavior on encapsulated scaffolds is required before implantation due to the possibility of created wear debris causing a pathological response to the implanted body (Di Puccio & Mattei, 2015). In lubricated and dry circumstances, in vitro wear, experiments often use pin-on-disk (Wahyudi et al., 2020), pin-on-plate (Ranuša et al., 2022), ball-on-disk (Shankar et al., 2022), and ball-on-plate (Wang et al., 2022) tribometers. In this scenario, one material acts as the tested material and the other as the counterface. Sometimes the same material is used for both parts (like a pin and a plate) to test how prepared materials wear when they rub against each other.

The resulting wear debris causes severe pathological reactions in the host body, including inflammation, bone resorption, osteolysis, tissue necrosis, and aseptic loosening (Costa et al., 2023). They truly promote implant failure, which leads to revision surgery; therefore, dealing with this wear debris is a critical responsibility for orthopedic surgeons (Reyes Rojas et al., 2023b). In this regard, the causes for wear debris creation, implications, and treatment strategies for extending the durability of artificial hip joints are comprehensively presented in this chapter.

11.2 PRINCIPLE OF FRICTION AND WEAR

Friction and wear are irresistible and complicated processes of materials opposing one another, such as in sliding or rolling movements. They are determined solely by the elements present, surface attributes, and surface textures (Arulkumar et al., 2023). The outer boundary of components is generally considered a surface, which has evolved due to the preparation procedures and operational settings. The surface characteristics of the component may differ marginally or completely from their bulk properties. Surface texture is another significant factor for constructing friction and wear qualities, which are defined by varying amplitudes and frequencies of surface irregularities, referred to as "surface topography" (Arulkumar et al., 2023).

The profilometer measures these surface imperfections and is classified into two categories based on the present profiles: roughness and waviness. Roughness refers to the inherent imperfections of the surfaces that form throughout the manufacturing process, while waviness refers to the superimposed roughness of the surfaces (Arnell, 2010). Surface roughness assessment is the most important responsibility during wear testing studies (before and after testing), since it determines the possibility of implant wear debris developing after implantation. Surface roughness is typically determined using the roughness average Ra and the root mean square deviation Rq, as shown in Equations (11.1) and (11.2).

$$Ra = \frac{1}{N} \sum_{n=1}^{N} \left| X_n \right|''$$ (11.1)

$$Rq = \sqrt{\frac{1}{N} \sum_{n=1}^{N} X_n^{2''}}$$ (11.2)

N represents the total number of readings, and X_n represents the distance between the nth reading and the center line. The development of stresses between two mating surfaces significantly impacts friction and wear behavior. Several key factors influence stress concentration on components, such as surface asperities and shapes, surface roughness, and elastic and plastic properties; so, before implantation, the effective surface properties followed by wear evaluation are most important for successful various clinical applications (Joshi et al., 2022).

11.3   WEAR MEASUREMENT LAWS AND MECHANISMS

Continuous rubbing causes the mating surfaces to undergo permanent deformation and wear, widening the chasm between them. Wear laws and the material removal rate are often used to assess the impact of wear depth profiles, which may be measured in terms of the mass of removed materials, the volume of removed materials, and the decrease in the bodies' dimensions (Niemczewska-Wójcik, 2017). The Archard wear law, which is fully detailed next, is widely used to assess wear depth.

11.3.1   Archard Wear Law

The friction and wear range of mating surfaces is determined by sliding conditions (normal pressure and sliding velocity) and the materials' qualities. The wear equation was first developed by Holm in 1946; it relates the volume of material withdrawn (W) in the sliding distance (S) to their actual contact areas. Nevertheless, the wear equation, as stated by Archard in 1953, is now universally recognized (Zmitrowicz, 2006). According to the Archard law, the volume of material removed (W) is directly proportional to the normal pressure (PN), sliding distance (S), and wear coefficients (K) and indirectly proportional to the worn away surface hardness (H).

The Archard equation is:

$$W = K \frac{P_N S}{H}$$ (11.3)

In recent years, wear is directly related to the load (W), the volume of materials removed (Δ_V), and sliding distance (D), as represented in Equation (11.4).

$$K = \frac{\Delta_V}{WD} \qquad (11.4)$$

11.3.2 Wear Mechanisms (Patterns)

The removal of surface material due to relative motion between the bodies included a number of mechanisms and influenced factors, as shown in Figures 11.2 and 11.3.

11.3.2.1 Abrasive Wear

Abrasive wear is one of the most prevalent forms of wear caused by harder surfaces rubbing against softer surfaces. In general, two forms of abrasive wear have been found in hip implants: abrasion of two bodies and abrasion of three bodies. Normally, three-body abrasion can cause serious damage to the host body (Wang et al., 2019). These effects depend on the hardness and roughness of the surfaces, the size and shape of the abrasive particles, and the pressure and speed of the rubbing motion (Varga et al., 2023). This abrasive wear reduction or removal is the most important duty for artificial joints. It will naturally decrease owing to bodily fluid lubrication, and the surface coating on implants is another viable technique for reducing abrasive wear.

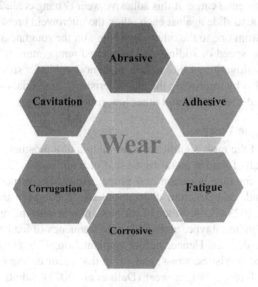

FIGURE 11.2   Wear mechanisms of artificial hip joints.

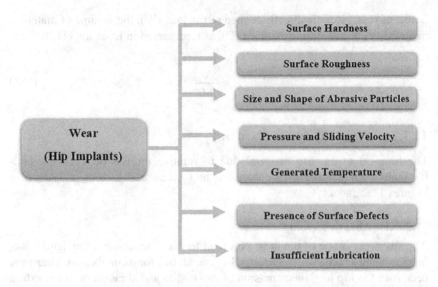

FIGURE 11.3   Major factors determining wear on artificial hip implants.

11.3.2.2   Adhesive Wear

Adhesive wear is a complex phenomenon of artificial implants that may substantially influence their reliability and longevity. This form of wear is often characterized by material transfer from one surface to another, resulting in surface damage and eventually implant deterioration. The production of microwelds between the mating surfaces, caused by high contact pressure and distortion of surface asperities, is the fundamental cause of this adhesive wear (Zhang et al., 2023). When the surfaces continue to slide against each other, the microweld breaks, and the material transitions from one to the other, depending on the roughness of the surfaces, contact pressure, speed of sliding, and generated temperature (Cui et al., 2020). As a result, the mitigation of this wear is most noticeable for successful implants, which are enabled by improving the characteristics of materials and their surface coating (diamond-like carbon and other low-friction coatings).

11.3.2.3   Fatigue Wear

Fatigue is one of the most significant wear factors of a prosthetic joint; this form of wear is typically found in metal-based scaffolds and is induced by cyclic stress, which leads to fracture initiation and propagation. Microstructural alterations, such as slip bands and structure dislocation, also accompany this kind of wear (Beadling et al., 2023). A multitude of variables may impact the severity of fatigue wear, including material type, magnitude, and frequency of loading, and the presence of surface defects. Hence, before implantation, it is feasible to measure the material characteristics, stress, and strain that occur during cyclic loading to understand and forecast fatigue wear (Dalli et al., 2022). Additionally, considerable computational analysis is necessary before material selection to check the complicated interaction between surfaces, leading to an estimate of fatigue wear before implantation. Under these conditions, it is critical to eliminate or reduce fatigue wear, which is accomplished by designing innovative alloys with strong fatigue resistance, a range of surface treatments, and improved coatings over the implant's surfaces (Bian et al., 2023).

11.3.2.4 Corrosive Wear

Corrosive wear may have serious consequences for the function and safety of hip implants. When exposed to a corrosive environment, the implant can undergo chemical reactions with the surrounding tissues and body fluids (Gessner et al., 2019). The corrosive environment within the human body can be highly acidic or alkaline, and the presence of enzymes and other biological compounds can motivate the corrosive process. This can lead to metal ion leaching. The released ions can be poisonous and cause hypersensitive reactions, such as inflammation and tissue damage over time, which can cause implants to fail and lead to revision surgeries (Ricciardi et al., 2016). Controlling corrosive wear is an important task for successful implantation. This is possible because corrosion-resistant materials with good biocompatibility with human tissues and surface treatments and coatings significantly impact corrosion resistance, ensuring the durability and effectiveness of the implants.

11.3.2.5 Corrugation Wear

Corrugation wear is a kind of material deterioration characterized by the creation of grooves and ridges on the surfaces of implants, which accelerates high friction and wear. Two distinct causes determine the creation of grooves and ridges: the presence of impurities and an inadequate lubrication system (Findik, 2020). These wear mechanisms entail repetitive deformations and plastic flow of materials, which may cause damage to surrounding tissues and end in implant failure. Preventing corrugation wear on hip implants by choosing high wear-resistant implant materials with acceptable biocompatibility and maintaining an adequate lubrication system is another effective strategy to minimize or lessen these effects. Additionally, frequent monitoring may be very beneficial in detecting signs of wear or damage and allowing for prompt replacement and revision procedures (Kheradmandfard et al., 2018).

11.3.2.6 Cavitation Wear

Cavitation wear is a puzzling phenomenon often occurring in the biomedical prosthesis realm. These types of wear occur when cavitation shock waves collapse near implant surfaces, producing microscopic pits, fissures, and other types of surface deterioration (Li et al., 2021). These faults spread over time, resulting in material loss and degradation, which may eventually lead to implant failure. Moreover, cavitation wear is often aggravated by corrosion, fatigue, and fretting, which may further impair the stability of encapsulated implants. Thus dealing with this wear is tough. However, it is possible with specialized coatings like DLC, titanium nitride (TiN) coating, and surface treatments such as shot peening, laser texturing,

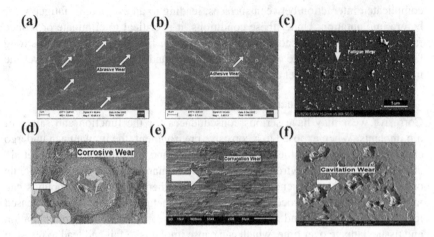

FIGURE 11.4   Different wear mechanism on artificial hip joints: (a) abrasive wear on GO-HA-PEEK-stainless steel, (b) adhesive wear on HA-PEEK-stainless steel, (c) fatigue wear on polyethylene-stainless steel (adapted from Dalli et al., 2022), (d) corrosive wear on Co-Cr-polyethylene (adapted from Ricciardi et al., 2016), (e) corrugation wear on titanium implants (adapted from ref (Kheradmandfard et al., 2018), (f) cavitation wear on metal implants (adapted from Jasionowski et al., 2016). Copyright Permission received for all figures.

and feasible implant designs (Skjöldebrand et al., 2022). Figure 11.4 showcases the different wear mechanisms that appeared in various hip implant materials.

11.4   TRIBOLOGICAL NATURE OF BIOIMPLANTS

The tribological characteristics of materials influence the performance, lifespan, and comfort of infected patients; hence, researchers should pay attention to their tribological natures and their reactivity with bodily fluids prior to implantation. Previous medical research indicates that the three various uppermost materials considerably help to lessen sufferers' tragedies, as shown in Figure 11.5. The tribological characteristics of implant materials and strategies for enhancing such characteristics are discussed in detail next.

11.4.1   METALS-BASED ARTIFICIAL HIP JOINTS

Due to their diverse physical properties, metals and their alloys are the key materials for several physiological applications. Nevertheless, wear and corrosion are significant negative consequences of metals, contributing to implant failure and further revision surgery (Heneghan et al., 2012). The materials connected with hip implants are shown in Figure 11.5.

The presence of carbide in the Co-based alloys gives them outstanding wear resistance compared to other metals. Nevertheless, the phase transformation (from metastable to martensitic) might have a detrimental impact on wear.

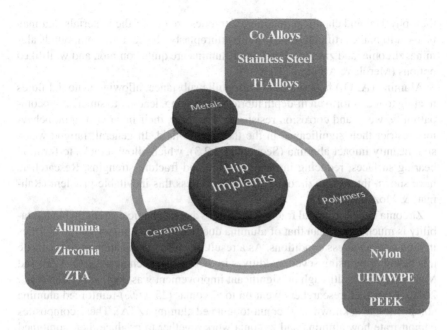

FIGURE 11.5 Effective materials for artificial hip joints.

In artificial hip joints, the femoral head is often exposed to a high wear rate; hence co-alloys are more desirable for use in the femoral head, although their Ni components strongly stimulate allergic responses in the impregnated body. In addition, compared to human cortical bone, the stress simulation value is significantly higher, leading to aseptic loosening and bone or implant fractures (Matusiewicz & Richter, 2022). Stainless steels of medical grade are another potentially useful metallic compound for prosthetic hip joints, although the Ni compounds they contain are the source of unpleasant effects. In addition, stainless steel hip implants have been shown to exhibit signs of very intense stress corrosion, including crevices and pitting (Marquez et al., 2023). In recent years, titanium-based alloys have occupied a prominent place in the medical market due to their mechanical and biological behaviors. On the other hand, the tribological behaviors of this element are not at a remarkable level due to low work hardening, low protection exerted by surface oxides, and low plastic shearing resistivity. Furthermore, the long-term presence of aluminum (Al) and vanadium (V) stimulates osteomalacia, neuropathy, and Alzheimer's disease. Hence, these all-metal implants, comprised of nickel, chromium, aluminum, and vanadium, develop allergic reactions on the host body, which shortens the lifespan of the artificial implants (Beadling et al., 2023).

11.4.2 Ceramics-Based Artificial Hip Joints

Ceramics are one of the inorganics, nonmetallic materials attracting the attention of medical scientists and orthopedic surgeons owing to the remarkable appeal of their physical and chemical qualities. Ceramics are one of the materials that may be used to make artificial joints. In hip arthroplasty, the ceramic compounds alumina, zirconia, and zirconia-toughened alumina are quite common and well-liked options (Merola & Affatato, 2019).

Alumina (Al_2O_3) behaves as a hydrophilic substance, allowing synovial fluids to cling to it and form an in-depth lubricating coating, leading to superior biocompatibility, wear, and corrosion resistance. However, their inherent fragile behaviors restrict their significance in the therapeutic field. In general, fatigue wears significantly impact alumina (Section 11.3.2.3), which allows cracks to form on bearing surfaces, reducing implants' tensile and fracture strengths. Researchers have shown interest in zirconia (ZrO_2) to address this inevitable problem (Rahmati & Mozafari, 2019).

Zirconia has exceptional fracture toughness and mechanical strength, but its stability is much lower than that of alumina due to its phase transformation abilities in high contact stress conditions. As a result, the researchers attempt to eradicate this behavior by using several additives in their study, such as Y_2O_3 (Y-TZP) and MgO (Mg-PSZ), although no significant improvement was obtained (Chen et al., 2016). After that, researchers went on to zirconia- (25 wt.%)-reinforced alumina composites, also known as zirconia-toughened alumina (ZTA). These composites demonstrate how alumina and zirconia work together to produce their combined effects, such as excellent resistance to the onset and propagation of cranking, a high level of toughness, an extraordinary level of wear resistance, and raised levels of chemical and hydrothermal stability, but, in long-term applications, it does not exhibit favorable responses in the host body (Reyes Rojas et al., 2023a).

11.4.3 POLYMER-BASED ARTIFICIAL HIP JOINTS

Polymers have become more popular as biomaterials in recent years because of their multiple desirable properties, including their low weight, high strength, resistance to corrosion and chemicals, flexibility, aesthetics, etc. In addition, it offers expanding structural characteristics, which are determined by their molecular weight, backbone structure, degree of cross-linking, entanglement density, and degree of crystallinity (Sathishkumar et al., 2022b). Polymers such as polytetrafluoroethylene (PTFE), ultra-high-molecular-weight polyethylene (UHMWPE) and polyether ether ketone (PEEK) are typically some of the most common types of polymers used in a variety of hip repair applications (Sankar et al., 2023).

Nylon is a more stable and hydrophobic material. However, it has no known notable wear resistance properties, with an estimated 0.5 mm wear rate per month, and it issues a large number of amorphous materials into the host body, which may cause serious adverse responses. Researchers tried using glass fiber (GF) inclusion to speed up nylon's wear behavior, but the results were unimpressive; the material still released a high volume of abrasive particles, which might contribute to an increase of 20% in infection and 57% in implant loosening.

UHMWPE is another promising polymer with intriguing uses. In short-term applications, these polymers' outstanding fracture toughness, low friction, and high wear resistance shine. However, in the long term, the creation of wear debris restricts the polymer's wear behavior. As a solution, UHMEPE is subjected to a thermally induced cross-linking process (like annealing) that produces the material's expected wear resistance at the expense of its stiffness, toughness, and tensile strength. Researchers have recently shifted their focus to PEEK polymers (Affatato et al., 2015). PEEK is a high-performance, biocompatible element with excellent mechanical and wear properties. Clinical data suggest that adding carbon fiber (CF) and carbon nanotubes (CNTs) to PEEK increases the material's wear resistance; several researchers are now striving to enhance and improve the longevity of PEEK-based polymers used in artificial hip applications (Sathishkumar et al., 2022a).

11.5 WEAR DEBRIS IMPACT ON HOST BODY

The primary cause of implant failure is the formation and accumulation of wear debris, which has a devastating effect on human health. Allergenic reactions are triggered by these minute particles, which dissolve readily in bodily fluids. Figure 11.6 depicts the unavoidable problems that arise from wear debris on an enclosed body.

11.5.1 INFLAMMATION

Inflammation is a complex biological reaction of the human body's immune system to damaging stimuli such as pathogens, irritants, and cell damage, characterized by the release of proinflammatory elements such as cytokines and chemokines that may attract immune cells to wounded and infected areas (Sargeant & Goswami, 2006).

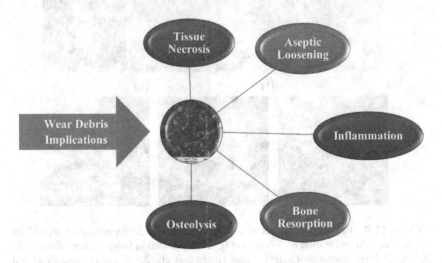

FIGURE 11.6 Wear Debris Impact on Artificial Hip Joints.

In general, the inflammatory reaction is split into two stages, which are shown in Figure 11.7. The acute stages occur within minutes to hours following infection or injury and include activating resident immune cells such as macrophages and mast cells. They are produced as pro-inflammatory cytokines, which increase vascular permeability, cause vasodilation, and activate other immune cells to address the issues, but the acute inflammatory phases are not always resolved owing to a low-grade immune response, which allows the chronic phase to take over.

Chronic inflammation is the process through which immune cells such as T-cells and macrophages infiltrate infected organs (Eltit et al., 2019). In our scenario, the wear debris surrounding the hip implant induces chronic phase inflammation, which adversely affects the implanted body. The wear debris generated by the articulating surfaces activates immune cells to degrade the wear particles, but this is not possible during the acute phase. Hence the chronic phases try to degrade the debris with the influence of cytokines and chemokines. However, these molecules cause tissue damage, fibrosis, and osteoclast activity, leading to bone resorption and implant loosening. Figure 11.8 indicates (a) the wear debris generation around the implant (b), as well as the infiltration of T-cells and (c) cell degradation.

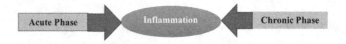

FIGURE 11.7   Phases of Inflammation.

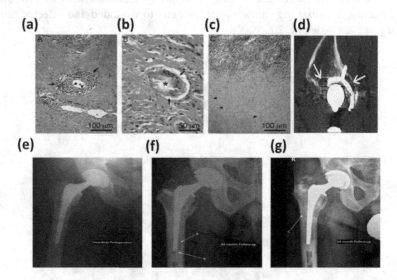

FIGURE 11.8   Pathological effects on wear debris: (a) wear debris generation around the implant (b). The infiltration of T-cells and (c) cell degradation (adapted from Eltit et al., 2019). (d) bone resorption (adapted from Holding et al., 2006). (e)–(g) osteolysis and aseptic loosening of the implant (adapted from Anil et al., 2022). Copyright permission received for all figures.

11.5.2 BONE RESORPTION

Bone resorption is a normal process in which osteoclasts break down and remove old or damaged bone tissue. A complex network of signaling pathways regulates bone resorption, including numerous hormones, cytokines, and growth factors (Sargeant & Goswami, 2006). RANKL, a signaling molecule generated by bone-forming cells called osteoblasts, activates osteoclasts. The binding of RANKL to its receptor on the surface of osteoclasts causes differentiation and activation, resulting in bone tissue destruction. Moreover, osteoclasts emit enzymes such as acid phosphatase and collagenase, which disintegrate the bone matrix and release minerals into the circulation, such as calcium and phosphate (Holding et al., 2006).

In the case of wear-debris-induced bone resorption in the hip joint, the inflammatory response elicited by the wear debris encourages the differentiation and activation of osteoclasts, resulting in the resorption of bone tissue around the implant. Figure 11.8d. depicts bone resorbed hip implant due to polyethylene wear. The wear debris particles trigger immune cells such as macrophages, which produce pro-inflammatory cytokines and chemokines, causing osteoclast activity and bone resorption. Moreover, wear debris may directly trigger osteoclast development and activation, leading to bone resorption. The process of bone resorption in the hip joint may result in the gradual degradation of bone tissue and implant loosening. When the bone tissue surrounding the implant resorbs, the implant becomes more unstable, resulting in discomfort and decreased joint motion. In extreme circumstances, the implant may entirely detach from the surrounding bone, causing major unpleasantness and disability (Restrepo-Noriega et al., 2022).

11.5.3 OSTEOLYSIS

Osteolysis is a pathological process characterized by excessive bone tissue resorption, resulting in bone mass and structural integrity loss. In reaction to the presence of wear debris, osteolysis includes the production of cytokines and chemokines such as tumor necrosis factor-alpha (TNF-) and interleukin-1 (IL-1). These signaling molecules stimulate immune cells like macrophages, which ingest the worn debris and create additional cytokines, triggering a chain reaction of inflammatory reactions (Sargeant & Goswami, 2006).

The inflammatory reaction causes osteoclasts to differentiate and activate, resulting in the disintegration of bone tissue surrounding the implant. The physical properties of the wear debris particles, such as their size and shape, might impact the severity of osteolysis in addition to the inflammatory response. Tiny particles have been demonstrated to be more efficient at triggering osteolysis than bigger particles because they are more easily phagocytosed by immune cells and may reach the bone tissue more quickly. Moreover, irregularly shaped particles, such as those created by abrasive wear, may harm bone tissue more than round or smooth particles (Eltit et al., 2019).

In the context of hip joint replacement surgery, osteolysis is closely connected with the accumulation of wear debris surrounding the implant, which causes inflammation and the activation of osteoclasts. Successful care of osteolysis in the hip joint requires a multifaceted strategy that tackles both the inflammatory response and the underlying mechanical causes that contribute to wear debris formation (Lin et al., 2022).

11.5.4 TISSUE NECROSIS

Tissue necrosis is a degenerative process that results in the death of cells and tissues as a consequence of a variety of circumstances such as trauma, infection, or ischemia. Tissue necrosis in the setting of hip joint replacement surgery may be induced by the buildup of wear particles surrounding the implant, resulting in inflammation and tissue destruction (Eltit et al., 2019). Tissue necrosis is caused by a complicated chain of events that includes disturbance of cellular metabolism, changes in ion homeostasis, and activation of apoptotic and necrotic cell death pathways. The development of worn debris surrounding the implant might activate immune cells, such as macrophages, which absorb the debris and generate additional cytokines, resulting in a cascade of inflammatory reactions. If the inflammatory reaction continues, tissue damage and cell death may occur, resulting in tissue necrosis (Xing et al., 2022).

The presence of wear debris may also disrupt the microvasculature, which decreases the quantity of blood that flows to the surrounding tissues and makes the damage to those tissues greater. The degree of tissue necrosis and the severity of the condition are both influenced by the nature and quantity of wear debris, as well as the reaction of the host to the debris. Necrosis of the tissues of the hip joint may have serious repercussions, including the failure of implants, increased joint discomfort, and decreased joint mobility. The necrotic tissue may secrete toxins that cause further harm to the tissues that are around the necrotic tissue as it dies. It is also possible for the necrotic tissue to serve as a location for bacterial infection, which may result in the implant becoming loose and the need for revision surgery (Eason et al., 2022).

11.5.5 ASEPTIC LOOSENING

Aseptic loosening is a seriously unfavorable disease defined by the separation of the prosthesis from the surrounding bone in the absence of infection. This disease is a frequent cause of failure in orthopedic surgery, especially hip joint replacement (Eltit et al., 2019). Aseptic loosening is mostly caused by wear debris produced by the implant's articulating surfaces, which causes an inflammatory reaction that leads to bone resorption and implant migration. The wear debris generated by the implant's articulating surfaces may vary in size from nanometers to micrometers. This debris may stimulate the immune system and induce a foreign body response, which sets off a chain of events that leads to bone resorption. Macrophages and other immune cells engulf and try to remove the debris, but they are unable to destroy the materials, resulting in persistent inflammation. The accumulating of wear debris, together with the inflammatory reaction, causes osteolysis and bone loss surrounding the implant (Holding et al., 2006). Figure 11.8d–g depicted the osteolysis and aseptic loosening of the hip implants.

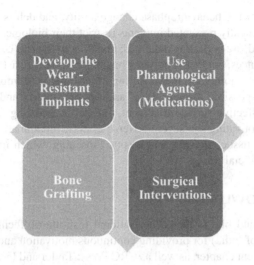

FIGURE 11.9 Effective methods for reduce wear implications.

The progressive process of aseptic loosening might take years to appear. Early symptoms may include mild pain and decreased joint mobility. When the situation worsens, the discomfort and movement restrictions intensify, and the implant becomes more unstable. In certain situations, the implant may entirely dislodge, causing severe suffering and dysfunction. Implant design, patient factors, and surgical technique are all factors that can lead to aseptic loosening. The design of an implant may have a substantial impact on wear debris formation and particle size. Patient variables, such as age, weight, and degree of activity, may potentially influence the rate of wear debris production. Implant stability and durability may be affected by surgical techniques, such as implant location and fixation. Thus careful control of wear debris is necessary. In order to increase the lifetime of artificial joints and give afflicted persons better quality of life, Figure 11.9 depicts a strategy for addressing and overcoming these debris responses on implanted bodies (Anil et al., 2022).

11.6 CONCLUSION

Wear management is a difficult assignment on biomedical implants that plays an important function in improving lifespan and ensuring patient comfort. The rate of wear of an implant material is determined by its surface hardness, surface roughness, abrasive particle size, shape, pressures, sliding velocity, generated temperature, presence of surface flaws, and lubrication level. Abrasive, adhesive, and fatigue wear significantly impact artificial joints. Metal-based implants have strong mechanical strength and wear resistance, but phase transition, Ni, Al, V, and Co emissions cause osteomalacia, neuropathy, and Alzheimer's disease, significantly reducing implant longevity. Ceramics offer short-term wear resistance.

However, their brittle behavior, phase change ability, and debris accumulation in long-term biologically presented implants restrict their biological use. Polymers, on the other hand, are appealing materials; however, nylon and UHMWPE display low wear resistances, but PEEK polymer has superior wear-resistant behaviors for artificial prosthetic joints. So the most important thing is to improve wear resistance, which is possible through novel and optimal matrix and reinforcements (composites), effective surface treatment, and surface coating methods that are capable of demotivating the severe adverse effects: inflammation, bone resorption, osteolysis, tissue necrosis, and aseptic loosening, which increases the longevity of the artificial joints.

11.7 ACKNOWLEDGMENTS

The authors would like to thank the National Institute of Technology Agartala (MHRD-Govt. of India) for providing continuous motivation and support in preparing this eminent chapter, as well as CRC Press: Taylor and Francis publication house for providing us with the wonderful opportunity to publish our chapter under the book title *Tribo-Behaviors of Biomaterials and Their Applications*.

11.7.1 CREDIT OF AUTHORSHIP CONTRIBUTION STATEMENT

S. Sathishkumar: Conceptualization, methodology, formal analysis, resources, investigation, data curation, writing–original draft
P. Jawahar: Supervision, editing
Prasun Chakraborti: Validation, project administration
M. Muthusivaramapandian: Editing, resources, and validation

11.7.2 DECLARATION OF COMPETING INTEREST

The authors declare that they have no known competing financial interests or personal relationships that could have appeared to influence the work reported in this chapter.

REFERENCES

Affatato, S., Ruggiero, A., & Merola, M. (2015). Advanced biomaterials in hip joint arthroplasty. A review on polymer and ceramics composites as alternative bearings. *Composites Part B: Engineering*, *83*, 276–283. https://doi.org/10.1016/j.compositesb.2015.07.019

Anil, U., Singh, V., & Schwarzkopf, R. (2022). Diagnosis and detection of subtle aseptic loosening in total hip arthroplasty. *The Journal of Arthroplasty*, *37*(8), 1494–1500. https://doi.org/10.1016/j.arth.2022.02.060

Arnell, D. (2010). Mechanisms and laws of friction and wear. In *Tribology and dynamics of engine and powertrain* (pp. 41–72). https://doi.org/10.1533/9781845699932.1.41

Arulkumar, M., Rangan, R. P., Ananth, M. P., Srividhyasakthi, V., & Aaditya, R. (2023). Experimental verification on the influence of surface texturing on biomaterials and study of its tribological characteristics. *Materials Today: Proceedings*. https://doi.org/10.1016/j.matpr.2023.01.172

Banoriya, D., Purohit, R., & Dwivedi, R. (2017). Advanced application of polymer based biomaterials. *Materials Today: Proceedings, 4*(2), 3534–3541. https://doi.org/10.1016/j.matpr.2017.02.244

Beadling, A. R., Neville, A., & Bryant, M. G. (2023). Degradation of metal hip implants. In I. Świątkowska (Ed.), *Biomarkers of hip implant function* (pp. 41–74). Elsevier. https://doi.org/10.1016/B978-0-12-821596-8.00006-9

Bian, Y., Cao, L., Zeng, D., Cui, J., Li, W., Yu, Z., & Zhang, P. (2023). The tribological properties of two-phase hard and soft composite wear-resistant coatings on titanium alloys. *Surface Coatings Technology, 456*, 129256. https://doi.org/10.1016/j.surfcoat.2023.129256

Bolognesi, M. P., & Ledford, C. K. (2015). Metal-on-metal total hip arthroplasty: Patient evaluation and treatment. *Journal of the American Academy of Orthopaedic Surgeons, 23*(12), 724–731. https://doi.org/10.5435/JAAOS-D-14-00183

Chen, Y.-W., Moussi, J., Drury, J. L., & Wataha, J. C. (2016). Zirconia in biomedical applications. *Expert Review of Medical Devices, 13*(10), 945–963. https://doi.org/10.1080/17434440.2016.1230017

Costa, M. D., Donner, S., Bertrand, J., Pop, O.-L., & Lohmann, C. H. (2023). Hypersensitivity and lymphocyte activation after total hip arthroplasty. *Die Orthopädie, 52*, 214–221. https://doi.org/10.1007/s00132-023-04349-7

Cui, W., Bian, Y., Zeng, H., Zhang, X., Zhang, Y., Weng, X., . . . Jin, Z. (2020). Structural and tribological characteristics of ultra-low-wear polyethylene as artificial joint materials. *Journal of the Mechanical Behavior of Biomedical Materials, 104*, 103629. https://doi.org/10.1016/j.jmbbm.2020.103629

Dalli, D., Buhagiar, J., Mollicone, P., & Wismayer, P. S. (2022). A novel hip joint prosthesis with uni-directional articulations for reduced wear. *Journal of the Mechanical Behavior of Biomedical Materials, 127*, 105072. https://doi.org/10.1016/j.jmbbm.2021.105072

Di Puccio, F., & Mattei, L. (2015). Biotribology of artificial hip joints. *World Journal of Orthopedics, 6*(1), 77. https://doi.org/10.5312/wjo.v6.i1.77

Eason, T. B., Cosgrove, C. T., & Mihalko, W. M. (2022). Necrotizing soft-tissue infections after hip arthroplasty. *Orthopedic Clinics, 53*(1), 33–41. https://doi.org/10.1016/j.ocl.2021.08.001

Eltit, F., Wang, Q., & Wang, R. (2019). Mechanisms of adverse local tissue reactions to hip implants. *Frontiers in Bioengineering, 7*, 176. https://doi.org/10.3389/fbioe.2019.00176

Findik, F. (2020). Recent developments of metallic implants for biomedical applications. *Periodicals of Engineering Natural Sciences 8*(1), 33–57. https://doi.org/10.21533/pen.v8i1.988.g487

Gessner, B. D., Steck, T., Woelber, E., & Tower, S. S. (2019). A systematic review of systemic cobaltism after wear or corrosion of chrome-cobalt hip implants. *Journal of Patient Safety, 15*(2), 97. https://doi.org/10.1097/PTS.0000000000000220

Goswami, C., Patnaik, A., Bhat, I., & Singh, T. (2021). Mechanical physical and wear properties of some oxide ceramics for hip joint application: A short review. *Materials Today: Proceedings, 44*, 4913–4918. https://doi.org/10.1016/j.matpr.2020.11.888

Heneghan, C., Langton, D., & Thompson. (2012). Ongoing problems with metal-on-metal hip implants. *BMJ Feature 344*. https://doi.org/10.1136/bmj.e1349

Holding, C. A., Findlay, D. M., Stamenkov, R., Neale, S. D., Lucas, H., Dharmapatni, A., . . . Howie, D. W. (2006). The correlation of RANK, RANKL and TNFα expression with bone loss volume and polyethylene wear debris around hip implants. *Biomaterials, 27*(30), 5212–5219. https://doi.org/10.1016/j.biomaterials.2006.05.054

Jasionowski, R., Polkowski, W., & Zasada, D. (2016). Destruction mechanism of ZnAl4 as cast alloy subjected to cavitational erosion using different laboratory stands. *Archives of Foundry Engineering*, *16*(1), 19–24. https://doi.org/10.1515/afe-2015-0096

Joshi, T., Sharma, R., Mittal, V. K., Gupta, V., & Krishan, G. (2022). Dynamic analysis of hip prosthesis using different biocompatible alloys. *ASME Open Journal of Engineering*, *1*. https://doi.org/10.1115/1.4053417

Kelmer, G., Stone, A. H., Turcotte, J., & King, P. (2021). Reasons for revision: Primary total hip arthroplasty mechanisms of failure. *Journal of the American Academy of Orthopaedic Surgeons*, *29*(2), 78–87. https://doi.org/10.5435/JAAOS-D-19-00860

Kheradmandfard, M., Kashani-Bozorg, S. F., Lee, J. S., Kim, C.-L., Hanzaki, A. Z., Pyun, Y.-S., . . . Kim, D.-E. (2018). Significant improvement in cell adhesion and wear resistance of biomedical β-type titanium alloy through ultrasonic nanocrystal surface modification. *Journal of Alloys Compounds*, *762*, 941–949. https://doi.org/10.1016/j.jallcom.2018.05.088

Li, H.-F., Huang, J.-Y., Lin, G.-C., & Wang, P.-Y. (2021). Recent advances in tribological and wear properties of biomedical metallic materials. *Rare Metals*, *40*(11), 3091–3106. https://doi.org/10.1007/s12598-021-01796-z

Lin, S., Wen, Z., Li, S., Chen, Z., Li, C., Ouyang, Z., . . . Ding, Y. (2022). LncRNA Neat1 promotes the macrophage inflammatory response and acts as a therapeutic target in titanium particle-induced osteolysis. *Acta Biomaterialia*, *142*, 345–360. https://doi.org/10.1016/j.actbio.2022.02.007

Marquez, A., Mencia, M., & Maharaj, C. (2023). Failure analysis of a stainless steel hip implant. *Journal of Failure Analysis Prevention*, *23*, 846–852. https://doi.org/10.1007/s11668-023-01622-x

Matusiewicz, H., & Richter, M. (2022). Metal ions release from metallic orthopedic implants exposed to tribocorrosion and electrochemical corrosion conditions in simulated body fluids: Clinical context and in vitro experimental investigations. *World Journal of Advanced Research 14*(2), 261–283. https://doi.org/10.30574/wjarr.2022.14.2.0438

Merola, M., & Affatato, S. (2019). Materials for hip prostheses: A review of wear and loading considerations. *Materials (Basel)*, *12*(3). https://doi.org/10.3390/ma12030495

Niemczewska-Wójcik, M. (2017). Wear mechanisms and surface topography of artificial hip joint components at the subsequent stages of tribological tests. *Measurement*, *107*, 89–98. https://doi.org/10.1016/j.measurement.2017.04.045

Rahmati, M., & Mozafari, M. (2019). Biocompatibility of alumina-based biomaterials–A review. *Journal of Cellular Physiology*, *234*(4), 3321–3335. https://doi.org/10.1002/jcp.27292

Ranuša, M., Čípek, P., Vrbka, M., Paloušek, D., Křupka, I., & Hartl, M. (2022). Tribological behaviour of 3D printed materials for small joint implants: A pilot study. *Journal of the Mechanical Behavior of Biomedical Materials*, *132*, 105274.

Restrepo-Noriega, V. E., Maya, I. D. S., Guzmán-Benedek, D. L., & Corrales-González, M. (2022). Total hip arthroplasty in a patient with Paget's disease. *Revista de la Asociación Argentina de Ortopedia y Traumatología*, *87*(5), 693–702. https://doi.org/10.15417/issn.1852-7434.2022.87.5.1660

Reyes Rojas, A., Aguilar Elguezabal, A., Porporati, A. A., Bocanegra Bernal, M., & Esparza Ponce, H. E. (2023a). Ceramics choice for implants. In *Performance of metals and ceramics in total hip arthroplasty* (pp. 59–87). Springer. https://doi.org/10.1007/978-3-031-25420-8_6

Reyes Rojas, A., Aguilar Elguezabal, A., Porporati, A. A., Bocanegra Bernal, M., & Esparza Ponce, H. E. (2023b). State of the art in orthopaedic implants. In *Performance of metals ceramics in total hip arthroplasty* (pp. 5–16). Springer. https://doi.org/10.1007/978-3-031-25420-8_2

Ricciardi, B. F., Nocon, A. A., Jerabek, S. A., Wilner, G., Kaplowitz, E., Goldring, S. R., . . . Perino, G. (2016). Histopathological characterization of corrosion product associated adverse local tissue reaction in hip implants: A study of 285 cases. *BMC Clinical Pathology, 16*, 1–17. https://doi.org/10.1186/s12907-016-0025-9

Sankar, S., Paulraj, J., & Chakraborti, P. (2023). Fused filament fabricated PEEK based polymer composites for orthopaedic implants: A review. *International Journal of Materials Research, 114*(10–11), 980–988. https://doi.org/10.1515/ijmr-2022-0225

Sargeant, A., & Goswami, T. (2006). Hip implants: Paper V. Physiological effects. *Materials, 27*(4), 287–307. https://doi.org/10.1016/j.matdes.2004.10.028

Sathishkumar, S., Jawahar, P., & Chakraborti, P. (2022a). Synthesis, properties, and applications of PEEK-based biomaterials. In *Advanced materials for biomedical applications* (pp. 81–107). CRC Press. https://doi.org/10.1201/9781003344810.5

Sathishkumar, S., Jawahar, P., & Chakraborti, P. (2022b). Influence of carbonaceous reinforcements on mechanical and tribological properties of PEEK composites – A review. *Polymer-Plastics Technology and Materials, 61*(12), 1367–1384. https://doi.org/10.1080/25740881.2022.2061995

Sathishkumar, S., Paulraj, J., Chakraborti, P., & Muthuraj, M. (2023). Comprehensive review on biomaterials and their inherent behaviors for hip repair applications. *ACS Applied Bio Materials, 6*(11), 4439–4464. https://doi.org/10.1021/acsabm.3c00327

Shankar, S., Nithyaprakash, R., Abbas, G., Kumar, R. N., Pramanik, A., Basak, A. K., & Prakash, C. (2022). Tribological behavior of zirconia-toughened alumina (ZTA) against Ti6Al4V under different bio-lubricants in hip prosthesis using experimental and finite element concepts. *Materials Letters, 307*, 131107. https://doi.org/10.1016/j.matlet.2021.131107

Sivasankar, M., Arunkumar, S., Bakkiyaraj, V., Muruganandam, A., & Sathishkumar, S. (2016). A review on total hip replacement. *International Research Journal in Advanced Engineering Technology, 2*(2), 589–592.

Skjöldebrand, C., Tipper, J. L., Hatto, P., Bryant, M., Hall, R. M., & Persson, C. (2022). Current status and future potential of wear-resistant coatings and articulating surfaces for hip and knee implants. *Materials Today Bio, 15*, 100270. https://doi.org/10.1016/j.mtbio.2022.100270

Varga, M., Grundtner, R., Maj, M., Tatzgern, F., & Alessio, K.-O. (2023). Impact-abrasive wear resistance of high alumina ceramics and ZTA. *Wear, 522*, 204700. https://doi.org/10.21203/rs.3.rs-2440544/v1

Wahyudi, M., Ismail, R., & Jamari, J. (2020). Friction and wear analysis of UHMWPE material using pin-on-disc tester with lubricant and non-lubricant. *Journal of Physics: Conference Series, 1569*, 032057.

Wang, H., Zheng, J., Sun, X., & Luo, Y. (2022). Tribo-corrosion mechanisms and electromechanical behaviours for metal implants materials of CoCrMo, Ti6Al4V and Ti15Mo alloys. *Biosurface and Biotribology 8*(1), 44–51. https://doi.org/10.1049/bsb2.12031

Wang, J.-W., Yang, H., Wang, C.-T., & Jin, Z.-M. (2019). Wear and diagnostic analysis of clinical failures of artificial hip joints. In *UHMWPE biomaterials for joint implants: Structures, properties clinical performance, Springer series in biomaterials science and engineering* (pp. 317–339). https://doi.org/10.1007/978-981-13-6924-7_10

Xing, D., Li, R., Li, J. J., Tao, K., Lin, J., Yan, T., & Zhou, D. (2022). Catastrophic periprosthetic osteolysis in total hip arthroplasty at 20 years: A case report and literature review. *Orthopaedic Surgery, 14*(8), 1918–1926. https://doi.org/10.1111/os.13322

Zhang, X., Ma, X., Lin, Q., Xiao, L., Wang, S., Yang, H., . . . Song, J. (2023). Study on the friction and wear properties of PEEK against cortical bone tissue under different lubricating conditions. *Macromolecular Bioscience, 23*, 2200548,. https://doi. org/10.1002/mabi.202200548

Zhou, Z., & Jin, Z. (2015). Biotribology: Recent progresses and future perspectives. *Biosurface Biotribology, 1*(1), 3–24. https://doi.org/10.1016/j.bsbt.2015.03.001

Zmitrowicz, A. (2006). Wear patterns and laws of wear–a review. *Journal of Theoretical Applied Mechanics 44*(2), 219–253.

12 Surface Coating Influences on Tribo-Behaviors of Bioimplants

S Sathishkumar[1], P Jawahar[1], Prasun Chakraborti[1], M Muthusivaramapandian[1], S Indiran[2], P Sathishkumar[2], and Suchart Siengchin[2]

[1] National Institute of Technology
Agartala, Tripura, India
[2] King Mongkut's University of Technology
North Bangkok, Thailand

12.1 INTRODUCTION

Bioimplants replace or augment human tissues or organs and are typically made of metals, ceramics, or polymers. In recent years, several bioimplants have become strongly associated with human health for various reasons, as shown in Figure 12.1. The field of bioimplants has been revolutionized by the use of advanced surface coating technologies that enhance their tribological behavior (Gautam et al., 2022). However, improving the lifespan of implant scaffolds is daunting for orthopedic surgeons, as it depends on factors such as implant material behaviors, patient age, surgery methods, and surgeon experience (Li & Leung, 2023). Longer lifespan also strongly depends on tribological behavior, which refers to its ability to withstand mechanical stresses and wear and tear due to regular use (Sathishkumar et al., 2023).

Furthermore, inadequate material behaviors can lead to severe consequences on the implanted body, such as inflammation, osteolysis, bone resorption, tissue necrosis, and aseptic loosening, ultimately resulting in implant failure and necessitating revision surgery (Sudha et al., 2023). Hence, proper material characterization prior to implantation is essential to minimize these risks and ensure the long-term success of the bioimplant. The durability of bioimplants is significantly influenced by the tribological behaviors of materials, which can vary depending on a range of factors such as their nature, processing methods, materials used, the presence of coatings, and the types of surface treatments applied (Shen et al., 2022).

Surface coatings effectively improve the tribological behavior of bioimplants, thereby improving their durability, efficacy, and long-term success (Montazerian et al., 2022). Typically, the bioimplants are used to replace or augment body tissues or organs, and they are subject to a range of mechanical, chemical, and biological

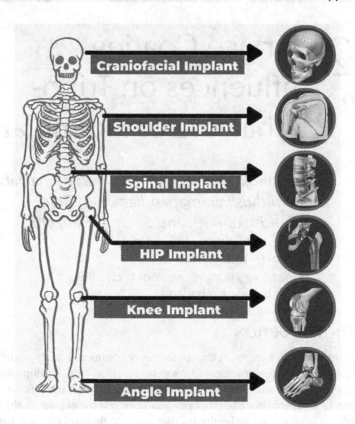

FIGURE 12.1 Bioimplants on the human body.

stresses in the body. So the surface coatings provide a protective layer on the implant's surface, which can prevent degradation, corrosion, and wear, thereby increasing the implant's lifespan and improving its biocompatibility (Amirtharaj Mosas et al., 2022). Surface coatings, such as physical vapor deposition (PVD: diamond-like carbon, titanium nitriding), chemical vapor deposition (CVD), electro deposition (ED), plasma spraying (PS), sol-gel deposition (SGD), and dip coating (DC), contribute greatly to reducing wear and extending the lifespan of the implants (Ralls et al., 2019). Another essential benefit of surface coatings is that they can improve the biocompatibility of the implant. In general, the surface coatings on implants are engineered to mimic the natural environment of the body tissues, thereby reducing the likelihood of an immune response or rejection. This also promotes tissue growth and integration around the implant, which can help to prevent implant loosening and improve long-term performance (Ching et al., 2014).

This chapter provides a detailed overview of the surface coating techniques used for bioimplants and their impact on tribological behavior. The chapter is divided into several sections that explore the various aspects of surface coatings for different bioimplants, including their types, properties, and applications.

12.2   IMPORTANCE OF TRIBOLOGICAL BEHAVIOR ON BIOIMPLANTS

Tribology plays a vital role in developing effective and safe bioimplants. It provides a framework for understanding surface interactions in relative motion and helps identify the critical factors influencing bioimplants' performance and durability (Mehta et al., 2022).

The tribological phenomena in bioimplants include friction, wear, corrosion, and lubrication. Friction is the force that opposes the motion between two surfaces in contact. In bioimplants, friction can cause wear, deformation, and damage to the implant surfaces, leading to pain, inflammation, and implant failure (Sahoo et al., 2019). Medical professionals use various surface coatings and surface treatments to reduce friction in bioimplants. Generally, wear is defined by material loss from the implant surfaces due to mechanical and chemical processes. Wear can cause the formation of debris particles that can lead to inflammation, osteolysis, and implant loosening. To minimize wear in bioimplants, medical professionals use wear-resistant materials and coatings, such as titanium, zirconia, and diamond-like carbon (Wei et al., 2022).

Corrosion is the degradation of the implant surfaces due to chemical reactions with the surrounding environment, such as body fluids and tissues. Corrosion can deteriorate implant performance and release metal ions into the body, leading to adverse effects such as tissue damage and inflammation. To minimize corrosion in bioimplants, medical professionals use corrosion-resistant materials, such as titanium alloys, ceramics, and polymer surface coatings over the implant surfaces (Thakur et al., 2022). Lubrication is the use of fluids or lubricants to reduce friction and wear in bioimplants. Synovial fluid lubricates joint surfaces in natural joints, reducing friction and wear. In bioimplants, medical professionals use lubricants like hyaluronic acid to lubricate the implant surfaces and reduce friction and wear (Wei et al., 2023).

In addition to the tribological phenomena, other factors such as surface roughness, implant geometry, loading conditions, and biological response also affect bioimplants' tribological behavior. The surface roughness of the implant surfaces affects the implant's friction, wear, and corrosion resistance. The implant geometry affects the stress distribution and wear patterns of the implant (Sankar et al., 2023). The loading conditions affect the mechanical stresses and strains in the implant and surrounding tissues. The biological response affects the healing process and tissue integration of the implants (Mehta et al., 2022).

12.3   SURFACE COATING TECHNIQUES FOR BIOIMPLANTS

Surface coatings on bioimplants have become increasingly important in recent years as they play an essential role in improving the implant's performance, durability, and success. Surface coatings can modify the surface properties of the implant, such as surface chemistry, roughness, and wettability, to enhance the interaction between the implant and the surrounding tissues. Generally, the choice

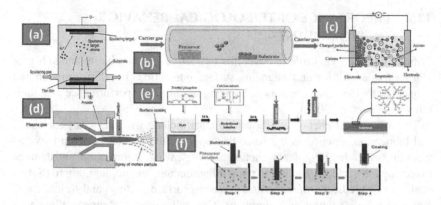

FIGURE 12.2 Significant surface coating techniques for bioimplants: (a) physical vapor deposition (Faraji et al., 2018), (b) chemical vapor deposition (Mittal et al., 2021), (c) electrodeposition (Yadav et al., 2020), (d) plasma spraying process (Devasia et al., 2021), (e) sol-gel deposition process (Tranquillo & Bollino, 2020), (f) dip coating process (Neacşu et al., 2016).

of surface coating technique depends on different factors, such as the type of material to be coated, the surface properties required, the coating thickness, and the manufacturing process of the implants (Zafar et al., 2020).

Various surface coating techniques can be used to modify the surface properties of bioimplants. Some of the commonly used surface coating techniques are represented in Figure 12.2.

12.3.1 PHYSICAL VAPOR DEPOSITION (PVD)

Physical vapor deposition (PVD) coating is a widely used surface coating technique in the field of bioimplants. It involves the deposition of a thin film of material onto the implant surfaces. PVD coating can be used to modify the surface properties of bioimplants, such as surface chemistry, roughness, and wettability, to enhance the interaction between the implant and the surrounding tissues (Ramoul et al., 2019).

The PVD coating process involves the use of a vacuum chamber, which is used to create a low-pressure environment. The implant is placed in the vacuum chamber, and a target material, such as titanium nitride (TiN), diamond-like carbon (DLC), or chromium nitride (CrN), is placed in the chamber as well. An electric current is applied to the target material, causing it to vaporize and deposit onto the implant surface. Figure 12.2a shows a detailed schematic view of the PVD process. One of the key advantages of PVD coating is that it can be used to deposit a thin film of material onto the implant surface, typically in the range of 1–5 μm. This thin film can modify the surface properties of the implant without significantly affecting its bulk properties. This is particularly important in the case of metallic implants, where changes to the bulk properties can have a significant impact on the implant's mechanical properties (Faraji et al., 2018).

PVD coating can be used to improve the wear resistance, corrosion resistance, and biocompatibility of bioimplants. TiN coatings are commonly used to improve wear resistance, as they are highly resistant to abrasion and have a low coefficient of friction (Uddin et al., 2019). DLC coatings are commonly used to improve both wear resistance and biocompatibility, as they have excellent biocompatibility and low friction properties (Rodríguez-Rojas et al., 2023). CrN coatings are commonly used to improve corrosion resistance, as they are highly resistant to corrosion in biological environments (Patnaik et al., 2021). Typically, the success of PVD coating on bioimplants depends on various factors, such as the quality of the coating, the thickness of the coating, and the manufacturing process of the implant. The coating should be uniform, adherent, and free from defects such as pores or cracks. The thickness of the coating should be carefully controlled to ensure that it has the desired properties without affecting the bulk properties of the implant. The manufacturing process of the implant should be carefully designed to ensure that the coating is not damaged during the manufacturing process (Grigoriev et al., 2023).

12.3.2 CHEMICAL VAPOR DEPOSITION (CVD)

Chemical vapor deposition (CVD) coating is another surface coating technique that has found widespread use in the field of bioimplants. CVD coating involves the deposition of a thin film of material onto the implant surface by a chemical reaction between gas-phase precursors and the implants. The resulting coating is highly conformal and can be used to modify the surface properties of bioimplants (Pandey & Sahoo, 2023).

The CVD coating process typically involves the use of a vacuum chamber, similar to that used in PVD coating. However, instead of a target material, gas-phase precursors are used, which react chemically with the implant surface to form a thin film. The precursors are typically introduced into the vacuum chamber in a gaseous state and then are activated by heat, plasma, or other means to initiate the chemical reaction. The resulting coating is deposited onto the implant surface in a highly conformal manner. Figure 12.2b shows the CVD coating process (Mittal et al., 2021).

One of the key advantages of CVD coating is its ability to produce highly conformal coatings, which can be used to modify the surface properties of complex-shaped implants, such as hip or knee implants. The resulting coatings are also highly uniform, adherent, and free from defects such as pores or cracks, which can improve the biocompatibility and durability of the implant. CVD coating can be used to improve the wear resistance, corrosion resistance, and biocompatibility of bioimplants. For example, diamond-like carbon (DLC) coatings can be deposited by CVD to improve wear resistance (Derakhshandeh et al., 2018), and titanium oxide (TiO_2) coatings can be deposited to improve corrosion resistance (Visentin et al., 2019). CVD can also be used to deposit hydrophilic or hydrophobic coatings onto the implant surface, which can improve the interaction between the implant and the surrounding tissues. The success of CVD coating on bioimplants depends on various factors, which is similar to the PVD coating.

12.3.3 ELECTRODEPOSITION (ED)

Electrodeposition (ED), also known as electroplating, is a surface coating technique used in the production of bioimplants. This method involves the use of an electric current to deposit a thin layer of metal onto the surface of the implant. During the electrodeposition process, the bioimplant is first cleaned and pretreated with a surface preparation solution to ensure proper adhesion of the coating. The implant is then immersed in an electrolyte solution containing the desired metal ions (Yadav et al., 2020). An electrical current is then applied to the solution, causing the metal ions to be attracted to the surface of the implant and deposit onto it. Figure 12.2c depicts the process of ED coating.

One advantage of electrodeposition is that it allows for precise control of the thickness and uniformity of the coating. The coating can also be tailored to achieve specific mechanical, chemical, and biological properties, making it an ideal method for producing bioimplants. In addition, electrodeposition can be used to deposit a variety of metals and alloys onto the implant surface, including titanium, gold, silver, and platinum. This allows for a wide range of coating options to meet the specific needs of each individual patient. ED coating is a relatively low-cost and environmentally friendly process compared to other coating methods, such as PVD and CVD (Drevet et al., 2019). However, one disadvantage of electrodeposition is that it may not be suitable for coating complex geometries or parts with narrow crevices or pores. Despite its limitations, electrodeposition remains a viable and effective method for producing bioimplants with enhanced functionality and durability (del Olmo et al., 2023).

12.3.4 PLASMA SPRAYING (PS)

Plasma spraying is a popular coating technique used in the production of bioimplants. It involves the use of a plasma torch to melt a material and then spray it onto the surface of the implant. The coating material can be a metal, ceramic, or polymer, depending on the desired properties of the implant (Hassan et al., 2023).

In general, the plasma spraying process, the coating material is fed into the plasma torch, where it is heated to extremely high temperatures and melts into a molten state. The molten material is then accelerated and sprayed onto the surface of the implant using a gas stream. As the molten material hits the surface of the implant, it rapidly cools and solidifies, forming a thin, uniform coating.

Primary advantage of plasma spraying is that it allows for the deposition of a wide range of materials onto the surface of the implant. This includes metals, ceramics, and polymers, which can provide different mechanical, chemical, and biological properties to the implant surface. Figure 12.2d elucidates process of PS in detail (Devasia et al., 2021). In addition, plasma spraying can be used to produce coatings with high porosity, which can promote osseointegration and cell growth, and it can produce coatings with high adhesion strength, which is important for ensuring the longevity of the implant. Plasma spraying can also be used to deposit coatings with varying thicknesses, allowing for precise control over the final coating properties (Mehta & Singh, 2023).

However, one disadvantage of plasma spraying is that it can be a relatively expensive process compared to other coating methods. It also requires specialized equipment and trained personnel to perform the process effectively. In addition, the plasma spraying process may generate heat that could potentially damage the implant material. Despite its limitations, plasma spraying remains a popular and effective coating technique for bioimplants due to its ability to produce coatings with a wide range of properties and high adhesion strength (Guo et al., 2023).

12.3.5 Sol-Gel Deposition (SGD)

Sol-gel coating is a popular technique for coating bioimplants. The process involves the transformation of a liquid precursor into a gel-like material that can be deposited onto the surface of the implant, which is represented in Figure 12.2e. The coating can be composed of a variety of materials such as ceramics, glasses, and polymers, depending on the intended application of the implant (Jaafar et al., 2020). The sol-gel coating process involves several stages, including hydrolysis, condensation, and aging. During the hydrolysis stage, the precursor materials are dissolved in a liquid solvent, typically water or alcohol, to create a colloidal solution. This solution is then subjected to condensation, where the precursor molecules react with one another to form a three-dimensional network. Finally, the aged sol is deposited onto the surface of the implant, and the coating is dried and cured to form a thin, uniform layer (Tranquillo & Bollino, 2020).

Normally, the sol-gel coating has the ability to produce coatings with a high level of control over the final properties. The thickness, porosity, and composition of the coating can be precisely controlled, allowing for the production of coatings with tailored mechanical, chemical, and biological properties. Additionally, the sol-gel coating process can be performed at relatively low temperatures, which reduces the risk of damage to the implant material. Another benefit is that sol-gel coatings are able to promote osseointegration and cell growth (Singh et al., 2022). The porous nature of the coatings allows for the infiltration of bone cells, promoting the formation of a strong bond between the implant and surrounding bone tissue. In addition, sol-gel coatings can be modified with bioactive molecules such as growth factors and peptides, which further promote cell attachment and differentiation (Ballarre & Ceré, 2022).

However, one disadvantage of sol-gel coatings is their susceptibility to degradation over time. The porous nature of the coatings can lead to the absorption of fluids, which can cause the coating to swell or degrade. This can lead to a loss of adhesion between the coating and the implant, reducing the lifespan of the implant. Nonetheless, sol-gel coating remains a popular and effective technique for coating bioimplants due to its ability to produce coatings with tailored properties that promote osseointegration and cell growth (Balestriere et al., 2020).

12.3.6 DIP COATING (DC)

Dip coating is a common technique used for coating bioimplants, in which the implant is dipped into a solution containing a coating material, and then withdrawn to allow the coating to dry and adhere to the surface (Zhu et al., 2022). This technique is used to create a thin, uniform layer of coating material on the surface of the implant, which can provide improved biocompatibility, wear resistance, and corrosion resistance. The dip coating process involves several steps. First, a solution containing the coating material is prepared. The solution may contain various types of materials, such as polymers, ceramics, or metals, depending on the desired properties of the coating (Neacşu et al., 2016). The implant is then dipped into the solution and held in place for a specified amount of time to allow the coating to adhere to the surface. Subsequently, the implant is then withdrawn from the solution, and the coating is allowed to dry and cure to form a thin, uniform layer. Figure 12.2f illustrates the dip coating process in detail.

Generally, dip coating is able to produce coatings with a high degree of control over thickness and uniformity. The thickness of the coating can be controlled by adjusting the viscosity of the coating solution, the duration of the dipping process, and the withdrawal speed. The uniformity of the coating can be improved by controlling the dipping process and ensuring that the implant is fully immersed in the coating solution. Another advantage of dip coating is its versatility; it can be used to coat implants made from a variety of materials, including metals, ceramics, and polymers. The coating material can also be tailored to provide specific properties, such as biocompatibility, corrosion resistance, or wear resistance (Tran et al., 2023). This allows for the development of coatings that can meet the specific needs of different implant applications.

However, one disadvantage of dip coating is its limited ability to produce coatings with complex geometries. The coating material tends to form a uniform layer on the surface of the implant, which may not adhere well to irregular or complex geometries. Additionally, the dip coating process can be time-consuming and may require multiple dips to achieve the desired coating thickness (Terranova, 2022). Table 12.1 summarizes the overall merits and drawbacks of various coating methods.

TABLE 12.1

Merits and Drawbacks of Coating Methods on Bioimplants

S. No.	Coating Method	Merits	Drawbacks
1	Physical vapor deposition	Low friction, high wear resistance, corrosion resistance, good aesthetics, and bio compatibility	High cost, thickness limitation, surface roughness, coating delamination
2	Chemical vapor deposition	High purity, good adhesion, thickness control, conformal coating	High processing temperature, surface roughness, high cost, complex processing and longer processing time
3	Electrodeposition	Cost-effective, excellent adhesion, uniform coating, high hardness, thickness control	Low effectiveness on complex shaped implants, surface roughness, risk of porosity, and complex process
4	Plasma spraying	Versatile materials can be used, good adhesion, thick coating, good thermal insulation	Limited coating uniformity, limited thin coating, surface roughness, and complex process
5	Sol-gel deposition	Thin and uniform coating, chemical stability, versatile materials can be used, good biocompatibility, and controlled drug delivery	Surface roughness, limited mechanical durability, possible for cracking, delamination, limited thickness
6	Dip coating	Cost-effective, uniform coating, versatile materials can be used, and able to customize the coating	Low effectiveness on complex shaped implants, surface roughness, limited coating thickness, possible for high porosity and delamination.

12.4   INFLUENCE OF SURFACE COATING ON TRIBO-BEHAVIORS OF BIOIMPLANTS

Longevity is primary consideration in artificial implants. Myriad factors contribute greatly in determining the performance and durability of encapsulated prosthesis. The surface coating is an effective preventive method for reducing the implant degradation and failure. Several surface coating methods have been developed over the years, as illustrated in preceding section, and their influences on tribo-behaviors are discussed next.

12.4.1   Dental Implants

Dental implants are a significant advancement in dental technology, providing patients with a long-lasting, comfortable, and natural-looking solution for missing teeth. As dental implant technology continues to evolve, it is likely that they will

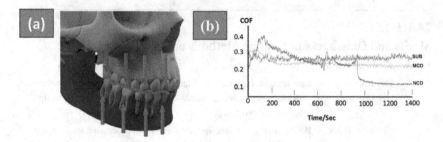

FIGURE 12.3 (a) Dental implant (Osak et al., 2022), (b) COF acquired in different grain diamond coating (Wang et al., 2014).

become even more important in the dental landscape of the future. The Figure 12.3a depicted the use of dental implants. Over past two decades, several materials have become closely associated with dental implantation for improving patients' health: titanium (Ti), stainless steel (3l6L), cobalt-chromium (Co-Cr), zirconia (ZrO_2), and polyether ether ketone (PEEK) (Souza et al., 2020).

The wear behaviors of these dental implants are most effective in improving performances, like reduced wear and tear, fewer bacterial infections, improved biocompatibility, osteointegration, and aesthetics (Chavan et al., 2022). Generally, dental materials are intensively affected and identified by the following wear mechanisms: attrition, abrasion, corrosion, fatigue, and fretting wear. Corrosion is the primary significant attribute for metal dental materials, depending on purity, processing methods, rate of metal ion emission, and patient food habits. Furthermore, fretting wear is also frequently identified by clinicians due to low amplitude frictions. According to appearance, durability, chemical and wear behaviors, ceramics are adoptable subtrates for dental implantation. Despite their brittle nature, abrasives generation effectively limits their contributions in the dental domain (Saha & Roy, 2023).

On the other hand, the internal porosity and surface defects are major reasons for high wear rate, which makes acidic/alkalic attack and intrinsic diseases on ceramics surfaces possible. In recent years, PEEK polymers are used for various dental applications, but their wear resistivity is obviously inadequate, and there are no successful clinical records for long-term dental applications (Sathishkumar et al., 2022b). Therefore, improving the tribo-behaviors of dental materials is the predominant task, which will be achievable by surface coating over the implant's surfaces. Hussein et al. investigated the impact of TiN (titanium nitride) coating on Ti-20Nb-13Zr (TNZ) alloy based on their mechanical, in vitro corrosion and tribological behaviors. The TiN coating was produced by cathodic arc physical vapor deposition method. This study indicated that the TiN coating influenced tribo-behaviors of TNZ alloy much more than uncoated substances, due to their high hardness (23.5 GPa) and lower coefficient of friction (0.4 μ). In addition, the coating developed a protective layer on the alloy surfaces, which significantly reduced the contact between the mating materials. Additionally, the TiN coating possessed an excellent adhesion strength, which largely prevented delamination and cracking from wear.

The result reported, the wear rate of TiN-coated samples was greatly reduced, estimated from $3.9 \pm 0.8 \times 10^{-5} mm^3/Nm$ to $0.62 \pm 0.07 \times 10^{-5} mm^3/Nm$. The TiN coating improved the wear resistivity more than 80% on TNZ alloys, and the study identified the uncoated samples infected by abrasive wear and adhesive wear for coated alloys. Furthermore, the TiN coating also built excellent corrosive resistivity due to the formation of a protective layer on the surface of the alloy. This coating acted as a barrier to prevent the diffusion of aggressive ions, which reduced the corrosion rate of the alloy. XPS analysis showed that the surface of the alloy contained mostly the TiN element rather than TiO_2 and TiO_3, indicating that the coating enabled high resistivity against oxidation and corrosion (Hussein et al., 2020).

The microcrystalline (MCD) and nanocrystalline (NCD) diamond coating also exhibit the high-resolution tribological, corrosion, and physiological behaviors of Ti 6A l4V (TC4) alloys. Wang et Al, tried to identify the dental implant failure possibilities and determined that the continuous wear of the fixing screws is one of the major reasons for the loosening of the implant. So he and his team were highly motivated to elevate the tribological, anticorrosive behaviors by means of MCD and NCD coating. The hot filament deposited chemical vapor deposition (HFCVD) method was used to deposit the film on TC4 alloy surfaces, and tribology testing was carried out with a ball-on-disk tribometer with artificial saliva lubrication. Through this extensive tribological examination, the author reported that the diamond coating highly improved the wear resistivity of implant surfaces and measured the coefficient of friction of uncoated TC4, MCD-coated TC4, and NCD-coated TC4, followed by 0.28, 0.2, and 0.1, as shown in Figure 12.3b. The outcome of this examination implies that the wear characteristics of TC4 were enhanced, based on its high hardness and low coefficient of friction, which can eliminate the generation of wear debris on implants, along with their adverse reactions on host's body. In addition, the author evaluated the corrosive behaviors of TC4 by the anodic polarization technique, and the results showed that the diamond coating reduced the corrosion rate due to its high hardness and chemical stability. Compared to MCD, NCD exhibited more favorable tribo-results on TC4 dental implants (Wang et al., 2014).

The ceramic coating on metal dental implants is another viable strategy for achieving feasible tribo-behaviors. Generally, the zirconia and zirconia-based substances have been employed in various dental applications since early 2000. Zambrano et al. conducted computational and experimental studies to explore the mechanical, tribological, and corrosive properties of Zr, ZrN (zirconia nitride), and Zr/ZrN coated stainless steel (SS304) dental implants. The coating imposed by a PVD magnetron sputtering method, wear and corrosive behaviors were extensively analyzed. According this report, Zr and Zr-based coatings can potentially diminish the rate of wear better than uncoated materials in the four wear mechanism categories of abrasion, scratching, plastic deformation, and adhesion.

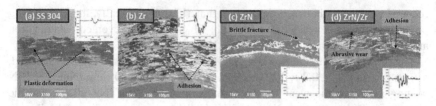

FIGURE 12.4 SEM images for uncoated and Zr-coated SS 304 dental implants. (Zambrano et al., 2023.)

Figure 12.4a–d shows the SEM images of the worn surfaces. Comparatively, in these three coatings, the ZrN coating, acting as a base for the superficial Zr thin film, exhibited remarkable impact on wear resistance because the ZrN coating acted as a barrier layer and reduced the contact between the ceramic thin film and counterface. Additionally, these bilayer coatings elevate the mechanical behaviors, like elastic modulus and hardness better than a Zr ceramics thin layer.

The corrosion characteristics were also inspected with potentiodynamic instruments with artificial physiological mediums (saliva and blood plasma), indicating that the Zr/ZrN coating effectively generates the double layers, which potentially controls the electrolytic diffusion and passivation, thus leading to improvement in the resistivity against corrosion agents. This elaborate investigation confirmed that the Zr/Zr ceramic coating is an energetic candidate for functionalizing and protecting the SS 304 dental prosthesis (Zambrano et al., 2023). Table 12.2 summarizes the surface coating impacts on various dental implants.

12.4.2 Orthopedic Implants

The need for orthopedic implants has emerged because human health has deteriorated for various inevitable reasons, such as osteoarthritis, rheumatoid arthritis, post-traumatic arthritis, osteonecrosis, and accidents. Extending the lifespan of these implants is most imperative, and doing so will depend on the features of the materials used. Figure 12.5 shows some significant bioimplants. Among them, tribology is crucial and considerable protocol is spent on orthopedic materials. Generally, the orthopedic implants, such as joint replacements, are subjected to repetitive loading and sliding motions. This can result in wear and material loss at the implant interface. The wear debris and friction-induced heat can contribute to implant failure (Sivasankar et al., 2016).

Furthermore, excessive wear, friction, and associated complications can lead to implant loosening and escalate the need for revision surgeries. Therefore, understanding and optimizing the tribological behavior of implant materials can help reduce wear and minimize the release of debris into the surrounding tissues, thereby extending the lifespan of the implant. The optimal tribological behavior

TABLE 12.2
Surface Coating Implication on the Tribo-Behaviors of Dental Implants

S. No.	Base Material	Coating Material	Coating Method	Results		Ref.
				Tribology	Corrosion	
1	Titanium grade:4	Amorphous calcium phosphate	Electrochemically assisted deposition	ACP coating highly encourages the wear resistivity of Ti due to its extensive improvement of surface roughness, local contact potential, and surface wettability by artificial saliva lubrication.	-	Osak et al., 2022
2	Zirconia-titanium	*Streptococcus salivarius*	—	Wear rate was reduced on zirconia-titanium tribo-couple due to formation of a mature *S. salivarius* biofilm between the sliding surfaces. Especially, the titanium wear significantly decreased, and no wear was identified on the zirconia substrate.	Biofilm highly influenced the rate of corrosion due to low OCP (open circuit potential) value of tribo-film.	Figueiredo-Pina et al., 2019
3	Ti-6Al-4V	Tantalum carbide (Ta2C) and multiwall carbon nanotube (MW-CNT)	Electron beam physical vapor deposition	Ta2C followed by MWCNT coating significantly improved the tribo-behaviors of Ti, by the enhancement of mechanical properties, such as hardness, fracture toughness, and elevated resistance of plastic deformation. In addition, the high roughness of MWCNT highly influenced the cell growth and adhesion of dental prosthesis.	Ti-Ta2C/MW-CNT surface showed corrosion resistance due to their high hardness and a reduction in the amount of harmful ions released. The Ta2C/MW-CNT coating layer can prevent implant failure and implant loosening.	Esmaeili et al., 2022

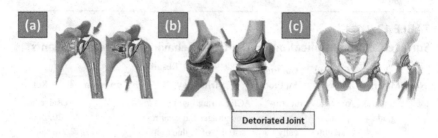

FIGURE 12.5 Significant orthopedic implants for biomedical application: (a) shoulder implant, (b) knee implant, and (c) hip implant.

facilitates smooth and effortless movement at the joint interface, restoring mobility and functionality for patients (Gupta et al., 2022). Implants with superior tribological properties contribute to reduced pain, increased range of motion, and improved overall quality of life for individuals with joint disorders, all of which can be enabled by the coating on the implant surfaces. Section12.3 discussed various coating techniques, along with their various biomedical applications.

Tuten et al. studied the microstructural and tribological behaviors of equimolar TiTaHfNbZr high-entropy alloy (HEA) thin films deposited on the biomedical Tie6Ale4V substrates by RF magnetron sputtering (PVD). The findings demonstrate that the TiTaHfNbZr HEA forms a homogeneous and dense coating mechanically compatible with the Tie6Ale4V substrates and provides enhanced surface protection against wear and cracking due to its homogeneous surface topography with a fine-grained amorphous structure, which provides a significant enhancement of the mechanical properties. Specifically, the significant increase of hardness and elastic modulus of the surface coating led to an enhancement of the tribological properties, such as wear resistance and coefficient of friction, which dictate the suitability of coatings for orthopedic applications (Tüten et al., 2019).

Similarly, the hybrid layer coatings are another viable strategy for developing the remarkable wear resistivity of Ti implants. Gobar and his team utilized the combination of PVD and MAO (micro-arc oxidation) coating technology and deposited the ZrTi and ZrSi oxides layers on Ti alloys. This hybrid coating showed the best wear resistance properties, with the outer layer being minimally abraded at the point of friction. The chemical compositions in the middle of the wear trace and on the outside of the wear trace were compared, and it was found that the composition was unchanged on the outside of the wear trace.

The Figure 12.6a shows the observed wear rate of this metal alloy, and these results suggest that the hybrid coatings have the potential to improve wear resistance due to their high hardness and excellent adhesion strength with the Ti alloys. In addition, the individual ceramic coatings also extend the utility of metals on orthopedic implantationfor superior wear behaviors (Gabor et al., 2022). Berni et al. reported the yttria-stabilized-zirconia- (YSZ-) coated titanium reduced the wear rate of their contact pair UHMEPE (ultra-high-molecular-weight polyethylene) for hip joint applications (metal-polymer). The pulsed-plasma-deposited YSZ coating was evaluated using a ball-on-disc tribometer in dry and lubricated

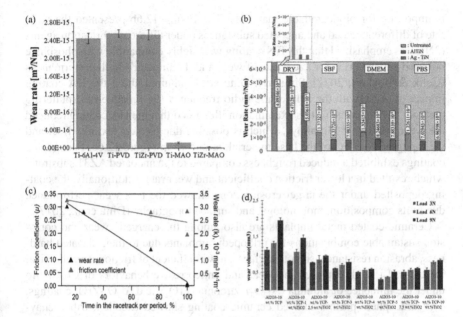

FIGURE 12.6 Wear rate and COF observed in different coatings: (a) Zr-Ti and Zr-Si coating on Ti alloys (Gabor et al., 2022), (b) TiN-based PVD coating on Mg alloy (AZ31) in a different lubrication medium (Çelik & Bozkurt, 2022), (c) RF-based hydroxyapatite coating on Mg alloy (AZ31) (Dinu et al., 2017), (d) (β-TCP) and titania powder (TiO2) coating over the alumina orthopedic implants (Barkallah et al., 2021).

conditions, up to an overall distance of 10 km. The YSZ coating significantly reduced UHMWPE wear rate and friction in dry conditions, with an overall difference of about 40% compared to the uncoated balls due to the reduction of plastic deformation in the sliding contact area, which was suggested by the lower number of ripples observed on the UHMWPE surface. However, in wet conditions, the friction values were found to be comparable between coated and uncoated materials, mainly due to a premature delamination of the coating. So further extensive investigation is highly advisable before implantation.

In the orthopedic industries, the magnesium-based alloys (AZ31) also occupy the essential priorities for successful applications due to their eminent physiological behaviors. Investigating this concern, Celik et al. evaluated the AZ31 surface characteristics by the influence of two different effective TiN-based PVD coatings, specifically AlTiN and Ag doped TiN films. The tribological behaviors of the AZ31 alloy were improved by the TiN-based PVD coatings due to their ability to reduce the wear rate and coefficient of friction. The XRD analysis showed that the coatings had a significant effect on the surface properties of the AZ31 alloy, which contributed to improved tribological performance.

The AlTiN- and Ag-doped TiN films were able to provide a protective layer on the surface of the AZ31 alloy, which reduced the contact between the implant and the surrounding tissue. This reduced the wear and corrosion of the implant, which is important for biodegradable materials. The Figure 12.6b presented the wear rate of different coated and uncoated substances under different lubrication agents (3N). It is emphasized that the TiN coating was highly compatible with phosphate buffered saline (PBS) for a low rate of wear and the implant's high performances (Çelik & Bozkurt, 2022). Similarly, Dinu et al. inquired about the HA coating impact on AZ31with the help of the radio frequency (RF) magnetron sputtering method. The outcome of this examination illustrated that the HA coating reduced the wear affinity of Mg alloys, which is possible due to their texture effect and the topography effect of the base material, as shown in Figure 12.6c. Further, the coatings exhibited a reduced roughness compared to the uncoated AZ31 substrate, which resulted in a lower friction coefficient and wear rate. Additionally, the coating deposited under the target erosion zone showed the best wear performance due to its composition, morphology, and surface topography (Dinu et al., 2017).

Ceramic-coated metal implants are also among the energetic wear and corrosion sustainable combinations for orthopedic implants due to their elevated hardness, abrasion resistance, smooth surfaces, low coefficient of friction, and chemical inertness. Li et al. explored the wear and anticorrosive behaviors of Co-Cr-Mo under the influence of alumina (Al_2O_3), zirconia (ZrO_2), and Al_2O_3-ZrO_2 coatings. The atmosphere-plasma-sprayed ceramic coating showed excellent tribo-behaviors, and the results indicate that the Al_2O_3-ZrO_2 composite coating has better corrosion and wear resistance compared with the ceramic coating (Al_2O_3, ZrO_2) and the Co-Cr-Mo substrate. The excellent adhesion strength (238Mpa), highly dense microstructure, fewer microcracks, and the amorphous phases are deterministic factors responsible for the superior tribological and corrosion performance of the Al_2O_3-ZrO_2 composite coating (Li et al., 2021). On other hand, Barkallah et al. investigated the mechanical and tribological progress of tricalcium phosphate (β-TCP) and titania-powder- (TiO_2-) coated Al_2O_3 orthopedic implants. The result showed the Al_2O_3-10 wt.%-TCP-5 wt.%-TiO_2 combination possesses superior wear resistivity under dry conditions. Figure 12.6d shows that the addition of TCP and TiO_2 to Al_2O_3 amplified the hardness and fracture toughness of the alumina, which contributed to supportive wear behavior (Barkallah et al., 2021). Table 12.3 summarizes the surface coating impacts on orthopaedic implants.

Since the 2000s, the polymers are highly utilized materials for various orthopedic applications. The polymer and their composite coating develop reasonable impact on tribo-behaviors of metal and ceramic implants. Mahmoodi et al. evaluated the biotribological and corrosion behavior of medical-grade tantalum (Ta) material with the influence of GO-reinforced HA electrophoretic deposition coating. The tribology test results indicated that the GO/HA composite coating on the Ta substrate upgraded the wear behavior, plastic deformation, and fracture toughness of the substrate. The stiffness of GO/HA-coated Ta was 8-fold higher than that of the uncoated Ta. The friction coefficient of GO/HA-coated Ta was lower than that of the uncoated Ta. This means that the coating can diminish the wear and tear on the implant and improve its durability. Nevertheless, during the corrosion test, the GO/HA-coated Ta showed significantly higher corrosion current density compared to the uncoated Ta. So it is indicating the samples

TABLE 12.3

Surface Coating Implication on Tribo-Behaviors of Orthopedic Implants

S. No.	Base Material	Coating Material	Coating Method	Results		Ref.
				Tribology	Corrosion	
1	Ti-6Al-4V	GO based hydrogel	Dip coating	GO-based hydrogel greatly extended the wear behaviors of Ti alloys, which is reduced to 80% of the wear rate of uncoated Ti. Especially the 0.5 wt.% of GO encapsulated hydrogel (PVA/PAA/0.5GO/PDA yielded remarkable outcomes due to their viscoelastic properties and reduced microhardness of hydrogel.	This investigation proved that that the Ti alloy corrosion resistivity was potentially enhanced by the GO-powered hydrogel coating due to that corrosion-inhibiting barrier and effective physical separation between the sheltered substrate and aggressive medium.	Wang et al., 2023
2	SS316L	Titanium/ baghdadite	Cold spray	Ti/10BG coating more significantly protected the wear damages on SS316L than did Ti/15BG, Ti/25BG due to its elevated micro-hardness characteristics and in lubrication conditions (Hank's solution) that provided the notable wear-resistive behaviors due to their micro hardness, excellent scratch adhesion, and high contact angle.	—	Kumar et al., 2021
3	Ti-6A-14V	Fe_3O_4/HA	Dip coating	Fe_3O_4/HA coating on Ti alloy exhibited excellent wear behaviors in dry and wet conditions compared to uncoated and HA-coated Ti alloys because of their changing wear mechanism (sliding to rolling), which leads to a falloff of spherical ferro/ferric oxide particles.	Fe_3O_4/HA has a larger radius of curvature than uncoated and HA-coated samples, which indicates their slowest electro-chemical reaction and outstanding corrosion resistive behaviors.	Tian et al., 2022

(Continued)

TABLE 12.3 (Continued)

S. No.	Base Material	Coating Material	Coating Method	Results Tribology	Corrosion	Ref.
4	Ti-6A-14V	TiN-Cu	Electroless copper plating process	Wear rate of Ti alloy was effectively reduced due to synergetic effects (high hardness and elastic modulus) between its hard coating (TiN) and (Cu) soft coating.	—	Bian et al., 2023
5	Ti-6A-14V	MWCNT	Electro-chemical deposition	The MWCNT self-lubrication behavior and their involvement on molecular bearings between friction pairs effectively and reduced the COF and wear volume of Ti alloys in the dry condition. In a wet atmosphere, (SBF) is exposed to unfavorable wear performances due to the presence of a hydrogen bond between the coating substance and SBF solution.	—	Cao et al., 2023
6	PEEK	nHA-rGO	Dip coating	The inclusion of rGO with HAp accelerates friction and wear behavior due to the carbonaceous films generated between the composite surfaces and counter body acted as solid lubricating films, resulting in a low COF. In addition, these agents help to increase the hydrophobicity of the coating. However, the fact that rGO increases the interstitial bonding strength between PEEK and HAp is one of the promising reasons for good wear performances.		Baligidad et al., 2023

might have the poor corrosion resistivity, and further studies are most essential for further utilization (Mahmoodi et al., 2021). Likewise, Awaja et al. reported the tribological performance of plasma-treated hybrid layers (GO-DLC) coating on PEEK polymer (Sathishkumar et al., 2022a) in order to identify the potential plasma coating method.

The tribological behavior of the plasma-treated hybrid layers of PEEK-GO-DLC improved due to the use of DLC coatings, which have shown good adhesion on PEEK polymer. The author identified the most effective and promising plasma treatments to ensure stable coating and found that, when an intermediate GO layer is present, a DLC deposition in H2-rich environment is to be preferred to treatments including N2, since the former gives rise to better coating quality and mechanical stability, while N2 induces the formation of defects and cracking during the scratch test even at relatively low applied normal loads. Therefore, these studies emphasized that the surface coating on the medical implants showed remarkable improvement in their tribological behaviors, which leads to excellent performances and augmented implant longevity, ultimately to a better life for suffering people (Awaja et al., 2022).

12.5 SUMMARY AND CONCLUSION

The tribo-functions of implants are the most important aspects affectin their lifespan and comfort. Over the last five decades, researchers have tried various ways to increase bioimplants' longevity. Among them, surface coating is a potential method for achieving superior wear and corrosion resistance. The tribo-properties of biomaterials are generally determined by their surface roughness, implant design, loading scenario, and biological reactions. PVD and CVD coatings are prevalent surface coating technologies for implants, with coating thickness, coating quality, and implant production procedures influencing success rates. The ED coating technology is less expensive and more ecologically friendly than PVD and CVD coatings. However, it could be better for intricate geometrical implants. Porosity is important for implants because it promotes osseointegration and cell proliferation in the host body. The porosity coating can be done by plasma spraying, but the high costs restrict their contribution to the medical industry. On other hand, sol-gel and dip coating are simple, cost-efficient approaches for improving tribal and biological behaviors. However, their susceptibility leads to deterioration, and the complicated geometry does not provide beneficial outcomes in terms of effects on life. Metal-based alloys are frequently employed in numerous dental and orthopedic applications in the clinical sector. The nanocrystalline TiN, CP, CNT, and Fe_3O_3 coating over Ti alloys and ZrN-coated SS 304 alloys, as well as TCP- and ZrN-based Co-Cr-Mo alloys, exhibit excellent tribological effects on bioimplants. TCP-coated Al_2O_3, GO-HA-coated TA subtract, and GO-coated PEEK polymer offer supporting properties for various orthopedic applications. Nonetheless, stress shielding and metal ion emission in long-term physiological environments have been observed in certain circumstances, suggesting that developing polymer-based implants and polymer-coated polymer composites are candidates for future clinical uses.

12.5.1 ACKNOWLEDGMENTS

The authors would like to thank the National Institute of Technology Agartala (MHRD-Govt. of India) for providing continuous motivation and support in preparing this eminent chapter, as well as CRC Press: Taylor and Francis publication house for providing us with the wonderful opportunity to publish our chapter under the book title *Tribo-Behaviors of Biomaterials and Their Applications*.

12.5.2 CREDIT OF AUTHORSHIP CONTRIBUTION STATEMENT

S. Sathishkumar: Conceptualization, methodology, formal analysis, resources, investigation, data curation, writing
Original draft by P. Jawahar: Supervision, writing—review and editing, resources
Prasun Chakraborti: Validation, project administration
M. Muthusivaramapandian: Editing, resources, and validation

12.5.3 DECLARATION OF COMPETING INTEREST

The authors declare that they have no known competing financial interests or personal relationships that could have appeared to influence the work reported in this chapter.

REFERENCES

Amirtharaj Mosas, K. K., Chandrasekar, A. R., Dasan, A., Pakseresht, A., & Galusek, D. (2022). Recent advancements in materials and coatings for biomedical implants. *Gels*, 8(5), 323. https://doi.org/10.3390/gels8050323

Awaja, F., Guarino, R., Tripathi, M., Fedel, M., Speranza, G., Dalton, A. B., . . . Nogler, M. (2022). Tuning the tribological performance of plasma-treated hybrid layers of PEEK-GO-DLC. *Tribology International*, 176. https://doi.org/10.1016/j.triboint.2022.107915

Balestriere, M., Schuhladen, K., Seitz, K. H., Boccaccini, A. R., Cere, S. M., & Ballarre, J. (2020). Sol-gel coatings incorporating borosilicate bioactive glass enhance anti corrosive and surface performance of stainless steel implants. *Journal of Electroanalytical Chemistry*, 876, 114735.

Baligidad, S. M., T, A., Thodda, G., & Elangovan, K. (2023). Fabrication of HAp/rGO nanocomposite coating on PEEK: Tribological performance study. *Surfaces and Interfaces*, 38. https://doi.org/10.1016/j.surfin.2023.102865

Ballarre, J., & Ceré, S. (2022). Sol-gel coatings for protection and biofunctionalization of stainless-steel prosthetic intracorporeal devices in Latin-America. *Journal of Sol-Gel Science*, 102(1), 96–104. https://doi.org/10.1007/s10971-021-05658-z

Barkallah, R., Taktak, R., Guermazi, N., Elleuch, K., & Bouaziz, J. (2021). Mechanical properties and wear behaviour of alumina/tricalcium phosphate/titania ceramics as coating for orthopedic implant. *Engineering Fracture Mechanics*, 241, 107399. https://doi.org/10.1016/j.engfracmech.2020.107399

Bian, Y., Cao, L., Zeng, D., Cui, J., Li, W., Yu, Z., & Zhang, P. (2023). The tribological properties of two-phase hard and soft composite wear-resistant coatings on titanium alloys. *Surface Coatings Technology 456*, 129256. https://doi.org/10.1016/j.surfcoat.2023.129256

Cao, H., Tian, P., Deng, J., Li, Y., Wang, C., Han, S., & Zhao, X. (2023). Electrochemical deposition multi-walled carbon nanotube coatings on the surface of Ti6Al4V alloy for enhancing its biotribological properties. *Journal of the Mechanical Behavior of Biomedical Materials*, *142*, 105825. https://doi.org/10.1016/j.jmbbm.2023.105825

Çelik, A., & Bozkurt, Y. B. (2022). Improvement of tribological performance of AZ31 biodegradable alloy by TiN-based PVD coatings. *Tribology International*, *173*. https://doi.org/10.1016/j.triboint.2022.107684

Chavan, A. B., Gawade, S. S., & Bhosale, D. G. (2022). Tribo-corrosion behaviour and characterization of biocompatible coatings. In *Handbook of research on tribology in coatings and surface treatment* (pp. 245–269). IGI Global. https://doi.org/10.4018/978-1-7998-9683-8.ch011

Ching, H. A., Choudhury, D., Nine, M. J., & Abu Osman, N. A. (2014). Effects of surface coating on reducing friction and wear of orthopaedic implants. *Science and Technology of Advanced Materials*, *15*(1), 014402. https://doi.org/10.1088/1468-6996/15/1/014402

del Olmo, R., Czerwiński, M., Santos-Coquillat, A., Dubey, V., Dhoble, S. J., & Michalska-Domańska, M. (2023). Nano-scale surface modification of dental implants: Fabrication. In *Surface modification of titanium dental implants* (pp. 83–116). Springer.

Derakhshandeh, M. R., Eshraghi, M. J., Hadavi, M. M., Javaheri, M., Khamseh, S., Sari, M. G., . . . Mozafari, M. (2018). Diamond-like carbon thin films prepared by pulsed-DC PE-CVD for biomedical applications. *Surface Innovations*, *6*(3), 167–175. https://doi.org/10.1680/jsuin.17.00069

Devasia, R., Painuly, A., Devapal, D., & Sreejith, K. (2021). Continuous fiber reinforced ceramic matrix composites. In *Fiber reinforced composites* (pp. 669–751). Elsevier. https://doi.org/10.1016/B978-0-12-821090-1.00022-3

Dinu, M., Ivanova, A. A., Surmeneva, M. A., Braic, M., Tyurin, A. I., Braic, V., . . . Vladescu, A. (2017). Tribological behaviour of RF-magnetron sputter deposited hydroxyapatite coatings in physiological solution. *Ceramics International*, *43*(9), 6858–6867. https://doi.org/10.1016/j.ceramint.2017.02.106

Drevet, R., Zhukova, Y., Dubinskiy, S., Kazakbiev, A., Naumenko, V., Abakumov, M., . . . C. (2019). Electrodeposition of cobalt-substituted calcium phosphate coatings on Ti22Nb6Zr alloy for bone implant applications. *Journal of Alloys Compounds*, *793*, 576–582. https://doi.org/10.1016/j.jallcom.2019.04.180

Esmaeili, M. M., Mahmoodi, M., Mokhtarzade, A., & Imani, R. (2022). In vitro corrosion and tribological behavior of multiwall carbon nanotube-coated Ti-6Al-4V/tantalum carbide surface for implant applications. *Journal of Materials Engineering and Performance*, *31*(9), 7719–7733. https://doi.org/10.1007/s11665-022-06766-9

Faraji, G., Kim, H. S., & Kashi, H. T. (2018). *Severe plastic deformation: Methods, processing and properties*. Elsevier. https://doi.org/10.1016/B978-0-12-813518-1.00020-5

Figueiredo-Pina, C. G., Guedes, M., Sequeira, J., Pinto, D., Bernardo, N., & Carneiro, C. (2019). On the influence of Streptococcus salivarius on the wear response of dental implants: An in vitro study. *Journal of Biomedical Materials Research Part B: Applied Biomaterials*, *107*(5), 1393–1399. https://doi.org/10.1002/jbm.b.34231

Gabor, R., Cvrček, L., Doubková, M., Nehasil, V., Hlinka, J., Unucka, P., . . . Bačáková, L. (2022). Hybrid coatings for orthopaedic implants formed by physical vapour deposition and microarc oxidation. *Materials & Design*, *219*. https://doi.org/10.1016/j.matdes.2022.110811

Gautam, S., Bhatnagar, D., Bansal, D., Batra, H., & Goyal, N. (2022). Recent advancements in nanomaterials for biomedical implants. *Biomedical Engineering Advances*, *3*, 100029. https://doi.org/10.1016/j.bea.2022.100029

Grigoriev, S., Sotova, C., Vereschaka, A., Uglov, V., & Cherenda, N. (2023). Modifying coatings for medical implants made of titanium alloys. *Metals*, *13*(4), 718. https://doi.org/10.3390/met13040718

Guo, T., Scimeca, J.-C., Ivanovski, S., Verron, E., & Gulati, K. (2023). Enhanced corrosion resistance and local therapy from nano-engineered titanium dental implants. *Pharmaceutics*, *15*(2), 315. https://doi.org/10.3390/pharmaceutics15020315

Gupta, M. K., Etri, H. E., Korkmaz, M. E., Ross, N. S., Krolczyk, G. M., Gawlik, J., . . . Pimenov, D. Y. (2022). Tribological and surface morphological characteristics of titanium alloys: A review. *Archives of Civil Mechanical Engineering*, *22*(2), 72. https://doi.org/10.1007/s43452-022-00392-x

Hassan, S., Nadeem, A. Y., Qaiser, H., Kashif, A. S., Ahmed, A., Khan, K., & Altaf, A. (2023). A review of carbon-based materials and their coating techniques for biomedical implants applications. *Carbon Letters*, 1–18. https://doi.org/10.1007/s42823-023-00496-1

Hussein, M. A., Adesina, A. Y., Kumar, A. M., Sorour, A. A., Ankah, N., & Al-Aqeeli, N. (2020). Mechanical, in-vitro corrosion, and tribological characteristics of TiN coating produced by cathodic arc physical vapor deposition on Ti20Nb13Zr alloy for biomedical applications. *Thin Solid Films*, *709*. https://doi.org/10.1016/j.tsf.2020.138183

Jaafar, A., Hecker, C., Árki, P., & Joseph, Y. J. B. (2020). Sol-gel derived hydroxyapatite coatings for titanium implants: A review. *Bioengineering*, *7*(4), 127.

Kumar, A., Kant, R., & Singh, H. (2021). Tribological behavior of cold-sprayed titanium/baghdadite composite coatings in dry and simulated body fluid environments. *Surface and Coatings Technology*, *425*. https://doi.org/10.1016/j.surfcoat.2021.127727

Li, D. T. S., & Leung, Y. Y. (2023). Patient-specific implants in orthognathic surgery. *Oral Maxillofacial Surgery Clinics*, *35*(1), 61–69. https://doi.org/10.1016/j.coms.2022.06.004

Li, H. Q., Guo, H., Shen, F. L., Lou, D. J., Xia, W. L., & Fang, X. Y. (2021). Tribological and corrosion performance of the plasma-sprayed conformal ceramic coating on selective laser melted CoCrMo alloy. *Journal of the Mechanical Behavior of Biomedical Materials*, *119*, 104520. https://doi.org/10.1016/j.jmbbm.2021.104520

Mahmoodi, M., Hydari, M. H., Mahmoodi, L., Gazanfari, L., & Mirhaj, M. (2021). Electrophoretic deposition of graphene oxide reinforced hydroxyapatite on the tantalum substrate for bone implant applications: In vitro corrosion and bio-tribological behavior. *Surface and Coatings Technology*, *424*. https://doi.org/10.1016/j.surfcoat.2021.127642

Mehta, A., & Singh, G. (2023). Consequences of hydroxyapatite doping using plasma spray to implant biomaterials. *Journal of Electrochemical Science Engineering*, *13*(1), 5–23. https://doi.org/10.5599/jese.1614

Mehta, S., Singh, G., Singh, H., & Saini, A. (2022). A review of tribological behavior of different bio-implant materials. *ECS Transactions*, *107*(1), 5147. https://doi.org/10.1149/10701.5147ecst

Mittal, M., Sardar, S., & Jana, A. (2021). Nanofabrication techniques for semiconductor chemical sensors. In *Handbook of nanomaterials for sensing applications* (pp. 119–137). Elsevier. https://doi.org/10.1016/B978-0-12-820783-3.00023-3

Montazerian, M., Hosseinzadeh, F., Migneco, C., Fook, M. V., & Baino, F. (2022). Bioceramic coatings on metallic implants: An overview. *Ceramics International*, *48*(7), 8987–9005. https://doi.org/10.1016/j.ceramint.2022.02.055

Neacşu, I. A., Nicoară, A. I., Vasile, O. R., & Vasile, B. Ş. (2016). Inorganic micro-and nanostructured implants for tissue engineering. In *Nanobiomaterials in hard tissue engineering* (pp. 271–295). Elsevier. https://doi.org/10.1016/B978-0-323-42862-0.00009-2

Osak, P., Maszybrocka, J., Kubisztal, J., & Łosiewicz, B. (2022). Effect of amorphous calcium phosphate coatings on tribological properties of titanium grade 4 in protein-free artificial saliva. *Biotribology*, *32*, 100219. https://doi.org/10.1016/j.biotri.2022.100219

Pandey, A., & Sahoo, S. (2023). Progress on medical implant: A review and prospects. *Journal of Bionic Engineering*, *20*(2), 470–494.

Patnaik, L., Maity, S. R., & Kumar, S. (2021). Mechanical and tribological assessment of composite AlCrN or aC: Ag-based thin films for implant application. *Ceramics International*, *47*(5), 6736–6752. https://doi.org/10.1016/j.ceramint.2020.11.016

Ralls, A., Kumar, P., Misra, M., & Menezes, P. L. (2019). Material design and surface engineering for bio-implants. *JOM*, *72*(2), 684–696. https://doi.org/10.1007/s11837-019-03687-2

Ramoul, C., Beliardouh, N. E., Bahi, R., Nouveau, C., Djahoudi, A., & Walock, M. J. (2019). Surface performances of PVD ZrN coatings in biological environments. *Tribology-Materials, Surfaces*, *13*(1), 12–19. https://doi.org/10.1080/17515831.2018.1553820

Rodríguez-Rojas, F., Kovylina, M., Pinilla-Cienfuegos, E., Borrero-López, Ó., Bendavid, A., Martin, P. J., & Hoffman, M. (2023). Effect of a DLC film on the sliding-wear behaviour of Ti6Al4V: Implications for dental implants. *Surface Coatings Technology*, *460*, 129409. https://doi.org/10.1016/j.surfcoat.2023.129409

Saha, S., & Roy, S. (2023). Metallic dental implants wear mechanisms, materials, and manufacturing processes: A literature review. *Materials*, *16*(1), 161. https://doi.org/10.3390/ma16010161

Sahoo, P., Das, S. K., & Davim, J. P. (2019). Tribology of materials for biomedical applications. In *Mechanical behaviour of biomaterials* (pp. 1–45). Elsevier. https://doi.org/10.1016/B978-0-08-102174-3.00001-2

Sankar, S., Paulraj, J., & Chakraborti, P. (2023). Fused filament fabricated PEEK based polymer composites for orthopaedic implants: A review. *International Journal of Materials Research*, *114*(10–11), 980–988. https://doi.org/10.1515/ijmr-2022-0225

Sathishkumar, S., Jawahar, P., & Chakraborti, P. (2022a). Synthesis, properties, and applications of PEEK-based biomaterials. In *Advanced materials for biomedical applications* (pp. 81–107). CRC Press. https://doi.org/10.1201/9781003344810.5

Sathishkumar, S., Jawahar, P., & Chakraborti, P. (2022b). Influence of carbonaceous reinforcements on mechanical and tribological properties of PEEK composites – A review. *Polymer-Plastics Technology and Materials*, *61*(12), 1367–1384. https://doi.org/10.1080/25740881.2022.2061995

Sathishkumar, S., Paulraj, J., Chakraborti, P., & Muthuraj, M. (2023). Comprehensive review on biomaterials and their inherent behaviors for hip repair applications. *ACS Applied Bio Materials*, *6*(11), 4439–4464. https://doi.org/10.1021/acsabm.3c00327

Shen, G., Zhang, J., Culliton, D., Melentiev, R., & Fang, F. (2022). Tribological study on the surface modification of metal-on-polymer bioimplants. *Frontiers of Mechanical Engineering*, *17*(2), 26. https://doi.org/10.1007/s11465-022-0682-6

Singh, P., Dixit, K., & Sinha, N. (2022). A sol-gel based bioactive glass coating on laser textured 316L stainless steel substrate for enhanced biocompatability and anticorrosion properties. *Ceramics International*, *48*(13), 18704–18715.

Sivasankar, M., Arunkumar, S., Bakkiyaraj, V., Muruganandam, A., & Sathishkumar, S. (2016). A review on total hip replacement. *International Research Journal in Advanced Engineering Technology*, *2*(2), 589–592.

Souza, J. C., Apaza-Bedoya, K., Benfatti, C. A., Silva, F. S., & Henriques, B. (2020). A comprehensive review on the corrosion pathways of titanium dental implants and their biological adverse effects. *Metals*, *10*(9), 1272. https://doi.org/10.3390/met10091272

Sudha, T. S., Varghese, A. M., Kumar, Z. N., Sasanka, K. K., Hari, T. S., & Thangaraju, P. (2023). Implants and prosthetics. In *Medical devices* (pp. 94–125). CRC Press. https://doi.org/10.1201/9781003220671

Terranova, M. L. (2022). Key challenges in diamond coating of titanium implants: Current status and future prospects. *Biomedicines*, *10*(12), 3149. https://doi.org/10.3390/biomedicines10123149

Thakur, A., Kumar, A., Kaya, S., Marzouki, R., Zhang, F., & Guo, L. (2022). Recent advancements in surface modification, characterization and functionalization for enhancing the biocompatibility and corrosion resistance of biomedical implants. *Coatings*, *12*(10), 1459. https://doi.org/10.3390/coatings12101459

Tian, P., Zhao, X., Sun, B., Cao, H., Zhao, Y., Yan, J., . . . Wang, C. (2022). Enhanced anticorrosion and tribological properties of Ti6Al4V alloys with Fe3O4/HA coatings. *Surface and Coatings Technology*, *433*. https://doi.org/10.1016/j.surfcoat.2022.128118

Tran, D.-T., Chen, F.-H., Wu, G.-L., Ching, P. C. O., & Yeh, M.-L. (2023). Influence of spin coating and dip coating with gelatin/hydroxyapatite for bioresorbable Mg alloy orthopedic implants: In vitro and in vivo studies. *ACS Biomaterials Science Engineering*, *9*(2), 705–718. https://doi.org/10.1016/B978-0-323-42862-0.00009-2

Tranquillo, E., & Bollino, F. (2020). Surface modifications for implants lifetime extension: An overview of sol-gel coatings. *Coatings*, *10*(6), 589. https://doi.org/10.3390/coatings10060589

Tüten, N., Canadinc, D., Motallebzadeh, A., & Bal, B. (2019). Microstructure and tribological properties of TiTaHfNbZr high entropy alloy coatings deposited on Ti 6Al 4V substrates. *Intermetallics*, *105*, 99–106. https://doi.org/10.1016/j.intermet.2018.11.015

Uddin, G. M., Jawad, M., Ghufran, M., Saleem, M. W., Raza, M. A., Rehman, Z. U., . . . Waseem, B. (2019). Experimental investigation of tribo-mechanical and chemical properties of TiN PVD coating on titanium substrate for biomedical implants manufacturing. *International Journal of Advanced Manufacturing Technology*, *102*, 1391–1404. https://doi.org/10.1007/s00170-018-03244-2

Visentin, F., Galenda, A., Fabrizio, M., Battiston, S., Brianese, N., Gerbasi, R., . . . El Habra, N. (2019). Assessment of synergistic effects of LP-MOCVD TiO2 and Ti surface finish for dental implant purposes. *Applied Surface Science*, *490*, 568–579. https://doi.org/10.1016/j.apsusc.2019.06.067

Wang, C., Zhu, K., Gao, Y., Han, S., Ju, J., Ren, T., & Zhao, X. (2023). Multifunctional GO-based hydrogel coating on Ti-6Al-4 V Alloy with enhanced bioactivity, anticorrosion and tribological properties against cortical bone. *Tribology International*, *184*. https://doi.org/10.1016/j.triboint.2023.108423

Wang, J., Zhou, J., Long, H. Y., Xie, Y. N., Zhang, X. W., Luo, H., . . . Tang, Z. G. (2014). Tribological, anticorrosive properties and biocompatibility of the micro- and nano-crystalline diamond coated Ti6Al4V. *Surface and Coatings Technology*, *258*, 1032–1038. https://doi.org/10.1016/j.surfcoat.2014.07.034

Wei, Q., Liu, H., Zhao, X., Zhao, W., Xu, R., Ma, S., & Zhou, F. (2023). Bio-inspired hydrogel-polymer brush bi-layered coating dramatically boosting the lubrication and wear-resistance. *Tribology International*, *177*, 108000. https://doi.org/10.1016/ j.triboint.2022.108000

Wei, X., Zhang, Y., Feng, H., Cao, X., Ding, Q., Lu, Z., . . . Engineering. (2022). Biotribology and corrosion behaviors of a Si-and N-incorporated diamond-like carbon film: A new class of protective film for Ti6Al4V artificial implants. *ACS Biomaterials Science*, *8*(3), 1166–1180. https://doi.org/10.1021/acsbiomaterials.1c01370

Yadav, V., Sankar, M., & Pandey, L. (2020). Coating of bioactive glass on magnesium alloys to improve its degradation behavior: Interfacial aspects. *Journal of Magnesium and Alloys*, *8*(4), 999–1015. https://doi.org/10.1016/j.jma.2020.05.005

Zafar, M. S., Fareed, M. A., Riaz, S., Latif, M., Habib, S. R., & Khurshid, Z. (2020). Customized therapeutic surface coatings for dental implants. *Coatings*, *10*(6), 568. https://doi.org/10.3390/coatings10060568

Zambrano, D. F., Hernández-Bravo, R., Ruden, A., Espinosa-Arbelaez, D. G., González-Carmona, J. M., & Mujica, V. (2023). Mechanical, tribological and electrochemical behavior of Zr-based ceramic thin films for dental implants. *Ceramics International*, *49*(2), 2102–2114. https://doi.org/10.1016/j.ceramint.2022.09.176

Zhu, Y., Liu, W., & Ngai, T. (2022). Polymer coatings on magnesium-based implants for orthopedic applications. *Journal of Polymer Science*, *60*(1), 32–51. https://doi.org/10.1002/pol.20210578

13 Machine Learning Approaches in Metal-Based Additive-Manufactured Wear-Resistant Bioimplants

T Archana Acharya[1], Anandakrishnan V[2], Ravi Kumar Kottala[3], and Bharat Kumar Chigilipalli[1]

[1] Vignan's Institute of Information Technology
Visakhapatnam, Andhra Pradesh, India

[2] National Institute of Technology
Tiruchirappalli, Tamil Nadu, India

[3] M V G R College of Engineering (A)
Vizianagaram, Andhra Pradesh, India

13.1 INTRODUCTION

In medical science, there is a growing need for transplants of organs as organ donations are stagnated with long waiting time, while the condition of the sufferers is deteriorating and inching toward mortality. This mismatch between the need for transplants and the supply of organs is addressed with regenerative medicine, a biocompatible material used for building required organs or tissue structure models using 3D bioprinters. Thus AM helps in developing complex fabrication and functional organ structures with regular machining and joining processes [1]. The computational advancements are now aiding the development of data-driven models that enhance not only the quality of the product but also productivity from process parameters to optimizing design and performance [2–4]. The output of the enhancement is a physic-based data-driven surrogate model [5].

Globally there is a high requirement to save lives and prevent disability especially in low- and middle-income countries. Around 143 million people are in need of additional surgical procedures [7]. The applications of 3D printing are distributed across many fields in general, but in particular, it is gaining prominence in the health care field [8, 9]. Earlier traditional practices and methods, such as casting

DOI: 10.1201/9781003384847-13

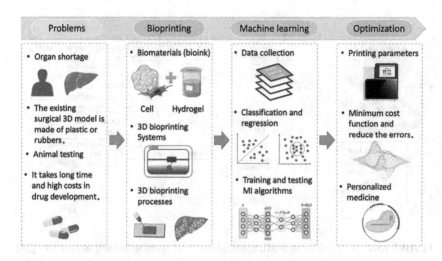

FIGURE 13.1 AI and ML in bioimplant applications [6].

[10], composites [11], welding [12, 13], joining [14] and machining, are all now supplanted by 3D printing practices for production. The 3D printing technologies are fused deposition molding (FDM), stereo lithography appearance (SLA), digital light processing (DLP), and inkjet 3D printing [15]. For example, SLA technology gives high-precision, large, and transparent models of heart and blood vessels that are used for education, training, and flow testing [16]. The flexibility point in this application is the creation of complex models like printing human organs with various dimensional features of shapes, sizes, etc. [17]. These features are accelerating the process of product development and further building a prospective future potential for specific organ model manufacturing and providing an opportunity for preoperative physicians training who have little experience in surgery.

To reduce high-risk medical practice—mortality of patients, procedure time, and complications—the prerequisite is for highly skilled and trained surgeons. Though high-precision models can be developed, the lack of training models and simulated clinical procedures in surgeons is the shortcoming. Artificial intelligence (AI) and machine learning are fulfilling these gaps effectively [4, 11], which is illustrated in Figure 13.1. Researchers used the optimization methods to do the surface characteristics optimization for biocompatible products made with titanium [18]. They have optimized the parameters using response surface methodology (RSM). Kumar et al. have studied parameters optimization for 3D printing of Inconel alloys [18]. Cheepu et al. have studied defect analysis using ML during the 3D printing deposition [19]. Chigilipalli et al. have successfully implemented neuro-fuzzy modeling for predicting deposition geometry, which helps researchers to identify the required dimensions with a limited number of experiments [1,20]. Biswal et al. have studied the wear and corrosion studies for biocompatible materials [21]. Korkmaz et al. have studied ML models for online detection of friction and wear behavior of biomedically graded SS316L under

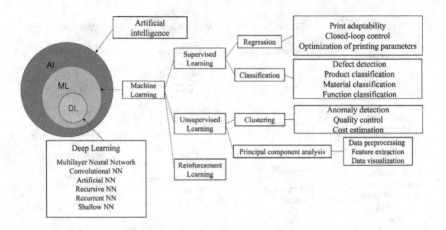

FIGURE 13.2   Classification of ML applications in 3D printing and neural networks [24].

lubricating conditions [22]. However, the research work in these areas is confined to a small portion where the time required to process the images, the lack of precision in processing the images, and the errors that occur during the printing process affect the quality of the printed models [19].

Literature reviews indicate that many researchers have utilized statistical optimization methods like RSM, Taguchi approach, and neural network methods to optimize the wear characteristics of biocompatible materials. There is a considerable research gap in effectively optimizing the wear behavior of such materials by harnessing bioinspired optimization algorithms, including particle swarm optimization, grey wolf algorithm, genetic algorithm, ANT colony algorithm, teacher learning-based algorithms, random forest, decision tree, etc.

13.2   SIGNIFICANCE OF ARTIFICIAL INTELLIGENCE AND MACHINE LEARNING IN 3D PRINTING

The applications of AI and ML using 3D printing to produce organ models are in their infancy but have wide potential scope. The characteristics include in situ corrections, image processing, and process monitoring, which enable rapid generation models, correction of printing errors, and generation of customized models that are introducing innovations and greater convenience. High-quality printed models with high-throughput aspects are the advantages of these applications [23, 24]. The preparation simulations carried out by clinicians are the limitation. Figure 13.2 shows the additive manufacturing applications using ML, AI, and DL.

13.3   OPTIMIZATION OF WEAR-RESISTANCE PROPERTIES OF BIOCOMPATIBLE MATERIALS

This section discusses the significance of enhancing wear properties in a variety of materials used frequently in joint prosthesis, such as titanium and its alloys, cobalt-chromium alloys, biocompatible ceramics, and bioactive materials using optimization techniques. The application of various optimization techniques in the context of biocompatible materials is thoroughly discussed in the section. It then dives into current advancements in this field.

To improve the performance and endurance of metal components in a variety of applications, optimization is crucial to the study of metal wear [25]. This optimization takes into account factors including material choice, surface improvement, lubrication, design improvement, tribological testing, wear modeling, material innovation, cost-efficiency considerations, and minimizing environmental effect. Overall, optimization efforts seek to increase the functioning and longevity of metal components while reducing the negative impacts of wear. The use of titanium alloys in technical applications is increasing due to their unique capabilities to combine high strength, lightweight properties, and corrosion resistance. Several industries, including aerospace, automotive, nuclear, chemical, marine, and biomedicine, use these alloys.

Saravanan et al. [26] fabricated the titanium-nitride- (TiN-) based alloy for artificial hip joints. The prepared specimens are tested under various parameters such as load, sliding velocity, and slide distance. The response surface methodology (RSM) optimization technique has been effectively employed to find the best findings about the appropriate wear and friction parameters. Using RSM, the input parameters of a 4 N load, 0.5 m/s sliding velocity, and 1000 m of sliding distance were optimized to produce the results with the lowest specific wear rate and coefficient of friction (COF). Sivaprakasam et al. [27] investigated the use of AlTiN-based physical vapor deposition on titanium alloy. They used the response surface methodology (RSM) to examine wear mass loss and the coefficient of friction as response parameters while analyzing important input components such as load, sliding speed, and sliding distance. According to the study's findings, AlTiN is a potential option for covering titanium implants in biomedical applications since it has exceptional wear resistance qualities. Notably, the study showed that, with an applied force of 15 N, a sliding speed of 0.5 m/s, and a sliding distance of 500 m, the minimal wear mass loss and coefficient of friction were attained. Palanikumar et al. [28] developed an innovative stochastic optimization method called the teaching-learning-based optimizer to improve parameters related to cutting force and surface finish. Extensive experimental testing and comparison with other active optimizers validated the anticipated results. They concluded that the application of this novel approach has the potential to significantly reduce production waste within the machining of titanium-based alloys. Soori et al. [29] conducted research on the significance of reducing cutting tool wear during drilling operations, particularly when working with difficult materials like Ti-6Al-4V alloy. Tool wear can adversely influence tool life as well as the accuracy and surface quality of the finished product. A virtual machining system that predicts and reduces cutting tool wear is introduced in a study to address this problem. To achieve this, it computes cutting forces and temperatures, predicts wear using finite element analysis, and optimizes drilling settings using a response surface analysis algorithm based on the Taguchi method. The system's usefulness is experimentally validated, showing that it can increase drilling efficiency and precision for Ti-6Al-4V alloy.

Cobalt-chromium (Co–Cr) alloys are preferred in industries where the lubrication of sliding interfaces is not feasible due to their excellent wear resistance and favorable frictional properties, outperforming other materials in these conditions. With the help of optimization techniques, it is possible to gain understanding of how modifications to material parameters and component geometry affect material wear rates. Aherwar et al. [30] examines the density, microhardness, and sliding wear behavior of Co–30Cr alloys. The addition of molybdenum increases density and hardness, with significant improvements observed as the molybdenum content increases. Also, they optimize the sliding wear behavior of the Co–30Cr alloy with molybdenum for use in implants. Taguchi experimental design techniques are applied to study the impact of normal loads, sliding velocities, sliding distances, and molybdenum content on wear behavior. The Taguchi experimental analysis revealed the best set of control factors, resulting in S/N ratios of −9.777 for wear loss and 6.670 for the friction coefficient. Aherwar et al. [31] fabricated the cobalt-chromium alloy material (Co-30Cr-4Mo-1Ni) using a high-temperature vacuum casting induction furnace. Mechanical properties were tested using a microhardness tester and compression testing machine, while wear performance was assessed using a pin-on-disk tribometer under various conditions at room temperature. The study initially conducted steady-state experiments to determine volumetric wear loss and friction coefficients by varying sliding velocity and normal load. Subsequently, Taguchi experimental design was employed to optimize wear response.

For long-term uses or to be used as permanent implants in the body, biocompatible ceramics and bioactive materials must demonstrate outstanding resistance to wear. Small abnormalities or pieces of artificial joint debris can enter the patient blood circulation during wear and tear, causing significant inflammation, osteolysis, and other issues that may eventually call for an early revision operation. To mitigate these problems, surfaces of implants are coated with durable biocompatible coatings that can withstand wear and corrosion within the body. Patnaik et al. [32] fabricated AlCrN-coated medical-grade 316LVM stainless steel for medical applications. They used a response surface methodology and Box–Behnken design to optimize and assess the effects of independent parameters such as applied load, sliding velocity, and sliding distance on various wear responses including surface roughness, friction coefficient, disk mass loss, wear depth, and hardness. The RSM model demonstrated a good fit with high R^2 values. The wear debris produced during dry sliding exhibited typical characteristics of fatigue wear particles with irregular and sharp peripheries.

Typically, dental implants made of zirconium are preferred because of their biocompatibility and resistance to corrosion, which is attributable to the development of a native zirconia layer [33]. Improving their bioactivity and therapeutic potential, particularly for patients with impaired diseases, is a major area of focus. Solanke et al. [34] conducted the wear characterization of titanium grade 2 and titanium grade 5 materials at room temperature under simulated bodily fluid circumstances. The Taguchi design of trials using an L18 orthogonal array was employed to examine the tribological qualities, in particular weight reduction, as the subject of the study. The applied normal load, which contributed 91.17% on an individual basis, was found to be the most important factor determining weight loss by the analysis of variance. This implies that the applied normal load has the biggest impact on weight reduction. The signal-to-noise ratio study revealed that titanium grade 5 material saw the best weight loss at 5 N of applied normal load, 0.05 m/s of sliding velocity, and 100 m of sliding distance. The findings revealed that weight loss increased with increasing applied normal load and sliding velocity.

13.4 CONCLUSION

Machine learning models that are used to predict outcomes with the available existing data are highly helpful in predicting critical things in the medical field. The medical field is witnessing remarkable advancements with the commencement of additive manufacturing using machine learning. Particularly, researchers can predict the wear resistance of implanted materials before implantation into the human body. This will reduce the life risk possibility of patients who are undergoing surgery and hence give researchers more scope to work in the field. These new innovative models are revolutionizing the research direction to open new windows of machine learning algorithms and artificial intelligence combined with 3D printing to achieve optimization. The features of the ML technique—high flexibility and adaptability—result in excellent prediction.

REFERENCES

1. Chigilipalli BK, Veeramani A. An experimental investigation and neuro-fuzzy modeling to ascertain metal deposition parameters for the wire arc additive manufacturing of Incoloy 825. CIRP Journal of Manufacturing Science and Technology. 2022, 38:386–400.
2. Kottala RK, Balasubramanian KR, Jinshah BS, Divakar S, Chigilipalli BK. Experimental investigation and machine learning modelling of phase change material-based receiver tube for natural circulated solar parabolic trough system under various weather conditions. Journal of Thermal Analysis and Calorimetry. 2023:1–24.
3. Kottala RK, Chigilipalli BK, Mukuloth S, Shanmugam R, Kantumuchu VC, Ainapurapu SB, Cheepu M. Thermal degradation studies and machine learning modelling of nano-enhanced sugar alcohol-based phase change materials for medium temperature applications. Energies. 2023, 16(5):2187.
4. Kumar KR, Balasubramanian KR, Kumar GP, Bharat Kumar C, Cheepu MM. Experimental investigation of nano-encapsulated molten salt for medium-temperature thermal storage systems and modeling of neural networks. International Journal of Thermophysics. 2022, 43(9):145.
5. Ma L, Yu S, Xu X, Amadi SM, Zhang J, Wang Z. Application of artificial intelligence in 3D printing physical organ models. Materials Today Bio. 2023:100792.
6. Shin J, Lee Y, Li Z, Hu J, Park SS, Kim K. Optimized 3D bioprinting technology based on machine learning: a review of recent trends and advances. Micromachines. 2022, 13(3):363.

7. Meara JG, Leather AJ, Hagander L, Alkire BC, Alonso N, Ameh EA, Bickler SW, Conteh L, Dare AJ, Davies J, Mérisier ED. Global Surgery 2030: evidence and solutions for achieving health, welfare, and economic development. International Journal of Obstetric Anesthesia. 2016, 25:75–8.

8. Bogue R. 3D printing: the dawn of a new era in manufacturing?, Assembly Automation. 2013, 33(4):307–11.

9. Ramola M, Yadav V, Jain R. On the adoption of additive manufacturing in healthcare: a literature review. Journal of Manufacturing Technology Management. 2019, 30(1):48–69.

10. Kandpal BC, Johri N, Kumar L, Tyagi A, Joshi V, Gupta U. Stir casting technology for magnesium-based metal matrix composites for bio-implants-a review. Materials Today: Proceedings. 2022, 62:4519–25.

11. Ramam RS, Pujari S, Chigilipalli BK, Naik BD, Kottala RK, Kantumuchu VC. Fabrication and optimization of acoustic properties of natural fiber reinforced composites. International Journal on Interactive Design and Manufacturing. 2023:1–9.

12. Babu KT, Muthukumaran S, Kumar CB, Narayanan CS. A study on influence of underwater friction stir welding on microstructural, mechanical properties and formability in 5052-O aluminium alloys. In Materials Science Forum 2019 (Vol. 969, pp. 27–33). Trans Tech Publications Ltd.

13. Sarila V, Koneru HP, Cheepu M, Chigilipalli BK, Kantumuchu VC, Shanmugam M. Microstructural and mechanical properties of AZ31B to AA6061 dissimilar joints fabricated by refill friction stir spot welding. Journal of Manufacturing and Materials Processing. 2022, 6(5):95.

14. Babu KT, Muthukumaran S, Kumar CB. The role of material location on the first mode of metal transfer and weld formation in dissimilar friction stir welded thin sheets. Transactions of the Indian Institute of Metals. 2019, 72:1589–92.

15. Jin Z, Li Y, Yu K, Liu L, Fu J, Yao X, Zhang A, He Y. 3D printing of physical organ models: recent developments and challenges. Advanced Science. 2021, 8(17):2101394.

16. Wang DD, Qian Z, Vukicevic M, Engelhardt S, Kheradvar A, Zhang C, Little SH, Verjans J, Comaniciu D, O'Neill WW, Vannan MA. 3D printing, computational modeling, and artificial intelligence for structural heart disease. Cardiovascular Imaging. 2021, 14(1):41–60.

17. Liu D, Jiang P, Wang Y, Lu Y, Wu J, Xu X, Ji Z, Sun C, Wang X, Liu W. Engineering tridimensional hydrogel tissue and organ phantoms with tunable springiness. Advanced Functional Materials. 2023, 33(17):2214885.

18. Dikshit MK, Singh S, Pathak VK, Saxena KK, Agrawal MK, Malik V, Hazim Salem K, Khan MI. Surface characteristics optimization of biocompatible Ti6Al4V with RCCD and NSGA II using die sinking EDM. Journal of Materials Research and Technology. 2023, 24:223–35.

19. Kumar CB, Anandakrishnan V. Experimental investigations on the effect of wire arc additive manufacturing process parameters on the layer geometry of Inconel 825. Materials Today: Proceedings. 2020, 21:622–7.

20. Cheepu M. Machine learning approach for the prediction of defect characteristics in wire arc additive manufacturing. Transactions of the Indian Institute of Metals. 2023, 76(2):447–55.

21. Biswal S, Tripathy S, Tripathy DK. Machining performance analysis for PMEDM of biocompatible material Ti-6Al-7Nb alloy: a machine learning approach. Materials Letters. 2022, 320:132337.

22. Korkmaz ME, Gupta MK, Singh G, Kuntoğlu M, Patange A, Demirsoz R, Ross NS, Prasad B. Machine learning models for online detection of wear and friction behavior of biomedical graded stainless steel 316L under lubricating conditions. The International Journal of Advanced Manufacturing Technology. 2023:1–8.
23. Chigilipalli BK, Veeramani A. A machine learning approach for the prediction of tensile deformation behavior in wire arc additive manufacturing. International Journal on Interactive Design and Manufacturing. 2023, 17:1–3.
24. Ladani LJ. Applications of artificial intelligence and machine learning in metal additive manufacturing. Journal of Physics: Materials. 2021, 4(4):042009.
25. Haribabu S, Cheepu M, Devuri V, Kantumuchu VC. Optimization of welding parameters for friction welding of 304 stainless steel to D3Tool steel using response surface methodology. In Techno-Societal 2018: Proceedings of the 2nd International Conference on Advanced Technologies for Societal Applications-Volume 2 2020 (pp. 427–37). Springer International Publishing.
26. Saravanan I, Elaya Perumal A, Vettivel SC, Selvakumar N, Baradeswaran A. Optimizing wear behavior of TiN coated SS 316L against Ti alloy using response surface methodology. Materials & Design. 2015, 67:469–82.
27. Sivaprakasam P, Kirubel A, Elias G, Maheandera Prabu P, Balasubramani P. Mathematical modeling and analysis of wear behavior of AlTiN coating on titanium alloy (Ti-6Al-4V). Advances in Materials Science and Engineering. 2021, 2021:1–9.
28. Palanikumar K, Nithyanandam J, Natarajan E, Lim WH, Tiang SS. Mitigated cutting force and surface roughness in titanium alloy-multiple effective guided chaotic multi-objective teaching learning-based optimization. Alexandria Engineering Journal. 2023, 64:877–905.
29. Soori M, Arezoo B. Cutting tool wear minimization in drilling operations of titanium alloy Ti-6Al-4V. Proceedings of the Institution of Mechanical Engineers, Part J: Journal of Engineering Tribology. 2023, 237(5):1250–63.
30. Aherwar A, Singh A, Patnaik A. A study on mechanical behavior and wear performance of a metal–metal Co–30Cr biomedical alloy with different molybdenum addition and optimized using Taguchi experimental design. Journal of the Brazilian Society of Mechanical Sciences and Engineering. 2018, 40:1–19.
31. Aherwar A, Bahraminasab M. Biocompatibility evaluation and corrosion resistance of tungsten added Co-30Cr-4Mo-1Ni alloy. Bio-Medical Materials and Engineering. 2017, 28(6):687–701.
32. Patnaik L, Maity SR, Kumar S. Modeling of wear parameters and multi-criteria optimization by Box-Behnken design of AlCrN thin film against gamma-irradiated Ti6Al4V Counterbody. Ceramics International. 2021, 47(14):20494–511.
33. Chopra D, Jayasree A, Guo T, Gulati K, Ivanovski S. Advancing dental implants: bioactive and therapeutic modifications of zirconia. Bioactive Materials. 2022, 13:161–78.
34. Solanke SG, Gaval VR. Optimization of wet sliding wear parameters of titanium grade 2 and grade 5 bioimplant materials for orthopedic application using Taguchi method. Journal of Metals, Materials and Minerals. 2020, 30(3).

Index

Note: Page numbers in *italics* indicate figures, and page numbers in **bold** indicate tables in the text.